Dear Professor M

Please accept this as a
small momento of your Paris
Trip in July 08.

It was our pleasure to spend
this in your company and
hear. so much about your travels.

Mark,

Controversies
in the management of
salivary gland disease

Controversies
in the management of
salivary gland disease

Edited by

Mark McGurk MD FRCS FDS DLO

Professor of Oral and Maxillofacial
Surgery, Guy's, King's and St Thomas'
Schools of Medicine, Dentistry and
Biomedical Sciences, London, UK

and

Andrew G. Renehan

PhD FRCS FDS

Senior Research Fellow, Department
of Surgery, Christie Hospital NHS
Trust and Paterson Institute for
Cancer Research, Manchester, UK

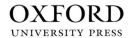

OXFORD
UNIVERSITY PRESS

OXFORD

UNIVERSITY PRESS

Great Clarendon Street, Oxford OX2 6DP

Oxford University Press is a department of the University of Oxford.
It furthers the University's objective of excellence in research, scholarship,
and education by publishing worldwide in

Oxford New York

Auckland Bangkok Buenos Aires Cape Town Chennai
Dar es Salaam Delhi Hong Kong Istanbul Karachi Kolkata
Kuala Lumpur Madrid Melbourne Mexico City Mumbai
Nairobi São Paulo Shanghai Taipei Tokyo Toronto
with associated companies in Berlin

Oxford is a registered trade mark of Oxford University Press
in the UK and in certain other countries

Published in the United States
by Oxford University Press Inc., New York

A catalogue record for this title is available from the British Library

Library of Congress Cataloging in Publication Data
Controversies in the management of salivary gland disease/edited by Mark McGurk,
Andrew G. Renehan.
Includes bibliographical references.
1. Salivary glands–Diseases–Treatment   2. Salivary glands–Tumours–Treatment
I. McGurk, Mark   II. Renehan, Andrew G.
[DNLM: 1. Salivary Gland Diseases–therapy   2. Salivary Gland Diseases–diagnosis.
3. Salivary Gland Neoplasms–diagnosis   4. Salivary Gland Neoplasms–therapy.
WI 230 C764 2001]
RC815.5.C66 2001   616.3'16–dc21   2001033911
ISBN 0 19 263278 7 (Hbk)
10 9 8 7 6 5 4 3 2 1

Typeset by EXPO Holdings, Malaysia
Printed on acid-free paper in Hong Kong

Preface

Neoplastic and non-neoplastic diseases of the major and minor salivary glands of the upper aerodigestive tract are, on the whole, relatively uncommon, yet they ignite interest in clinicians and scientists from many backgrounds. The list includes surgeons (general, otolaryngological, plastic, maxillofacial, and paediatric), oncologists, pathologists, radiologists, rheumatologists, and clinical immunologists. This book is based on an international symposium on salivary gland disease held recently at Guy's and St Thomas' Hospital in London, the primary aim of which was to bring together a group of contributors from many of these fields to discuss area of controversies in the management of patients with salivary gland diseases.

This book represents a re-evaluation of a considerable amount of pathological and clinical data relating to salivary gland disease. Historically the difficulties have been the relative rarity of these disorders together with the protracted natural histories in many cases. Individual surgical experience has been small and therefore pathologists were the first to collect information on the subject. Consequently, there has been an understandable reliance on pathological evidence to explain clinical events. Clinical based evidence revealing the natural course of events has been slower to accumulate because careful record keeping and long-term follow-up is required. What is new is that sufficient clinical data of adequate quality are now available to provide a clearer picture. In some situations, the clinical findings support the historical concepts, in others there are conflicts of evidence. The intention of this book is to highlight these discrepancies where they occur and if possible resolve them. Many of the topics have been addressed from opposing points of view, so at the end of each chapter the editors have attempted to summarize the evidence and where possible provide a clear perspective. The method used was to accept the pathological evidence (or premise), work out the logical consequences, and then relate them to the observed clinical course of events. This approach is intended to be systematic and scientific, and the editors accept (and expect) that as new evidence accumulates, revision of these 'new' concepts will be required. However this is no reason not to express a clear opinion on the evidence available now.

We are indebted to all of our contributors.

Mark McGurk and Andrew G. Renehan

Contents

List of contributors

Emilio Arzoz, Hospital Virgin del Camino, Servico de Cirga Maxillofacial, Navarra, Spain.

B. Malcolm Bailey, Consultant Surgeon, Department of Oral and Maxillofacial Surgery, Roehamptom, London, UK.

Andrew W. Barrett, Department of Oral Pathology, Eastman Dental Institute, London, UK.

Pasquale Berloco, Institute of Otolaryngology and Head and Neck Surgery, Florence, Italy.

Patrick Bradley, Consultant Surgeon, Department of Otolaryngology and Head and Neck Surgery, Queens Medical Centre, Nottingham, UK.

Bernadette M. Brennan, Consultant Paediatric Oncologist, Royal Manchester Children's Hospital, Manchester, UK.

Jacqueline Brown, Department of Dental Radiology, Guy's and St Thomas' Hospital, London, UK.

Luca Bruschini, Institute of Otolaryngology and Head and Neck Surgery, Florence, Italy.

Pasquale Capaccio, Departmento di Scienze Otorhinolaringologiche, Milano, Italy.

Nicholas Drage, Department of Dental Radiology, Guy's and St Thomas' Hospital, London, UK.

Michael Escudier, Salivary Service Unit, Guy's and St Thomas' Hospital, London, UK.

John W. Eveson, Reader on Oral Pathology, University of Bristol, Bristol, UK.

Robert A. Frankenthaler, Consultant Otolaryngologist, Joint Centre for Otolaryngology, Boston, USA.

Oreste Gallo, Institute of Otolaryngology and Head and Neck Surgery, Florence, Italy.

Brian D. Hancock, Consultant Surgeon, Department of Surgery, Wythenshawe Hospital, Manchester, UK.

Philip Katz, Maxillofacial Unit, Thedore de Banville, Paris, France.

John Langdon, Professor of Oral and Maxillofacial Surgery, King's College Hospital, London, UK.

Mark McGurk, Professor of Oral and Maxillofacial Surgery, Guy's and St Thomas' Hospital, London, UK.

Oded Nahleili, Department of Oral and Maxillofacial Surgery, Tel Aviv, Israel.

Ketil Natvig, Professor, ENT Department, National Hospital, Oslo, Norway.

Christopher J. O'Brien, Clinical Professor, Royal Prince Alfred Hospital, Newtown, Australia.

Andrew G. Renehan, Senior Research Fellow, Department of Surgery, Christie Hospital NHS Trust, Manchester, UK.

Nicholas J. Slevin, Consultant, Department of Clinical Oncology, Christie Hospital NHS Trust, Manchester, UK.

Gordon B. Snow, Professor of Otolaryngology and Head and Neck Surgery, Academisch Ziekenhuis, Amsterdam, The Netherlands.

Paul Speight, Professor of Oral Pathology, Eastman Dental Institute, London, UK.

Ronald H. Spiro, Head and Neck Surgeon, Memorial Sloan-Kettering Cancer Center, New York, USA.

J. Meirion Thomas, Consultant Surgeon, Royal Marsden Hospital, Chelsea and Westminister Hospital, London, UK.

Isaac van der Waal, Professor of Oral Pathology, Academisch Ziekenhuis, Amsterdam, Netherlands.

John C. Watkinson, Consultant Surgeon, Department of Otolaryngology and Head and Neck Surgery, Queen Elizabeth's Hospital, Birmingham, UK.

A. John Webb, Senior Research Fellow and formerly Consultant Surgeon, Department of Surgery, Bristol Royal Infirmary, Bristol, UK.

Andrew Yeudall, Molecular Biologist, Department of Oral Biology, Guy's and St Thomas' Hospital, London, UK.

SECTION ONE
Salivary Neoplasms – General Factors

CHAPTER 1

General epidemiology and statistics in a defined UK population

Patrick Bradley

General epidemiology

Incidence

Population incidence data for salivary gland tumours, in the past, have been incomplete for two reasons: (i) population data were not routinely collected for benign neoplasms, the commonest tumour group; and (ii) minor gland carcinomas were coded with other upper aerodigestive tract malignancies, and hence were indeterminable. Thus, incidences for all salivary tumours ranging from 0.4 to 13.5 per 100 000 have been reported in population studies from Uganda (Davies *et al.* 1964), Malaya (Loke 1967), Malawi (Thomas *et al.* 1980), Scotland (Lennox *et al.* 1978), and Greenland (Wallace *et al.* 1963). It is difficult to distinguish whether these variations are due to errors of registration or represent real demographic differences due to local factors.

Salivary cancers

For salivary cancers arising in the major glands, the incidence in England and Wales has been approximately 0.7 per 100 000 for the past decade (Cancer Statistics Registrations for 1986–1993 from the Office of Population Censuses and Surveys 1991, 1993, 1994*a,b*; Office for National Statistics 1997*a,b*, 1998, 1999). Cancer incidences increase with age and are more common in males (Fig. 1.1). Among European and American Caucasian populations, it is generally held that incidences of major gland cancers are similar (Parkin *et al.* 1992). In contrast, relatively larger numbers of the rare undifferentiated salivary carcinoma account for high incidences among Inuit Eskimos of northern Canada and Greenland, and populations of southern Chinese (Wallace *et al.* 1963).

A recent study of 3305 patients, from the Swedish Cancer Registry, is noteworthy as it is the largest population-based study to date that includes minor gland carcinomas (Ostman *et al.* 1997). The study reported an age-standardized incidence rate of 1.32 per 100 000 population, 0.5% of all newly diagnosed cancers.

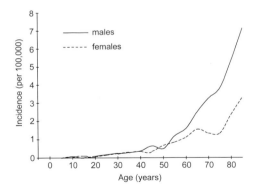

Fig. 1.1 Incidence rates (per 100 000 population) for major salivary gland sites (ICD 9th revision, number = 142) shown for males and females. Data for England and Wales 1983–1993 (Office of Population Censuses and Surveys 1991, 1993, 1994a,b; Office for National Statistics 1997a,b, 1998, 1999).

Three studies have suggested that the incidence of salivary gland cancers may be increasing, but this may simply reflect improved histological coding (Horn Ross *et al.* 1991; Rippin and Potts 1992; Zheng *et al.* 1997).

Benign salivary tumours

Institutional series demonstrate that benign neoplasms are the commonest salivary tumours. In the Christie series, for all sites, benign histologies accounted for 80% (940/1194) of tumours (Renehan *et al.* 1996). Of the benign group, the two commonest histological types are pleomorphic adenoma and Warthin's tumour (Fig. 1.2).

Population-based data for incidences of benign tumours are lacking. Gunn and Parrott (1988) estimated, based on pathology reports, an incidence of 1.6 per 100 000 for parotid pleomorphic adenomas within the North East region of England. Warthin's tumour is male dominant and largely in an older age group than pleomorphic adenoma. Its exact incidence in the population is not known but there may be demographic variations, notably uncommon among African and American Blacks (Yoo *et al.* 1994), but with an increased incidence in Singapore Chinese (Chung *et al.* 1999).

Site distributions

Salivary tissue is distributed widely in the mucosa of the upper aerodigestive tract as well as being concentrated in three major salivary glands. It is a popular belief that for every 100 parotid tumours there are 10 submandibular, 10 minor salivary, and one

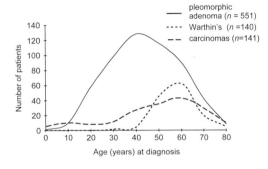

Fig. 1.2 Distributions of the three main salivary tumour groups (pleomorphic adenoma, Warthin's tumour, and carcinoma) by age at diagnosis in the Christie series (1948–1992) (Data courtesy of Mr A. Renehan).

sublingual gland tumour (Spiro 1998). It is also widely believed that the probability of encountering a malignant neoplasm is less than 25% in patients with parotid gland tumours, about 50% in those with submandibular gland tumours, more than 80% in those with minor salivary gland lesions, and virtually 100% in those few patients with a sublingual gland tumour (Eveson and Cawson 1985).

It is important to remember that most statistics on the anatomical distribution of salivary gland tumours and the proportion of malignant to benign are derived from clinicians who have a particular interest in salivary gland tumours and, consequently, are likely to contain a degree of bias due to case selection. For example, only patients who undergo surgery are normally included in these series.

Statistics in a defined UK population

The incidence of salivary gland tumours, both benign and malignant, presenting at a secondary care facility in the UK has not been reported in a fixed population to date. Such an investigation was undertaken recently in a discrete stable population over a 10-year period, 1988–1997, to clarify the incidence of these neoplasia.

The Nottingham population

Nottingham Health Authority provides primary and secondary health care for a fixed population of 642 000 (Nottingham Health Authority 1996). This population receives hospital care, free on the National Health Service (NHS), on referral by letter from their general practitioners to a hospital-based specialist. In Nottingham, this service is provided by two NHS hospitals both based within the city of Nottingham, i.e. Nottingham University Hospital Queen's Medical Centre and The City Hospital, and by two private facilities. The pathology service for all four hospitals is provided by the pathology laboratories based at the two NHS hospitals. The records have been computerized since 1987. This work is provided on a 'fee per item of service' basis, and salivary neoplasms were reported in accordance with the WHO classifications (Chapter 2).

This made it simple to gather data on salivary gland disease in the local population. The histopathology records were scrutinized for patients who had salivary specimens or associated tissue analysed in the period January 1988–December 1997. Those patients with a neoplasm of salivary origin were then analysed further. Included in these data were patients who had undergone a fine needle aspiration cytology (FNAC) biopsy of a salivary neoplasm. Data collected nationally by disease type were used for comparison. This was possible because in the NHS all in-patient hospital activity in an NHS hospital is recorded routinely by the Department of Health. Each patient's admission and subsequent treatment of a particular illness by a particular consultant is recorded as a finished consultant episode (FCE). There may be multiple FCEs for a single illness if there are repeated admissions to hospital, but this is uncommon with salivary tumours because surgery is a single event. FCEs should therefore represent a reasonable approximation of activity in the NHS. These data are collated annually and are made available to central government through the Department of Health. A similar system of data collection is not available in the private sector.

Table 1.1 The proportions of benign and malignant salivary gland tumours by anatomic site - Nottingham 1988-1997

		Benign	Malignant	Total
Major salivary glands	Parotid gland	397	26 (6)	423
	Submandibular gland	35	12 (34)	47
	Sublingual gland	0	5 (100)	5
Minor salivary glands		32	10 (24)	42
Total		**464**	**53**	**517**

Values in parentheses are percentages.

Tumour site distribution

In total, 517 patients were identified with a diagnosis of a salivary gland tumour between January 1988 and December 1997. Sixty-six were cases treated in the private sector. The site distributions, and the benign and malignant categories are shown in Table 1.1. In this series, 82% of neoplasms occurred in the parotid, 9% in the submandibular, and 8% in the minor salivary glands, confirming the 10:1:1 rule of tumour distribution. Approximately 1% of tumours were sited in the parapharyngeal space (5/517), and all proved to be pleomorphic adenomas. Five patients (1%) had tumours arising from the sublingual glands, and all these were malignant (three adenoid cystic carcinomas, two mucoepidermoid carcinomas).

Notably, the benign:malignant ratio of tumours at each site did not conform to standard teaching. Overall, 10% of salivary gland tumours were malignant. The proportions for the three main sites, parotid, submandibular, and minor glands, were 6, 34, and 24%.

Histological types

When analysed by histological type, the most common benign neoplasm was the pleomorphic adenoma (71% or 331/464) followed by Warthin's tumour (22% or 102/464) (Table 1.2). The other histological types together only comprised 7% of benign neoplasms. The data suggest that about 52 pleomorphic and 16 Warthin's tumours can be expected annually per million population.

In the malignant tumours, three histological types were equally represented in the mouth and major salivary glands: adenoid cystic (30% or 16/52), mucoepidermoid (25% or 14/52), and adenocarcinoma (21% or 11/52). The next most frequent type was acinic cell (7/52), whereas the remaining histological varieties only occurred sporadically, and collectively represented 10% of all malignant tumour.

Incidences

The annual incidences for benign and malignant salivary tumours over the 10-year study period are shown in Table 1.3. The overall tumour incidence was 8.0 per

Table 1.2 The histological types by site in a Nottingham population (1988-97)

	Major salivary glands			Minor glands	Total
	Parotid	Submandibular	Sublingual		
Benign tumours					
Pleomorphic adenoma	275	31	–	27	**333**
Warthin's tumour	100	2	–	–	**102**
Oncocytoma	3	1	–	–	**4**
Monomorphic, NOS	9	1	–	–	**10**
Basal cell adenoma	6	1	–	–	**7**
Canalicular adenoma	–	–	–	3	**3**
Cystadenema	3	–	–	1	**4**
Myoepithelioma	1	–	–	–	**1**
Malignant tumours					
Mucoepidermoid carcinoma	7	3	2	2	**14**
Adenoid cystic carcinoma	6	5	3	2	**16**
Adenocarcinoma, NOS	7	1	–	3	**11**
Acinic cell carcinoma	5	–	–	2	**7**
LGP adenocarcinoma	–	–	–	1	**1**
Clear cell carcinoma	1	–	–	–	**1**
Carcinoma in-PA	–	1	–	–	**1**
Undifferentiated carcinoma	–	2	–	–	**2**

NOS: not otherwise specified. PA:pleomorphic adenoma. LGP: low-grade polymorphous adenocarcinoma.

Table 1.3 Annual incidence (per 100 000 population) of salivary gland neoplasms by site – Nottingham 1988–1997

	Benign	Malignant
Major salivary glands		
Parotid gland	6.2	0.4
Submandibular gland	0.55	0.19
Sublingual gland	0	0.08
Minor salivary glands	0.47	0.16
Total	7.2	0.8

100 000. The incidence of benign tumours for all sites was 7.2 per 100 000 population. The incidence for cancer was 0.8 per 100 000, and 0.6 per 100 000 for major glands, consistent with the National Cancer Registry.

Comparisons with Department of Health FCE data

The Department of Health FCE statistics for salivary tumours covering the financial years 1991–1997 inclusive were compared with manually collected NHS data for the same period to validate the data. The manually collected pathology data showed an annual rate of benign salivary gland tumours in the Nottingham population (642 000 individuals) of 39.5 against the official Department of Health figures of 28.5. The malignant salivary tumour rate was 3.8 against a Department of Health rate of 7.3. The manually derived figures for cancer compared almost exactly with cancer registry data, which suggests that the discrepancy is due to errors in FCE statistics.

The annual average incidence of malignant salivary tumours was 8.2 (per million population) and, if the private cases were excluded (5/53 cases), the figure was 7.5. The National Cancer Registry data report six cases per million population, but this figure would exclude minor salivary gland cancers which are included in the above calculations and constituted 28% of cancers in this series.

Surgical disciplines and the treatment of salivary tumours

One of the features highlighted by this analysis was the large numbers of surgical disciplines that undertook surgical treatment of salivary tumours (Table 1.4). Thirty-two clinical teams were involved in patient management of parotid tumours. In the 10-year study period, there were only eight surgeons who performed more than 10 operations. The median patient caseload of the 32 surgeons identified was four. In the management of submandibular salivary tumours, 16 surgical teams were identified; the median workload of this surgical group was one case over the same period.

Lessons from the Nottingham series

There are three main lessons learned from the Nottingham study listed in Box 1.1.

Problems of accurate data collection

In the UK, patients who are diagnosed with cancer are registered anatomically by the Regional Cancer Registry, which is forwarded to the Department of Health. Only malignant disease is reported to this registry. In addition, there is a second anatomical collection of data related to treatment in NHS hospitals by FCEs. In the past, this information has not been collected consistently, and surgeons who have kept their own

Table 1.4 Number of cases treated by different surgical disciplines within the Nottingham region (1988–1997)

	Orl-HNS	G Surg	Plastics	OMFS	Others*
Major salivary glands					
Parotid gland	234	104	50	31	4
Submandibular gland	26	9	3	8	1
Sublingual gland				5	
Minor salivary glands	9		4	26	3
Total	269	113	57	70	5

Orl-HNS, otolaryngology–head and neck surgery; G Surg, general surgery; OMFS, oral and maxillofacial surgery.

* One parotid lesion and two oral lesions were treated initially by dermatologists. The remainder of the 'others' were treated by paediatric surgeons.

Box 1.1 Lessons from the Nottingham population study

◆ There are marked problems in collection of actual population-based data. National data, such as Department of Health FECs may be significantly inaccurate.

◆ The overall incidence for all salivary gland tumours in the UK is approximately 8 per 100,000 population. This has probably been underestimated in the past.

◆ The 100:10:1:10 rule holds true for the ratios of tumours by site; parotid: submandibular: sublingual: minor salivary glands. But institutional series overestimate the proportions of malignancies, particularly in the parotid gland, and minor salivary glands.

tumour data register have questioned the accuracy of both official data sets. Some of the objectives of having a cancer registry are to assess the needs for cancer services at a local level, to evaluate quality of care within the population, and for research into epidemiology, health technology, and treatment outcomes (Trent Cancer Registry 1997). The incidence of salivary gland cancer recorded by the cancer registries (0.6), and the present manual exercise were essentially identical, but the FCE data grossly inflated estimates of disease.

Overall incidence has been underestimated

Gunn and Parrott (1988) collected figures for all new parotid tumours (benign and malignant) operated on in the North East of England over a 5-year period, and reported an incidence of 2.4 per 100 000 population. The Nottingham figure for operated parotid tumours was 7.21 per 100 000 population. Exclusion of the patients operated on in the private sector would still give an annual incidence figure of 6.4 per 100 000. A subanalysis of Gunn and Parrot's data suggests that the incidence of parotid pleomorphic adenoma was 1.5 per 100 000, whereas in the Nottingham population the overall figure was 4.28, and when the private patients were excluded it was 3.66 per 100 000 per year. The difference in incidence may represent a real population difference between these two communities or a change in incidence over time. However, the more likely explanation is incomplete data collection due to the difficulties of data retrieval from such a large geographical area.

Proportions by site

This population-based study has confirmed the 100:10:1:10 rule for the proportions of salivary tumours by the four main sites: parotid glands; submandibular glands; sublingual glands; and minor salivary glands. Comparison between this population-based study and large institutional series (both surgical and pathological) is shown in Table 1.5 (Eneroth 1971; Eveson and Cawson 1985; Seifert et al. 1986; Spiro 1986;

Table 1.5 The proportions of benign and malignant epithelial salivary gland tumours in different large series

	Population-based	Surgical series			Pathology series		
	Nottingham	Karolinska	SKMCC	Christie	Hamburg*	BSG Panel	AFIP*
Parotid gland							
Benign	397	1638	1062	722	1605	1498	2568
Malignant	26 (6)	345 (17)	354 (25)	141 (16)	329 (17)	258 (15)	1668 (39)
Submandibular gland							
Benign	35	100	92	21	194	162	309
Malignant	12 (34)	61 (38)	68 (43)	11 (34)	193 (50)	95 (37)	294 (49)
Sublingual gland†							
Benign	0	–	–	–	–	1	7
Malignant	5 (100)	–	–	–	–	6 (86)	21 (75)
Minor salivary glands							
Benign	32	93	72	25	129	180	978
Malignant	10 (24)	748 (44)	318 (82)	23 (48)	129 (50)	156 (46)	1176 (55)
Totals	517	2311	1966	943	2579	2410‡	7021
Ratios (P:SM:SL:M)	100:10:1:10	100:10:–:10	100:10:–:30	100:5:–:5	100:15:–:10	100:10:1:10	100:15:1:50

SKMCC, Sloan-Kettering Memorial Cancer Center; AFIP, Armed Forces Institute of Pathology; BSG, British Salivary Gland Panel; P, parotid; SM, submandibular; SL, sublingual; M. minor salivary glands.

Values in parentheses are the percentage malignant tumours per site.

* Included secondary referrals in the analysis.

† Sublingual gland tumours included within minor glands in four series.

‡ Unknown site in 54 cases.

Auclair *et al.* 1991; Renehan *et al.* 1996). This comparison highlights that these series have probably overestimated the proportion of malignancies, particularly for the parotid gland and the minor salivary glands. This has implications for cancer service resources.

REFERENCES

Auclair, P.L., Ellis, G.L., Gnepp, D.R., Wenig, B.M., and Janney, C.G. (1991) Salivary gland neoplasms: general considerations. In: *Surgical Pathology of the Salivary Glands*. pp. 135–64. (eds G.L. Ellis, P.L. Auclair, and D.R. Gnepp) W.B. Saunders Co., Philadelphia.

Chung, Y.F., Khoo, M.L., Heng, M.K., Hong, G.S., and Soo, K.C. (1999) Epidemiology of Warthin's tumour of the parotid gland in an Asian population. *Br J Surg*, **86**, 661–4.

Davies, J.N.P., Dodge, O.G., and Burkitt, D.P. (1964) Salivary gland tumours in Uganda. *Cancer*, **17**, 1310–22.

Eneroth, C.M. (1971) Salivary gland tumors in the parotid gland, submandibular gland, and the palate region. *Cancer*, **27**, 1415–8.

Eveson, J.W. and Cawson, R.A. (1985) Salivary gland tumours. A review of 2410 cases with particular reference to histological types, site, age and sex distribution. *J Pathol*, **146**, 51–8.

Gunn, A. and Parrott, N.R. (1988) Parotid tumours: a review of parotid tumour surgery in the Northern Regional Health Authority of the United Kingdom 1978–1982. *Br J Surg*, **75**, 1144–6.

Horn Ross, P.L., West, D.W., and Brown, S.R. (1991) Recent trends in the incidence of salivary gland cancer. *Int J Epidemiol*, **20**, 628–33.

Lennox, B., Clarke, J.A., Drake, F., and Ewen, S.W. (1978) Incidence of salivary gland tumours in Scotland: accuracy of national records. *Br Med J*, **1**, 687–9.

Loke, Y.W. (1967) Salivary gland tumours in Malaya. *Br J Cancer*, **21**, 665–74.

Nottingham Health Authority (1996) *1995/96 Annual Report, Review and Financial Statement*. Standard Court, Nottingham.

Office of Population Censuses and Surveys (1991) *Cancer Statistics Registrations 1986*. Series MB1 No. 19. HMSO, London.

Office of Population Censuses and Surveys (1993) *Cancer Statistics Registrations 1987*. Series MB1 No. 20. HMSO, London.

Office of Population Censuses and Surveys (1994a) *Cancer Statistics Registrations 1988*. Series MB1 No. 21. HMSO, London.

Office of Population Censuses and Surveys (1994b) *Cancer Statistics Registrations 1989*. Series MB1 No. 22. HMSO, London.

Office for National Statistics (1997a) *Cancer Statistics Registrations 1990*. Series MB1 No. 23. HMSO, London.

Office for National Statistics (1997b) *Cancer Statistics Registrations 1991*. Series MB1 No. 24. HMSO, London.

Office for National Statistics (1998) *Cancer Statistics Registrations 1992*. Series MB1 No. 25. HMSO, London.

Office for National Statistics (1999) *Cancer Statistics Registrations 1993*. Series MB1 No. 26. HMSO, London.

Ostman, J., Anneroth, G., Gustafsson, H., and Tavelin, B. (1997) Malignant salivary gland tumours in Sweden 1960–1989—an epidemiological study. *Oral Oncol*, **33**, 169–76.

Parkin, D.M., Muir, C.S., Whelan, S.L., Gao, Y.T., Ferlay, J., and Powell, J. (1992) *Cancer Incidence in Five Continents*, Vol. VI. pp. 906–7. IARC Scientific Publications No. 120, Lyon.

Renehan, A., Gleave, E.N., Hancock, B.D., Smith, P., and McGurk, M. (1996) Long-term follow-up of over 1000 patients with salivary gland tumours treated in a single centre. *Br J Surg*, **83**, 1750–4.

Rippin, J.W. and Potts, A.J. (1992) Intra-oral salivary gland tumours in the West Midlands. *Br Dent J*, **173**, 17–9.

Seifert, G., Miehlke, J., Haubrich, J., and Chilla, R. (1986) *Diseases of the Salivary Glands*. pp. 239–40. Georg Thime Verlag, Stuttgart.

Spiro, R.H. (1986) Salivary neoplasms: overview of a 35-year experience with 2,807 patients. *Head Neck Surg*, **8**, 177–84.

Spiro, R.H. (1998) Management of malignant tumors of the salivary glands. *Oncol Huntingt*, **12**, 671–80.

Thomas, K.M., Hutt, M.S., and Borgstein, J. (1980) Salivary gland tumors in Malawi. *Cancer*, **46**, 2328–34.

Trent Cancer Registry (1997) *First Report: 1996/97*. Weston Park Hospital, Sheffield.

Wallace, A.C., McDougal, J.T., Hildes, J.A., and Lederman, J.M. (1963) Salivary gland tumours in Canadian Eskimos. *Cancer*, **16**, 1338–53.

Yoo, G.H., Eisele, D.W., Askin, F.B., Driben, J.S., and Johns, M.E. (1994) Warthin's tumor: a 40-year experience at the Johns Hopkins Hospital. *Laryngoscope*, **104**, 799–803.

Zheng, T., Holford, T.R., Chen, Y., Ward, B., Liu, W., Flannery, J. *et al.* (1997) Are cancers of the salivary gland increasing? Experience from Connecticut, USA. *Int J Epidemiol*, **26**, 264–71.

Editorial comment

Only a rough estimate of the incidence of salivary gland tumour can be obtained from the literature, but the recent large Swedish study (Ostman *et al.* 1997) has helped substantially in establishing the true incidence in a European population. This differs from most other studies in that minor salivary gland cancers are included separately in the analysis rather than grouped with oropharyngeal cancer. The Nottingham study makes a significant contribution to this body of knowledge. In contrast to the Scandinavian study, the Nottingham data set is not large, but it is a comprehensive analysis of a well-defined population. Large quantities of relatively crude data allow only coarse-grain evaluation, whereas small but defined data sets provide the luxury of a fine-grain analysis. Mr Bradley knows the Nottingham area intimately and it is highly unlikely that a significant number of cases have been lost to analysis. As such, this chapter gives an authoritative insight into the incidence of both benign and malignant salivary neoplasms at various anatomical sites (parotid, submandibular, sublingual, and minor salivary glands) in the UK population. The data are unique because this is the first attempt to establish the incidence of benign salivary tumours for all sites. An interesting observation is that malignant disease may not be as common in the submandibular gland or mouth as is traditionally believed. The 100:10:10 ratio of tumours in the parotid, submandibular, and minor salivary glands holds true. The prominence of minor salivary gland cancer in the overall picture has not been widely appreciated nor has the high risk of malignancy in minor salivary gland tumours of the floor of the mouth.

CHAPTER 2

Aetiology and molecular changes in salivary gland tumours

Oreste Gallo

Aetiology

The aetiology of salivary gland neoplasms remains unknown; however, as for many other neoplasms, there is growing evidence to incriminate environmental factors and certain genetic abnormalities.

Environmental factors

A list of environmental aetiological factors is shown in Box 2.1.

Radiation

The strongest evidence for a link between high-dose ionizing radiation and salivary gland neoplasms is provided by studies of survivors who were exposed to radiation from the atomic bombs in Hiroshima and Nagasaki in 1945, and who have been monitored by both the Atomic Bomb Casualty Commission and Radiation Effects Foundations (Belsky *et al.* 1972, 1975; Takeichi *et al.* 1976; Land *et al.* 1996). A significantly higher incidence of salivary gland tumours was reported for the period 1957–1970 in persons exposed to radiation doses of ≤3 Gy. Recently, Saku and colleagues (1997) extended this work, analysing the same cohort, but now with a total period of observation of 37 years. These survivors had a higher radiation-related risk of developing both benign and malignant salivary gland tumours compared with the general population. The risk was dose related for both tumour types but was highest for malignant tumours, particularly mucoepidermoid carcinomas, rather than benign neoplasms. Interestingly, Warthin's tumour (WT) showed the highest dose–response-related risk for the latter group. The association has been supported by a study of 498 patients with histopathologically confirmed carcinoma of the salivary glands, 57 of whom had a history of radiation exposure and 49 who had been irradiated in a field encompassing the salivary gland area (Spitz *et al.* 1984). More interestingly, the same investigators also reported the potential risk of ultraviolet radiation exposure in the development of salivary gland tumours (Spitz *et al.* 1988).

Box 2.1 Environmental aetiological factors

High-dose radiation (atomic bomb survivors)

- Low-dose radiation
- dental and medical radiographs
- external radiotherapy for childhood benign diseases
- iodine[131] therapy
- ultraviolet radiation

Epstein–Barr virus is associated with:

- undifferentiated carcinoma
- Warthin's tumour
- salivary T-cell lymphoma in AIDS patients

Cigarette smoking is associated with:

- Warthin's tumour

Miscellaneous

- silica dust
- kerosene cooking fuel
- high cholesterol and low vitamins
- low intake of dark yellow vegetables

Several studies have also demonstrated associations between low-dose radiation expo-sure and the development of salivary gland tumours. Increased incidences of salivary gland tumours have been observed in individuals treated with ionizing radiation for benign lesions of the head and neck or chest (Ju 1968; Katz and Preston Martin 1984), including children treated for tinea capitis (Shore *et al.* 1976; Modan *et al.* 1998; Schweider *et al.* 1998), patients who received I[131] for hyperthyroidism (Hoffman *et al.* 1982), and patients exposed to repeated diagnostic radiation to the oral cavity (Preston Martin *et al.* 1988).

Viruses

There is circumstantial evidence to incriminate oncogenic viruses in the development of some salivary gland neoplasms. Epstein–Barr virus (EBV), cytomegalovirus, and human herpes virus have been implicated because they may replicate in salivary tissue; however, to date, convincing evidence for a role in salivary tumorigenesis has been reported only for EBV (Atula *et al.* 1998). Several studies have demonstrated a close association between undifferentiated carcinoma in tumours with lymphoid stroma, notably nasopharyngeal carcinoma and EBV (Saemundsen *et al.* 1982; Nagao *et al.* 1996; Tsai *et al.* 1996; Sheen *et al.* 1997). This is a rare cancer with a relatively high incidence among the Inuit of North America and Greenland, and the southern

Chinese. Lymphoepithelial carcinoma and undifferentiated carcinoma of the salivary gland in these populations may share a similar EBV-related pathogenesis. The detection of the virus in a clonal form and the expression of its viral oncoprotein in epithelial neoplastic cells from lymphoepithelial and undifferentiated carcinoma of the salivary gland further support this assertion (Iezzoni *et al.* 1995; Kuo and Hsueh 1997). The relative high incidence of these tumours among Eskimoes and southern Chinese may be the result of an enhanced oncogenic potential of an EBV strain or genetic susceptibility; however, we recently have reported the detection of EBV DNA in undifferentiated carcinomas of the parotid gland from Caucasian patients (Gallo *et al.* 1996). Others have detected a lytic EBV infection in non-malignant epithelial cells surrounded by an EBV-positive T-cell lymphoma (Wen *et al.* 1996, 1997). Taken together, these findings suggest a possible role for EBV in salivary gland disorders characterized by lymphoepithelial proliferation because EBV has the dual ability to infect both epithelial salivary gland cells (particularly ductal cells which express the C3d/EBV receptor of B cells) and B lymphocytes (Deacon *et al.* 1991).

The possible association of EBV with lymphoepithelial pathology prompted our group to investigate a potential role for EBV in the pathogenesis of Warthin's tumour (WT), a benign salivary gland tumour characterized by a lymphoepithelial proliferation. We reported the presence of EBV DNA sequences, using a non-radioactive biotinylated EBV DNA (*Bam*HI-W fragment) probe by an *in situ* hybridization technique in the cytoplasm of neoplastic oxyphilic cells in a significant number of patients with multiple or bilateral WT (87%), whereas the EBV genome was less common in solitary WT (17%) (Santucci *et al.* 1993; Gallo *et al.* 1994). Moreover, the EBV genome often was detected in the cytoplasm of ductal cells (75% bilateral and 33% of solitary WT) and occasionally acinar cells (17% of both multiple/bilateral and solitary WT). These findings have been confirmed by others using polymerase chain reaction (PCR) and immunohistochemistry but have not been identified in all reported series of WT (Taira *et al.* 1992; Takezawa *et al.* 1998; Tornoczky *et al.* 1998). The evidence for EBV in WT remains equivocal; however, WT is associated with some autoimmune diseases [relative risk (RR) = 8.69, $P < 0.0001$ in the WT population] and frequently those related to viral infections (supporting a viral pathogenesis), and suggests an association with immune disorders (Gallo and Bocciolini 1997). Moreover, in our WT population, we were able to identify a higher level of EBV-VCA-IgG and EBV-EA-IgG as well as a statistically significant association between HLA-DR6 antigen. As with other immune diseases, a specific HLA haplotype could be associated with a high risk of viral infection because of a decreased immune response. Recently, Chung *et al.* (1999) reported the apparent increased incidence of WT in the Chinese, a population well known for its endemic distribution of EBV infection (about 25% of all parotid tumours). These epidemiological data provide further indirect support for the pathogenic role of EBV in WT (Renehan *et al.* 1999).

Tobacco exposure

Tobacco use has been implicated in a number of studies (Ebbs and Webb 1986; Cadier *et al.* 1992; Chung *et al.* 1999) as a possible risk factor in the development of WT, but not for malignant salivary gland neoplasms. This association with WT has also been observed in our Italian population (Gallo and Bocciolini 1997) where 87% of our WT patients had a positive smoking history, compared with 38% in 409 patients with pleomorphic adenoma of the parotid gland (P <0.001). This strong association between WT and smoking seems to conform to the acknowledged tumorigenic properties of cigarettes, but the mechanism of pathogenesis may be different in salivary glands because there is no similar association with other histotypes, particularly malignant salivary gland tumours (Gallo 1994).

Other environmental factors

Occupational exposure to silica dust is associated with a 2.5-fold risk of salivary gland cancer (Hanna and Suen 1988), and there is a significantly increased risk among patients using kerosene as cooking fuel. There have also been reported associations with diet with high cholesterol and low vitamin intake (Zheng *et al.* 1996), and with low intake of dark yellow vegetables (Horn Ross *et al.* 1997).

Molecular changes

In recent years, extensive cytogenetic and molecular studies have revealed specific chromosomal abnormalities and gene mutations specific to benign and malignant salivary gland tumours that may, in due course, be useful in the diagnosis, therapy, and prognosis of salivary gland neoplasms. However, despite these developments, there are

---

Box 2.2 Molecular changes in salivary oncogenesis

Structural rearrangements
◆ Pleomorphic adenoma

      PLAG1 associated: 8q12–15★

      HMGIC associated: 12q13–15★

◆ Carcinomas

      6q23, 11q21, 17p13 (*p53* gene), trisomy 5

Allelic loss and loss of heterozygosity (LOH)

◆ chromosome 12p and 19q in mucoepidermoid carcinoma

◆ chromosome 8 in adenoid cystic carcinoma

◆ LOH at multiple chromosomal sites in malignant tumours

Oncogenes and tumour suppressor genes

◆ *p53*, c-*erb* 2, E-cadherin, p21^{ras}, c-*fos*

★*PLAG1*, pleomorphic adenoma gene 1; *HMG1C*, high-mobility gene 1 (see Guerts *et al.* 1997)

---

still no definitive data on the genetic mechanisms responsible for the development of salivary gland tumours. Those that have been demonstrated are listed in Box 2.2.

Structural rearrangement

Specific structural chromosome rearrangement has been noted in different histotypes of salivary gland neoplasms, usually characterized by translocation of genetic material involving chromosome 8 in pleomorphic adenomas, chromosome 11 in muco-epidemoid carcinoma and by a translocation on chromosome 6 in adenoid cystic carcinomas (Queimado *et al.* 1998). The largest and best characterized reciprocal translocation in salivary pleomorphic adenomas frequently occurs at t(3;8) (p21;q12) and involves band 8q12 (present in about 40% of adenomas) (Voz *et al.* 1998). This translocation involves a developmentally regulated zinc finger gene (*PLAG1*), while the level of β-catenin is reduced (Kas *et al.* 1997). This is postulated to be the pathogenic mechanism for induction of pleomorphic adenomas with the 8q12 translocation.

El Naggar and colleagues, at the M.D. Anderson Hospital (el Naggar *et al.* 1997) described a t(11,19) (q21;p3.1) translocation of mucoepidermoid carcinoma of the minor salivary glands, indicating that this rearrangement may be a primary event in at least a subset of these neoplasms. Similarly, in adenoid cystic carcinoma of the salivary glands, there is an increased frequency of t(6,9) (q23;p21) translocation (Nordkvist *et al.* 1994). Another possible regulator of salivary tumour growth may be interleukin-6 which we demonstrated to be an autocrine growth regulator of a cell line derived from a parotid pleomorphic adenoma (Gallo *et al.* 1992), and has been detected in most salivary gland tumours with prognostic significance (Gandour Edwards *et al.* 1995).

Monosomy and polysomy

Most benign and malignant salivary gland tumours have alterations in the number of chromosomes, and the loss of the Y chromosome has been described in malignant adenocarcinomas (Stenman *et al.* 1986). The M.D. Anderson group (el Naggar *et al.* 1994) have also described trisomy 5 as the only karyotypic abnormality in a primary mucoepidermoid carcinoma of the base of the tongue, and others have reported polysomy of chromosomes 3 and 17 occurring in salivary tumours, notably adenoid cystic carcinomas. In addition, monosomy of chromosome 17 has been implicated (Li *et al.* 1995), and has generated interest as the *p53* tumour suppressor gene is located on this chromosome.

Allelic loss and microsatellite instability

The analysis of genetic abnormalities has been facilitated by the identification of microsatellite repeats for most chromosomal regions and their suitability for amplification by polymerase chain reaction (PCR) (Sidransky 1995). In hereditary colon cancer, alterations in microsatellite sequence can serve as sensitive markers for detecting replicative errors and assessing genomic mutations. Two recent studies have used these techniques in benign and malignant salivary gland tumours with interesting clinical implications. The first study (Johns *et al.* 1996) demonstrated a high allele loss at chromosome 12p (35% of informative cases), and at chromosome 19q (40% of informative cases) in pleomorphic adenomas and in adenoid cystic carcinomas, and mucoepidermoid carcinomas showed 50% or greater loss at 2q, 5p, 12p and 16q. The second study, from the M.D. Anderson group (el Naggar *et al.* 1997), showed that most pleomorphic adenomas had allelic loss on the long arm of chromosome 8, while loss of heterozygosity (LOH) was demonstrated in 53% of malignant and 41% of benign tumours. Interestingly, the malignant tumours with LOH also demonstrated aggressive tumour characteristics, and the progression of benign pleomorphic adenoma to malignant mixed tumours frequently was associated with alterations on the short arm of chromosome 17. The focal regions of chromosomal damage or loss identified in salivary neoplasm may harbour tumour suppressor genes, and although some regions are shared with other tumour types (notably the putative site of the *p53* tumour suppressor gene), many appear unique to salivary gland tumours (such as loss on 8q), suggesting a distinct genetic pathway in salivary gland tumorigenesis.

Proto-oncogenes and tumour suppressor genes

The development and the progression of various benign and malignant neoplasms are known to be associated with activation of oncogenes and inactivation of tumour suppressor genes. A number of immunohistochemical and molecular studies have been undertaken to identify the genes involved in salivary gland tumorigenesis.

One of the best known tumour suppressor genes is *p53* which is located on human chromosome 17 (p13) at a site frequently altered in some benign and particularly malignant salivary gland tumours (Karja *et al.* 1997). The mutated *p53* gene product accumulates in the nucleus of neoplastic cells, and we detected it in three of 26 (11%) benign tumours and in 31 of 46 (67%) malignant parotid gland tumours. In our study, we first reported that *p53* aberration was statistically associated with regional and distant metastases ($P = 0.07$ and $P = 0.004$, respectively) and that patients whose cancers had moderate or high p53 protein expression had lower disease-free and actuarial survival rates than those with low or wild-type p53 expression ($P = 0.021$ and $P = 0.033$, respectively; Gallo *et al.* 1995*a,b*). These observations were supported by others who demonstrated *p53* mutations and/or p53 protein overexpression in most salivary gland neoplasms, including adenoid cystic carcinomas (Papadaki *et al.* 1996; Yamamoto *et al.* 1996), adenocarcinomas and salivary duct carcinomas (Kamio, 1996), pleomorphic adenomas, and carcinomas arising from pleomorphic adenomas (Li *et al.* 1995), as well as in mucoepidermoid and squamous cell carcinomas (Pignataro *et al.* 1998). The conclusion that can be drawn from this work is that the *p53* tumour suppressor gene seems to be involved in the transformation of some salivary gland cells to tumour cells, and the presence of the altered gene product is linked to clinical outcome. Increased or aberrant expression of p53 may also be associated with factors that favour angiogenesis (Doi *et al.* 1999). We have demonstrated recently that lack of or reduced E-cadherin expression is a sensitive prognostic maker in adenoid cystic carcinomas of the salivary glands, suggesting a role as a tumour suppressor gene (Franchi *et al.* 1999).

Historically, an association has been drawn between salivary gland and mammary gland tumours and this has prompted researchers to study the c-*erbB-2* (HER-2, neu) oncogene. The amplification of this proto-oncogene and overexpression of its protein have been demonstrated in almost 35% of carcinomas of the salivary glands with a clear correlation with tumour aggressiveness (Sugano *et al.* 1992; Press *et al.* 1994), particularly in adenoid cystic carcinomas and adenocarcinomas of the major salivary glands. Overexpression of c-erbB-2 has also been demonstrated in WT (47%) and in pleomorphic adenoma (33%) (Giannoni *et al.* 1995).

Another oncogene recently associated with salivary tumorigenesis is c-*fos*. Underexpression measured by *in situ* hybridization has been linked to loss of differentiation, particularly in poorly differentiated adenocarcinoma (Birek *et al.* 1993). Reduced expression of the cell cycle regulatory peptide, p27^{KAP1} is associated with increased metastases in adenoid cystic carcinoma (Takata *et al.* 1999).

REFERENCES

Atula, T., Grenman, R., Klemi, P., and Syrjanen, S. (1998) Human papillomavirus, Epstein–Barr virus, human herpesvirus 8 and human cytomegalovirus involvement in salivary gland tumours. *Oral Oncol*, **34**, 391–5.

Belsky, J.L., Tachikawa, K., Cihak, R.W., and Yamamoto, T. (1972) Salivary gland tumors in atomic bomb survivors, Hiroshima–Nagasaki, 1957 to 1970. *J Am Med Assoc*, **219**, 864–8.

Belsky, J.L., Takeichi, N., Yamamoto, T., Cihak, R.W., Hirose, F., Ezaki, H. *et al.* (1975) Salivary gland neoplasms following atomic radiation: additional cases and reanalysis of combined data in a fixed population, 1957–1970. *Cancer*, **35**, 555–9.

Birek, C., Lui, E., and Dardick, I. (1993) c-*fos* oncogene underexpression in salivary gland tumors as measured by *in situ* hybridization. *Am J Pathol*, **142**, 917–23.

Cadier, M., Watkin, G., and Hobsley, M. (1992) Smoking predisposes to parotid adenolymphoma. *Br J Surg*, **79**, 928–30.

Chung, Y.F., Khoo, M.L., Heng, M.K., Hong, G.S., and Soo, K.C. (1999) Epidemiology of Warthin's tumour of the parotid gland in an Asian population. *Br J Surg*, **86**, 661–4.

Deacon, E.M., Matthews, J.B., Potts, A.J., Hamburger, J., Bevan, I.S., and Young, L.S. (1991) Detection of Epstein–Barr virus antigens and DNA in major and minor salivary glands using immunocytochemistry and polymerase chain reaction: possible relationship with Sjogren's syndrome. *J Pathol*, **163**, 351–60.

Doi, R., Kuratate, I., Okamoto, E., Ryoke, K., and Ito, H. (1999) Expression of p53 oncoprotein increases intratumoral microvessel formation in human salivary gland carcinomas. *J Oral Pathol Med*, **28**, 259–63.

Ebbs, S.R. and Webb, A.J. (1986) Adenolymphoma of the parotid: aetiology, diagnosis and treatment. *Br J Surg*, **73**, 627–30.

el Naggar, A.K., Hurr, K., Kagan, J., Gillenwater, A., Callender, D., Luna, M.A. *et al.* (1997) Genotypic alterations in benign and malignant salivary gland tumors: histogenetic and clinical implications. *Am J Surg Pathol*, **21**, 691–7.

el Naggar, A.K., Lovell, M., Killary, A., and Batsakis, J.G. (1994) Trisomy 5 as the sole chromosomal abnormality in a primary mucoepidermoid carcinoma of the minor salivary gland. *Cancer Genet Cytogenet*, **76**, 96–9.

Franchi, A., Gallo, O., Bocciolini, C., Franchi, L., Paglierani, M., and Santucci, M. (1999) Reduced E-cadherin expression correlates with unfavorable prognosis in adenoid cystic carcinoma of salivary glands of the oral cavity. *Am J Clin Pathol*, **111**, 43–50.

Gallo, O. (1994) Is Warthin's tumor an Epstein–Barr virus-related disease? [letter]. *Int J Cancer*, **58**, 756–7.

Gallo, O. (1996) Increasing evidence that Epstein–Barr virus may be involved in the pathogenesis of undifferentiated carcinoma of the salivary glands [letter]. *Hum Pathol*, **27**, 1381.

Gallo, O. and Bocciolini, C. (1997) Warthin's tumour associated with autoimmune diseases and tobacco use. *Acta Otolaryngol Stockh*, **117**, 623–7.

Gallo, O., Bani, D., Toccafondi, G., Almerigogna, F., and Storchi, O.F. (1992) Characterization of a novel cell line from pleomorphic adenoma of the parotid gland with myoepithelial phenotype and producing interleukin-6 as an autocrine growth factor. *Cancer*, **70**, 559–68.

Gallo, O., Santucci, M., Calzolari, A., and Storchi, O.F. (1994) Epstein–Barr virus (EBV) infection and undifferentiated carcinoma of the parotid gland in Caucasian patients. *Acta Otolaryngol*, **114**, 572–5.

Gallo, O., Bianchi, S., Giovannucci Uzzielli, M.L., Santoro, R., Lenzi, S., Salimbeni, C. *et al.* (1995a) p53 oncoprotein overexpression correlates with mutagen-induced chromosome fragility in head and neck cancer patients with multiple malignancies. *Br J Cancer*, **71**, 1008–12.

Gallo, O., Franchi, A., Bianchi, S., Boddi, V., Giannelli, E., and Alajmo, E. (1995b) p53 oncoprotein expression in parotid gland carcinoma is associated with clinical outcome. *Cancer*, **75**, 2037–44.

Gandour Edwards, R., Kapadia, S.B., Gumerlock, P.H., and Barnes, L. (1995) Immunolocalization of interleukin-6 in salivary gland tumors. *Hum Pathol*, **26**, 501–3.

Geurts, J.M., Schoenmakers, E.F., Roijer, E., Stenman, G., and Van de Ven, W.J. (1997) Expression of reciprocal hybrid transcripts of HMGIC and FHIT in a pleomorphic adenoma of the parotid gland. *Cancer Res*, **57**, 13–7.

Giannoni, C., el Naggar, A.K., Ordonez, N.G., Tu, Z.N., Austin, J., Luna, M.A. *et al.* (1995) c-*erbB-2*/*neu* oncogene and Ki-67 analysis in the assessment of palatal salivary gland neoplasms. *Otolaryngol Head Neck Surg*, **112**, 391–8.

Hanna, E.Y. and Suen, J.Y. (1998) Neoplasms of the salivary glands. In: *Otolaryngology, Head and Neck Surgery*, 3rd edn. pp. 1255–1302 (ed. C.W. Cummings) W.B. Saunders, Philadelphia.

Hoffman, D.A., McConahey, W.M., Fraumeni, J.F., Jr, and Kurland, L.T. (1982) Cancer incidence following treatment of hyperthyroidism. *Int J Epidemiol*, **11**, 218–24.

Horn Ross, P.L., Morrow, M., and Ljung, B.M. (1997) Diet and the risk of salivary gland cancer. *Am J Epidemiol*, **146**, 171–6.

Iezzoni, J.C., Gaffey, M.J., and Weiss, L.M. (1995) The role of Epstein–Barr virus in lymphoepithelioma-like carcinomas. *Am J Clin Pathol*, **103**, 308–15.

Johns, M.M., 3rd, Westra, W.H., Califano, J.A., Eisele, D., Koch, W.M., and Sidransky, D. (1996) Allelotype of salivary gland tumors. *Cancer Res*, **56**, 1151–4.

Ju, D.M. (1968) Salivary gland tumors occurring after radiation of the head and neck area. *Am J Surg*, **116**, 518–23.

Kamio, N. (1996) Coexpression of p53 and c-erbB-2 proteins is associated with histological type, tumour stage, and cell proliferation in malignant salivary gland tumours. *Virchows Arch*, **428**, 75–83.

Karja, V.J., Syrjanen, K.J., Kurvinen, A.K., and Syrjanen, S.M. (1997) Expression and mutations of p53 in salivary gland tumours. *J Oral Pathol Med*, **26**, 217–23.

Kas, K., Voz, M.L., Roijer, E., Astrom, A.K., Meyen, E., Stenman, G. *et al.* (1997) Promoter swapping between the genes for a novel zinc finger protein and beta-catenin in pleiomorphic adenomas with t(3;8)(p21;q12) translocations [published erratum appears in Nat Genet 1997 Apr;15(4):411]. *Nat Genet*, **15**, 170–4.

Katz, A.D. and Preston Martin, S. (1984) Salivary gland tumors and previous radiotherapy to the head or neck. Report of a clinical series. *Am J Surg*, **147**, 345–8.

Kuo, T. and Hsueh, C. (1997) Lymphoepithelioma-like salivary gland carcinoma in Taiwan: a clinicopathological study of nine cases demonstrating a strong association with Epstein–Barr virus. *Histopathology*, **31**, 75–82.

Land, C.E., Saku, T., Hayashi, Y., Takahara, O., Matsuura, H., Tokuoka, S. *et al.* (1996) Incidence of salivary gland tumors among atomic bomb survivors, 1950–1987. Evaluation of radiation-related risk [published erratum appears in Radiat Res 1996 Sep;146(3):356]. *Radiat Res*, **146**, 28–36.

Li, X., Tsuji, T., Wen, S., Mimura, Y., Wang, Z., Sasaki, K. *et al.* (1995) A fluorescence *in situ* hybridization (FISH) analysis with centromere-specific DNA probes of chromosomes 3 and 17 in pleomorphic adenomas and adenoid cystic carcinomas. *J Oral Pathol Med*, **24**, 398–401.

Modan, B., Chetrit, A., Alfandary, E., Tamir, A., Lusky, A., Wolf, M. *et al.* (1998) Increased risk of salivary gland tumors after low-dose irradiation. *Laryngoscope*, **108**, 1095–7.

Nagao, T., Ishida, Y., Sugano, I., Tajima, Y., Matsuzaki, O., Hino, T. *et al.* (1996) Epstein–Barr virus-associated undifferentiated carcinoma with lymphoid stroma of the salivary gland in Japanese patients. Comparison with benign lymphoepithelial lesion. *Cancer*, **78**, 695–703.

Nordkvist, A., Gustafsson, H., Juberg Ode, M., and Stenman, G. (1994). Recurrent rearrangements of 11q14–22 in mucoepidermoid carcinoma [see comments]. *Cancer Genet Cytogenet*, **74**, 77–83.

Papadaki, H., Finkelstein, S.D., Kounelis, S., Bakker, A., Swalsky, P.A., and Kapadia, S.B. (1996) The role of p53 mutation and protein expression in primary and recurrent adenoid cystic carcinoma. *Hum Pathol*, **27**, 567–72.

Pignataro, L., Capaccio, P., Carboni, N., Pruneri, G., Ottaviani, A., Buffa, R. *et al.* (1998) p53 and cyclinX D1 protein expression in carcinomas of the parotid gland. *Anticancer Res*, **18**, 1287–90.

Press, M.F., Pike, M.C., Hung, G., Zhou, J.Y., Ma, Y., George, J. *et al.* (1994) Amplification and overexpression of HER-2/neu in carcinomas of the salivary gland: correlation with poor prognosis. *Cancer Res*, **54**, 5675–82.

Preston Martin, S., Thomas, D.C., White, S.C., and Cohen, D. (1988) Prior exposure to medical and dental X-rays related to tumors of the parotid gland. *J Natl Cancer Inst*, **80**, 943–9.

Queimado, L., Reis, A., Fonseca, I., Martins, C., Lovett, M., Soares, J. *et al.* (1998) A refined localization of two deleted regions in chromosome 6q associated with salivary gland carcinomas. *Oncogene*, **16**, 83–8.

Renehan, A., Gallo, O., and McGurk, M. (1999) Epidemiology of Warthin's tumour of the parotid gland in an Asian population [letter]. *Br J Surg*, **86**, 1480.

Saemundsen, A.K., Albeck, H., Hansen, J.P., Nielsen, N.H., Anvret, M., Henle, W. *et al.* (1982) Epstein–Barr virus in nasopharyngeal and salivary gland carcinomas of Greenland Eskimoes. *Br J Cancer*, **46**, 721–8.

Saku, T., Hayashi, Y., Takahara, O., Matsuura, H., Tokunaga, M., Tokunaga, M. *et al.* (1997) Salivary gland tumors among atomic bomb survivors, 1950–1987. *Cancer*, **79**, 1465–75.

Santucci, M., Gallo, O., Calzolari, A., and Bondi, R. (1993) Detection of Epstein–Barr viral genome in tumor cells of Warthin's tumor of parotid gland. *Am J Clin Pathol*, **100**, 662–5.

Schneider, A.B., Lubin, J., Ron, E., Abrahams, C., Stovall, M., Goel, A. *et al.* (1998) Salivary gland tumors after childhood radiation treatment for benign conditions of the head and neck: dose–response relationships. *Radiat Res*, **149**, 625–30.

Sheen, T.S., Tsai, C.C., Ko, J.Y., Chang, Y.L., and Hsu, M.M. (1997) Undifferentiated carcinoma of the major salivary glands. *Cancer*, **80**, 357–63.

Shore, R.E., Albert, R.E., and Pasternack, B.S. (1976) Follow-up study of patients treated by X-ray epilation for Tinea capitis; resurvey of post-treatment illness and mortality experience. *Arch Environ Health*, **31**, 21–8.

Sidransky, D. (1995) Molecular genetics of head and neck cancer. *Curr Opin Oncol*, **7**, 229–33.

Spitz, M.R., Tilley, B.C., Batsakis, J.G., Gibeau, J.M., and Newell, G.R. (1984) Risk factors for major salivary gland carcinoma. A case-comparison study. *Cancer*, **54**, 1854–9.

Spitz, M.R., Sider, J.G., Newell, G.R., and Batsakis, J.G. (1988) Incidence of salivary gland cancer in the United States relative to ultraviolet radiation exposure. *Head Neck Surg*, **10**, 305–8.

Stenman, G., Sandros, J., Dahlenfors, R., Juberg Ode, M., and Mark, J. (1986) 6q- and loss of the Y chromosome—two common deviations in malignant human salivary gland tumors. *Cancer Genet Cytogenet*, **22**, 283–93.

Sugano, S., Mukai, K., Tsuda, H., Hirohashi, S., Furuya, S., Shimosato, Y. *et al.* (1992) Immunohistochemical study of c-erbB-2 oncoprotein overexpression in human major salivary gland carcinoma: an indicator of aggressiveness. *Laryngoscope*, **102**, 923–7.

Taira, S., Okuda, M., Osato, T., and Mizuno, F. (1992) [Detection of Epstein–Barr virus DNA in salivary gland tumors]. *Nippon Jibiinkoka Gakkai Kaiho*, **95**, 860–8.

Takata, T., Kudo, Y., Zhao, M., Ogawa, I., Miyauchi, M., Sato, S. *et al.* (1999) Reduced expression of p27(Kip1) protein in relation to salivary adenoid cystic carcinoma metastasis. *Cancer*, **86**, 928–35.

Takeichi, N., Hirose, F., and Yamamoto, H. (1976) Salivary gland tumors in atomic bomb survivors, Hiroshima, Japan. I. Epidemiologic observations. *Cancer*, **38**, 2462–8.

Takezawa, K., Jackson, C., Gnepp, D.R., and King, T.C. (1998). Molecular characterization of Warthin tumor. *Oral Surg, Oral Med, Oral Pathol Oral Radiol Endod*, **85**, 569–75.

Tornoczky, T., Kelenyi, G., and Pajor, L. (1998) EBER oligonucleotide RNA *in situ* hybridization in EBV associated neoplasms. *Pathol Oncol Res*, **4**, 201–5.

Tsai, C.C., Chen, C.L., and Hsu, H.C. (1996) Expression of Epstein–Barr virus in carcinomas of major salivary glands: a strong association with lymphoepithelioma-like carcinoma. *Hum Pathol*, **27**, 258–62.

Voz, M.L., Astrom, A.K., Kas, K., Mark, J., Stenman, G. *et al.* (1998) The recurrent translocation t(5;8)(p13;q12) in pleomorphic adenomas results in upregulation of *PLAG1* gene expression under control of the LIFR promoter. *Oncogene*, **16**, 1409–16.

Wen, S., Shimizu, N., Yoshiyama, H., Mizugaki, Y., Shinozaki, F., and Takada, K. (1996) Association of Epstein–Barr virus (EBV) with Sjogren's syndrome: differential EBV expression between epithelial cells and lymphocytes in salivary glands. *Am J Pathol*, **149**, 1511–7.

Wen, S., Mizugaki, Y., Shinozaki, F., and Takada, K. (1997) Epstein–Barr virus (EBV) infection in salivary gland tumors: lytic EBV infection in nonmalignant epithelial cells surrounded by EBV-positive T-lymphoma cells. *Virology*, **227**, 484–7.

Yamamoto, Y., Kishimoto, Y., Virmani, A.K., Smith, A., Vuitch, F., Albores Saavedra, J. *et al.* (1996) Mutations associated with carcinomas arising from pleomorphic adenomas of the salivary glands. *Hum Pathol*, **27**, 782–6.

Zheng, W., Shu, X.O., Ji, B.T., and Gao, Y.T. (1996) Diet and other risk factors for cancer of the salivary glands: a population-based case–control study. *Int J Cancer*, **67**, 194–8.

Audience discussion

Professor O'Brien (Sydney, Australia): The relationship between Warthin's tumour and EBV is very interesting. It is recognized that the epithelial component of Warthin's tumour is oncocyctic; is there any evidence that EBV can induce oncocyctic change in any other tumours?

Dr Gallo: No. We have no information on this point, but several papers report molecular evidence of EBV inside the epithelial cells. But it seems not to be a question of full transformation by EBV but a supportive or facilitatory role with other factors. For example, *in vitro* these cells have an increasing proliferative rate which cannot be explained. Also, there is no information as to the clonality of the virus inside of the cells, so we cannot be sure about a direct pathogenetic role in Warthin's tumour, unlike nasopharyngeal carcinoma.

Professor van del Waal (Amsterdam, The Netherlands): Is there any explanation for the preference for men instead of women in relation to this Epstein–Barr virus?

Dr Gallo: It is possible smoking is the common factor; the incidence of Warthin's tumour in females has slowly increased in the last three decades as smoking has increased in this population. Smoking may lead to reactivation of the virus within the salivary gland, for we know that perhaps this tissue is a reservoir for the virus.

Editorial comment

The aetiology of salivary gland neoplasia remains largely unknown, a problem aggravated by the comparative rarity of these tumours and the dispersal of clinical experience between many disciplines and institutes. The problem is compounded by the diversity of histological types and the habit of studying the cellular and molecular biology of each separately. Self-evidently, the aetiological factors that bring about salivary gland tumours must be of a subtle order for if not we should have identified them over the last 100 years.

However, Dr Gallo and colleague have pointed to many advances over the past decade, but the only really indisputable contributory factor is radiation. Epidemiological studies need to be substantiated particularly in the associations with dietary and lifestyle factors. Our best hope seems to be the study of the molecular aspects of salivary gland tumours. Genetic defects may show affinities for certain aetiological factors and so direct attention to common environmental aetiological agents.

CHAPTER 3

The WHO histological classification of salivary gland tumours: is it overelaborate for clinical use?

A pathologist's view
John Eveson

A surgeon's view
John Watkinson

A pathologist's view   John Eveson

Salivary gland tumours are a varied and complex group of neoplasms, and their classification is difficult. This difficulty is reflected in the many classifications that have been proposed (for a review, see Ellis and Auclair 1991). Some oversimplify the groups and important clinicopathological differences are masked, while others are so complex they become almost unworkable in practice.

To many surgeons, some tumour classifications and taxonomy appear to be rather esoteric and academic exercises of limited practical value in the clinical situation. Therefore, it is important to understand the purpose of classifications. A logical classification ideally should be based on and contribute to our understanding of histogenesis and should be of value in assessing likely tumour behaviour. In many branches of surgery, treatment is becoming more tumour specific and this increases the clinician's expectation of precise diagnosis. However, it is important to remember that any classification is dynamic rather than static. At best it represents no more than the consensus of those individuals involved at the time of its formulation. Any tendency to regard a classification as immutable should be firmly resisted.

The surgical pathologist's primary function is to produce as precise a diagnosis as possible. It is only by evaluation of subsequent clinical experience of behaviour and responses to a variety of treatment protocols that the relative importance of the individual diagnosis can be established. It is in the area of precise diagnosis that the value of an extended classification of salivary gland tumours becomes most evident. Broad prognostic groupings and tumour gradings are of no help if the initial diagnostic category was inaccurate.

The 2nd edition World Health Organization (WHO) histological classification

The WHO histological classification of salivary tumours proposed by Thackray and Sobin (1972) was much simpler than earlier classifications such as those of Foote and Frazell (1953) and Evans and Cruikshank (1970). It received widespread acceptance, but by the late 1980s it was outdated. Thus, the term 'monomorphic adenoma' was seen to be inaccurate (Warthin's tumour was included as a monomorphic adenoma but is *biphasic*), and potentially masked important subgroups that could lead to diagnostic inaccuracies with significant clinical consequences. Mucoepidermoid and acinic cell 'tumours' were widely regarded as carcinomas, albeit with a variable range of behaviour, and were reclassified as such. In addition, there were an increasing number of newly described carcinomas that had important clinicopathological characteristics which could easily be masked by the term adenocarcinoma, as used in the earlier WHO classification.

These anomalies were considered by a reconstituted WHO panel, and a new classification formulated (Table 3.1) (Seifert and Sobin 1991). This was meant to be a practical classification, rather than a histogenetically based system because the precise histogenesis and morphogenesis of many of the tumours was then speculative (Seifert *et al.* 1990; Seifert and Sobin 1992), and remains so today (Dardick, 1998). Rare but clearly defined tumour entities were included. The resulting classification was considerably longer than its predecessor, and to justify its complexity some selected examples are given:

Adenomas

In the 1972 classification, under the adenoma group there was a category of 'other monomorphic adenomas'. In the 1991 classification, this was expanded to include many more types and subtypes (Box 3.1). On the face of it, this is a considerable extension of the diagnostic complexity of what are essentially benign tumours, so what was the point? The 1972 classification, and several standard pathological texts, illustrated a variant of 'other monomorphic adenomas' as a so-called *glycogen-rich adenoma* or *clear cell adenoma*. It is now realized that this neoplasm is malignant and it is known as an *epithelial–myoepithelial carcinoma*, a tumour which itself has a wide spectrum of morphological appearances. Criteria have been established to distinguish between the range of *basal cell adenomas* and the adenocarcinomatous variant, *basal cell adenocarcinoma*, that was first described in the late 1980s (Ellis and Wiscovitch 1990). In addition, it is important to distinguish between the solid variant of basal cell adenoma and the solid, or basaloid, variant of *adenoid cystic carcinoma* (Eveson 1992). *Canalicular adenoma* is easily mistaken for the cribriform variant of adenoid cystic carcinoma and, to add to the diagnostic confusion, it can also be multifocal. *Sialadenoma papilliferum*, although rare, can be mistaken for an adenocarcinoma, especially when the orientation of the specimen is less than ideal. These subcategories are not mere histopathological nuances but have a critical role in enabling the pathologist to reach an appropriate diagnosis.

Table 3.1 WHO histological classification of salivary gland tumours (2nd edition)

1	**Adenomas**	
	1.1	Pleomophic adenoma
	1.2	Myoepithelioma
	1.3	Basal cell adenoma
	1.4	Warthin's tumour (adenolymphoma)
	1.5	Oncocytoma (onocytic adenoma)
	1.6	Canalicular adenoma
	1.7	Sebaceous adenoma
	1.8	Ductal papilloma
	1.9	Cystadenoma
2	**Carcinomas**	
	2.1	Acinic cell carcinoma
	2.2	Mucoepidermoid carcinoma
	2.3	Adenoid cystic carcinoma
	2.4	Polymorphous low grade adenocarcinoma
	2.5	Epithelial–myoepithelial carcinoma
	2.6	Basal cell adenocarcinoma
	2.7	Sebaceous carcinoma
	2.8	Papillary cystadenocarcinoma
	2.9	Mucinous adenocarcinoma
	2.10	Oncocytic carcinoma
	2.11	Salivary duct carcinoma
	2.12	Adenocarcinoma, NOS
	2.13	Malignant myoepithelioma (myoepithelial carcinoma)
	2.14	Carcinoma in pleomorphic adenoma (malignant mixed tumour)
	2.15	Squamous cell carcinoma
	2.16	Small cell carcinoma
	2.17	Undifferentiated carcinoma
	2.18	Other carcinomas
3	**Non-epithelial tumours**	
4	**Malignant lymphomas**	
5	**Secondary tumours**	
6	**Unclassified tumours**	
7	**Tumour-like lesions**	
	7.1	Sialadenosis
	7.2	Oncocytosis
	7.3	Necrotizing sialometaplasia (Salivary gland infarction)
	7.4	Benign lymphoepithelial lesion
	7.5	Salivary gland cysts
	7.6	Chronic sclerosing sialadenitis of submandibular gland (Küttner tumour)
	7.7	Cystic lymphoid hyperplasia of AIDS

NOS, not otherwise specified; AIDS, acquired immunodeficiency syndrome.

> ## Box 3.1 The 2nd edition WHO classification of 'other monomorphic adenomas'
>
> Basal cell adenomas
>
> ◆ trabecular and tubular
>
> ◆ solid
>
> ◆ membranous (dermal analogue type)
>
> Canalicular adenoma
>
> Sebaceous adenoma
>
> Ductal papilloma
>
> ◆ inverted duct papilloma
>
> ◆ intraductal papilloma
>
> ◆ sialadenoma papilliferum
>
> Cystadenoma
>
> ◆ papillary cystadenoma
>
> ◆ mucinous cystadenoma

Adenocarcinomas

No other salivary gland tumour illustrates the importance of precise diagnosis more clearly than the *polymorphous low grade adenocarcinoma* (Merchant *et al.* 1996; Castle *et al.* 1999). This tumour initially was described independently by several groups of workers and was given a variety of names including *lobular carcinoma*, *terminal duct carcinoma*, and *polymorphous low grade adenocarcinoma of minor salivary gland* (they may also arise within the major salivary glands). The hallmark of this tumour is cytological uniformity and blandness together with morphological diversity. It is characterized by a relatively low malignant potential. Before the histological characterization of this tumour subtype, it would clearly have been called something else. The cribriform nature and neurotropism characteristic of some of these tumours would have led many pathologists towards a histological diagnosis of *adenoid cystic carcinoma*, while the morphological diversity could easily have resulted in a diagnosis of *carcinoma in pleomorphic adenoma*. Both of these alternatives carry a considerably worse prognosis. At best, the diagnostic confusion will have caused a distortion of clinicopathological studies into both of these tumour groups, and at worst has resulted in significant overtreatment.

Carcinoma in pleomorphic adenoma

The categorization of *carcinoma in pleomorphic adenoma* was refined in the WHO classification as shown in Box 3.2. One of the characteristic features of salivary gland pleomorphic adenomas is their propensity over time to progress from benign to malig-

> ## Box 3.2 The 2nd edition WHO classification subtypes of 'carcinoma in pleomorphic adenoma'
>
> ◆ Non-invasive carcinoma (*in situ* carcinoma, intracapsular carcinoma)
> ◆ Invasive carcinoma in pleomorphic adenoma
> ◆ Carcinosarcoma
> ◆ Metastasizing pleomorphic adenoma

nant (Chapter 9). During this progression, they may go through a phase where there are dysplastic histological features within the tumour (*in situ* carcinoma). If there is no invasion of the surrounding tissues, this variant does not appear to behave any differently from a conventional pleomorphic adenoma. The recognition of this variant helps to prevent overtreatment and also adds a note of possible caution to the interpretation of fine needle aspiration biopsy specimens.

Other classifications

In the American Forces Institute of Pathology morphological classification of salivary gland neoplasms (Ellis and Auclair 1991), the system is equally (if not more) comprehensive than that for the WHO. Tumours are grouped into low, intermediate, and high grade subtypes, and some clinicians find this refinement useful (see Mr Watkinson's discussion below). However, this results in some tumours such as *mucoepidermoid carcinoma* and *adenocarcinoma (NOS)* appearing in all three categories. My own feeling is that this system can be too rigid, as predicting the behaviour of some tumour types is difficult. In other cases, there is good evidence that tumour grading can be useful in determining prognosis; mucoepidermoid carcinoma is perhaps the best example. A number of investigators (Hicks *et al.* 1995; Goode *et al.* 1998) have shown clear differences in the prognosis of the various grades. However, clinicians should not be lulled into a false sense of security by such grading. Histologically high-grade mucoepidermoid carcinomas are certainly aggressive clinically, but low-grade tumours unpredictably can metastasize. Similarly, acinic cell carcinoma is generally regarded as low grade but the morphology does not correlate well with clinical behaviour.

Therefore, each tumour has to be judged on its own merits, and histopathology is only one of the wide variety of factors that has to be taken into account when assessing prognosis. In many cases, clinical features such as anatomical site, staging, or nerve involvement are more important when making therapeutic decisions.

A surgeon's view   John Watkinson

The first question that needs to be asked is why do we classify tumours histologically. First it provides the clinician with a diagnosis and a label. Secondly, it allows us to group tumours within certain types with similar biology and natural history so that physicians and surgeons can tailor their management accordingly. Sometimes this involves grouping tumours together histologically rather than with any reference to their behaviour. By doing this, it allows us to establish local, national, and international standards whereby treatments can be compared from centre to centre so that management strategies can be developed and advice can be given to patients regarding prognosis. One of the keys to understanding pathogenesis is by grouping together tumours with similar histological features which denote the same underlying genetic defect which must, by definition, allow research into pathogenesis. One of the problems with grouping tumours together is that one must be wary of describing the behaviour of one tumour group under the broad umbrella of one histological label, e.g. adenocarcinoma and bowel cancer. Surely it would be better to represent a spectrum of disease.

Histological grading

The definitions and systems of clinical staging and tumour grade for salivary gland tumours are dealt with in detail in Chapter 13. Suffice to say, at this time, that tumour grading may be confusing but is determined predominantly by histological factors. For salivary tumours, clinical stage is a composite of tumour size, local extension, and cervical nodal involvement. Spiro (Chapter 13) has elegantly shown, using univariate analysis, that stage is the most important predictor of survival and is more important than tumour grade. However, histological grade is still very important (Table 13.1), and assists in treatment options. A prognostic index combining stage, grade, and possibly other prognostic indicators, such as that suggested recently by Vander Poorton et al. (1999), and similar to the Nottingham Prognostic Index for breast cancer (Galea et al. 1992; O'Rourke et al. 1994), is ideal. I am a surgical oncologist; I not only perform the surgery for these patients but I must also coordinate other aspects of their management. Thus, histological type and grade help me to predict prognosis and help me to compare my results with others. Moreover, the histological grade is crucial in my decisions about post-operative radiotherapy in patients with salivary cancers, as most investigators agree that post-operative radiation therapy should be administered when the tumour is high stage or high grade (Chapter 15).

With histological grade and management decisions in mind, I feel that the AFIP classification of salivary carcinomas has many merits (Ellis and Auclair 1991). Unlike the WHO classification, salivary carcinomas are categorized specifically into low, intermediate, and high grade. I caution somewhat against the use of the term 'intermediate grade' as it is liable to lead to some confusion when several examples of the same entity of tumour appear in more than one grade. Furthermore, some studies have lumped all adenoid cystic carcinomas as 'intermediate grade' (Renehan et al. 1999) and, because of this, there is potential for confusion. I suggest a modification of the AFIP classification as shown in Table 3.2.

Table 3.2 Modification of WHO and AFIP classifications to denote grade

	Low-grade	High-grade
Acinic cell carcinoma	✔	
Polymorphous low grade adenocarcinoma	✔	
Basal cell adenocarcinoma	✔	
Sebaceous carcinoma	✔	
Papillary cystadenocarcinoma	✔	
Mucinous adenocarcinoma	✔	
Basal cell adenocarcinoma	✔	
Sebaceous carcinoma	✔	
Papillary cystadenocarcinoma	✔	
Mucinous adenocarcinoma	✔	
Malignant myoepithelialioma	✔	
Mucoepidermoid carcinoma	✔	✔
Adenoid cystic carcinoma	✔	✔
Adenocarcinoma, NOS	✔	✔
Epithelial–myoepithelial carcinoma		✔
Oncocytic carcinoma		✔
Salivary duct carcinoma		✔
Carcinoma in pleomorphic adenoma		✔
Squamous cell carcinoma		✔
Small cell carcinoma		✔
Undifferentiated carcinoma		✔

NOS, not otherwise specified.

REFERENCES

Castle, J.T., Thompson, L.D., Frommelt, R.A., Wenig, B.M., and Kessler, H.P. (1999) Polymorphous low grade adenocarcinoma: a clinicopathologic study of 164 cases. *Cancer*, **86**, 207–19.

Dardick, I. (1998) Mounting evidence against current histogenetic concepts for salivary gland tumorigenesis. *Eur J Morphol*, **36 Suppl**, 257–61.

Ellis, G.L. and Auclair, P.L. (1991) Calssification of salivary gland neoplasms. In: *Surgical Pathology of the Salivary Glands*. pp. 129–134. (eds G.L. Ellis, P.L. Auclair, and D.R. Gnepp) W.B. Saunders Co., Philadelphia.

Ellis, G.L. and Wiscovitch, J.G. (1990) Basal cell adenocarcinomas of the major salivary glands. *Oral Surg, Oral Med Oral Pathol*, **69**, 461–9.

Evans, R.W. and Cruikshank, A.H. (1970) *Epithelial Tumours of the Salivary Glands*. W.B. Saunders Co., Philadelphia.

Eveson, J.W. (1992) Troublesome tumours 2: borderline tumours of salivary glands. *J Clin Pathol*, **45**, 369–77.

Foote, F.W. and Frazell, E.L. (1953) Tumors of the major salivary glands. *Cancer*, **6**, 1065–113.

Galea, M.H., Blamey, R.W., Elston, C.E., and Ellis, I.O. (1992) The Nottingham Prognostic Index in primary breast cancer. *Breast Cancer Res Treat*, **22**, 207–19.

Goode, R.K., Auclair, P.L., and Ellis, G.L. (1998) Mucoepidermoid carcinoma of the major salivary glands: clinical and histopathologic analysis of 234 cases with evaluation of grading criteria. *Cancer*, **82**, 1217–24.

Hicks, M.J., el Naggar, A.K., Flaitz, C.M., Luna, M.A., and Batsakis, J.G. (1995) Histocytologic grading of mucoepidermoid carcinoma of major salivary glands in prognosis and survival: a clinicopathologic and flow cytometric investigation. *Head Neck*, **17**, 89–95.

Merchant, W.J., Cook, M.G., and Eveson, J.W. (1996) Polymorphous low-grade adenocarcinoma of parotid gland. *Br J Oral Maxillofac Surg*, **34**, 328–30.

O'Rourke, S., Galea, M.H., Morgan, D., Euhus, D., Pinder, S., Ellis, I.O. *et al.* (1994) Local recurrence after simple mastectomy. *Br J Surg*, **81**, 386–9.

Renehan, A.G., Gleave, E.N., Slevin, N.J., and McGurk, M. (1999) Clinico-pathological and treatment-related factors influencing survival in parotid cancer. *Br J Cancer*, **80**, 1296–300.

Seifert, G. and Sobin, L.H. (1991) *WHO International Histological Classification of Tumours. Histological Typing of Salivary Gland Tumours*, 2nd edn. Springer-Verlag, Berlin.

Seifert, G. and Sobin, L.H. (1992) The World Health Organization's Histological Classification of Salivary Gland Tumors. A commentary on the second edition. *Cancer*, **70**, 379–85.

Seifert, G., Brocheriou, C., Cardesa, A., and Eveson, J.W. (1990). WHO International Histological Classification of Tumours. Tentative histological classification of salivary gland tumours. *Pathol Res Pract*, **186**, 555–81.

Thackray, A.C. and Sobin, L.H. (1972) *Histological Typing of Salivary Gland Tumours*. World Health Organization, Geneva.

Vander Poorten, V.L., Balm, A.J., Hilgers, F.J., Tan, I.B., Loftus Coll, B.M., Keus, R.B. *et al.* (1999) The development of a prognostic score for patients with parotid carcinoma. *Cancer*, **85**, 2057–67.

Audience discussion

Professor McGurk (London, UK): I would like to try and crystallize this issue by first asking why we are using visual images as a method of classification. Why not use ultrasound, electrical stimuli, or extracellular matrix protein? The reason I suggest, is that vision has been important for man in evolutionary development and so we favour its use over the other senses. The investigation is not tumour specific and it is likely at some point to be fallible. I am concerned that what is happening is that pathologists are continuing to identify a range of tumour entities based on histological appearance (but not necessarily on natural history), while, from the surgeon's perspective, it is the natural biology which is all important, rather than appearance.

Professor O'Brien (Sydney, Australia): I think you have raised an interesting point. Certainly the prediction of clinical behaviour from histological appearance is not reliable and pathologists fall back on the basic nature of the family of tumours reported in textbooks. I think the point that you make is exactly right and I believe that the new WHO classification is too complex. One gets the impression that every pathologist who becomes involved with salivary pathology is tempted to find his own tumour. I am basically a 'lumper' and lump on the basis of what is relevant in terms of treatment and outcome. However, overall, I am also a precisionist, and would hate to think that we could fall back to the imprecise classifications of previous decades. There is a good argument for the classification to be linked with staging and clinically relevant factors.

Professor Spiro (New York, USA): I just want to echo what Chris (Professor O'Brien) has been saying. Dr John Batsakis would be the first to agree that the elaborate classification that we now see and which was so well presented really does not help the clinician very much. I do feel, however, that classification is absolutely essential to our understanding of histogenesis, and it may be helpful as we investigate aetiology. But from the standpoint of the clinician who is looking at the patient and has to decide on management, the classification tends to come *after* treatment discussion has taken place.

Professor Speight (London, UK): I have to stand up and defend the pathologists. First of all, I take exception to the description that we are just trying to match patterns. I think as John Eveson showed very well, if we were to match patterns we would have the diagnosis wrong probably 50% of the time when diagnosing salivary gland disease. The role of pathologists is to understand disease and to interpret the histological features in front of them, and, in addition, to take into account the clinical presentation, the staging, and any other information that is available. Nowadays that includes molecular biological data and, of course, immunohistochemistry. So I think it is a much more complicated picture than you are presenting. The classification which Dr Eveson showed is quite elaborate but it would be facile to suggest that the pathologist should write on the report 'the features are those of a salivary gland tumour'. The surgeon will come back and say 'well, which salivary gland tumour?' The surgeon can lump the diagnoses if he wishes into various clinicopathological entities which determine management; the pathologist role is always to classify the tumour precisely.

Dr Eveson: I think it is important to remember when we are talking about salivary tumours, we are not just talking about the parotid gland as there is a tacit assumption that we are. We accept that initial surgery for parotid tumours is without a prior histological diagnosis, however, in the lip and palate, initial surgery is frequently incisional biopsy. Thus, the subtleties which are present in the classification not only prevent misdiagnosis but also prevent overtreatment. I think it is important to keep that in mind and not just consider this to be a disease of the parotid gland.

Professor van der Waal (Amsterdam, The Netherlands): Two comments, if I may. First, I would be reluctant to put too much emphasis on the value of histological grading of salivary gland tumours as suggested by Mr Watkinson. Although there are reports in the literature of different grading systems, these have been based on series where parotid, submandibular, and intraoral tumours were analysed together. So I do not believe there is sufficient scientific evidence to use histological grading of a salivary gland tumour to predict behaviour and tailoring treatment in individual patients. I have made several mistakes by using the term *polymorphous low-grade adenocarcinoma* thinking that it was a relatively benign disease. In my experience, it is not, and so I am extremely careful to avoid label directed treatment of individual patients.

My second comment is that I fear that the WHO classification is elitist, okay for the specialist who sees a lot of salivary tumours. I would like to have a classification that has wider application, and which is not just understood by a few pathologist. It suggests to me that the present classification and definitions are not sufficently clear for widespread use.

Editorial comment

The question (is the WHO classification overelaborate?) arises out of the expansion of the classification from 15 epithelial tumour types in 1972 to 28 types (plus many subtypes) in 1991, and more categories are anticipated in the next WHO review. The two authors of this chapter have advanced a strong argument in favour of a detailed system, but the editors argue for a simpler system, with preference given to tumours with different discernible biological natures.

One of the authors' main points is that a surgeon cannot work without a diagnosis, and this statement is undeniable. At present, there is the tacit assumption that each histologically defined entity has a different natural history or nature. If so, they represent individual diagnostic entities. However, if the natural history is unknown or indistinguishable from other tumours, then the particular histological pattern is no more than a microscopic observation. Many of the 'entities' in the current WHO classification are histological observations, not distinct diagnoses.

In order to test groups of tumours with a recently recognized histological appearance are a distinct diagnostic entity, their natural history should be followed in large data sets of uniformly treated cases with well documented natural histories. There are now five or six of these data sets in existence. If they are combined (with representative specimens) then a valuable test resource would be available to sift out spurious entities. A plea is also made for tissue samples and patients' blood to be banked centrally to help identify biological markers and facilitate molecular studies in these relatively rare tumours.

CHAPTER 4

Investigation of salivary gland lumps

Clinical evaluation with a selective approach to the use of imaging and fine needle aspiration cytology

Mark McGurk and Nicholas Drage

Fine needle aspiration cytology: a 'surgical cytologist's' view

John Webb

Clinical evaluation with a selective approach to the use of imaging and fine needle aspiration cytology
Mark McGurk and Nicholas Drage

Technological advance, particularly in the field of investigative medicine, has had a significant impact on the management of many conditions, and the salivary glands are no exception. Once these tests are adopted widely by the profession they become by definition the 'norm', and anything less in terms of investigation is difficult to defend. The result of this process is the continual broadening of the investigative base. The situation is difficult to reverse or even rationalize as disorders of salivary glands, and in particular tumours, are uncommon, and experience in managing these entities is limited. For many clinicians, experience is gained vicariously, and the development of popular opinion or trends cannot be checked by personal experience. This chapter seeks to present a logical and defensible framework for investigation of the salivary gland lump, and emphasizes a policy towards reliance on clinical judgement.

A salivary lump

For the purposes of this discussion, we are focusing on the discrete salivary lump, as diffuse or bilateral salivary disease is usually the mark of a systemic disorder. Investigations may be broadly categorized into two classes: *descriptive* including radiological studies, and *diagnostic* such as biopsy in all its forms. In turn, the value of a test may be judged from two perspectives: its accuracy and more pertinently, its impact on management.

It is may be prudent to reiterate that a lump in the tail of the parotid or in the sub-mandibular gland both fall within the diagnosis of a 'lump in the neck'. The primary lesion may lie outside the gland itself. This is particularly the case in sunny climates where there is a risk of metastasis from melanotic or epithelial scalp lesions, and so a full head and neck evaluation is required (Chapter 20).

Testing clinical judgement versus histology

The merits of clinical evaluation of salivary tumours were investigated by treating 'clinical evaluation' as the 'test' versus final histological diagnosis using consecutive series of patients from three UK hospitals: Christie Hospital, Manchester; Hull Royal Infirmary, Yorkshire; and Guy's Hospital, London. The patient characteristics and the study periods for the three series are shown in Table 4.1. In all three series, management relied heavily on pre-operative assessment. Computerized tomography (CT) scans were not routinely available until the mid-1980s, and hence were limited to a few patients in the Christie and Hull series. Fine needle aspiration cytology (FNAC) was not routinely used in any series. Consistency in diagnostic evaluation was maintained throughout the study periods in the three studies: two consecutive surgeons in the Christie series, and a single person at Hull and Guy's, respectively. The accuracy of clinical examination predicting a benign histology was assessed for all three studies. In addition, for the Hull and Guy's series, diagnostic errors (defined as an error that adversely effected the course of the disease or led to inappropriate management) were identified.

Table 4.1 Patient characteristics of series from Christie, Hull, and Guy's Hospital; all are parotid gland tumours

	Christie	Hull/Guy's
No. of patients	855	114
Median age (range)	57 (5–92)	–
Male	342 (40)	67(59)
Malignant	141 (16)	17 (15)

Values in parentheses are percentages.

Table 4.2 Clinical assessment (the 'test') versus histological category for series from Christie, Hull, and Guy's

Test	Christie		Hull/Guy's	
	B	M	B	M
Clinically 'benign'	680	50	92	7
Clinically 'malignant'	6	91	5	10
Sensitivity	99%			
Specificity	65%			
PPV	93%			

B, benign histology; M, malignant histology; PPV, positive predictive value.

'Test' = The clinical assessment that the histology was benign.

The sensitivities, specificities, and positive predictive values for clinical assessment versus final histological diagnosis are shown in Table 4.2. The key message is that pre-operative clinical assessment correctly distinguished benign and malignant disease with a range from 93 to 96%, which equals or betters that for specialized tests such as scanning and FNAC (see below).

Imaging of the salivary mass

Plain radiology and sialography

Plain films are now obsolete in evaluating a salivary mass, except when an underlying bony lesion is suspected. Sialography is an excellent technique for demonstrating the ductal anatomy of the salivary glands (Chapter 25). Classically tumours produce a 'ball in the hand' appearance on sialography, where the intraglandular ducts are displaced and stretched by underlying mass. It has a very limited contribution to make in the descriptive evaluation of a mass as only relatively large lesions are discernible, and these are nearly always apparent on clinical examination.

Cross-sectional imaging

Cross-sectional imaging using CT or magnetic resonance imaging (MRI) is a powerful evaluation tool. CT has been used extensively to assess salivary abnormalities and has many advantages, being cheap, readily available, and with excellent resolution. It has several advantages over MRI, since it can be used in patients fitted with pacemakers or those with ferromagnetic foreign objects, and is far less claustrophobic. It is used to identify the position of the mass, i.e. whether it is intra- or extraglandular, and establish its relationship to adjacent structures. It is particularly useful in defining a deep lobe tumour, and for staging purposes. A major disadvantage when imaging the parotid is the risk of significant image degradation due to star artefacts from dental amalgam. In the past, CT sialography has been advocated to demonstrate margins of tumours more clearly but, with the advent of high-resolution scanners, this is no longer justified. Intravenous contrast can be used to distinguish blood vessels from lymph nodes and to aid in the delineation of tumour margins. The sensitivity of identifying a mass is nearly 100% (Bryan *et al.* 1982). CT is also very sensitive for the identification of calcification within a lesion. Vascular lesions often have a characteristic appearance on CT.

The facial nerve cannot be identified on CT scans but its position is judged indirectly from adjacent landmarks such as the styloid process, posterior belly of the digastric, and the retromandibular vein. Such information, however, is of little material value to the parotid surgeon because the identification of the nerve is a clinical procedure.

MRI is more expensive than CT but has several advantages. It does not use ionizing radiation and the images can be acquired in any plane. The soft tissue contrast is superior to CT and, due to the choice of pulse sequencing, contrast agents are not always required. However, slow acquisition times in MRI may lead to significant artefacts due to patient movement or swallowing. It is reported that MRI can be used to identify the facial nerve (Teresi *et al.* 1987; McGhee *et al.* 1993), but there is some disagreement as to whether low signal linear structures of T_1-weighted images are ducts rather than nerve branches (Thibault *et al.* 1993). Vessels can be identified as flow voids on the images, and the relationship between the mass and vessels can be delineated easily. Tumour spread along the facial nerve can be seen on MRI (Som and Curtin 1996) but in the vast majority of such cases this situation is heralded by dysfunction of the nerve. This itself forewarns the surgeon of impending risk to the facial nerve at surgery. Radiological evidence of a pathological enlarged facial nerve in the absence of motor dysfunction is useful when counselling the patient prior to surgery, but such a situation is uncommon. If nerve infiltration is suspected, it is reasonable to consider evaluation by MRI.

Ultrasonography

The main advantages of ultrasound (US) for the evaluation of salivary lumps are that it is quick, readily available, is relatively cheap, and has no morbidity. It can be used in the clinical setting but the procedure is operator dependent and the images are difficult for the inexperienced to interpret. The submandibular salivary gland and the superficial part of the parotid gland can be visualized with ease (Fig. 4.1) but the deep pole of the parotid is shielded by the ramus of the mandible. This does not detract from its use as over 90% of parotid masses arise in the superficial portion of the gland (Renehan *et al.* 1996). For those masses in the deep aspect of the gland, MRI or CT is a better investigation. It is possible to determine with confidence whether the mass is intra- or extraglandular (Zhao and Zong 1990; Wittich *et al.* 1985), and also if it is cystic or solid in nature (Zhao and Zhang 1990). The addition of colour Doppler allows vessels to be identified. Some authorities recommend US as the first line investigation for masses of the salivary glands (Rinast *et al.* 1989; Vanden Akker 1988 1988), and certainly the overall detection rate of salivary tumours is high (Gritzman 1989; Rineast 1989; Schemelzeisen *et al.* 1991), but most are detectable clinically. It may prove useful, however, for rare occasions when a small occult tumour presents with symptoms of pain. The authors feel that US is a useful first line investigation when applied selectively.

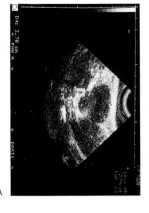
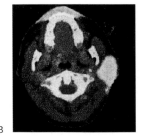

Fig. 4.1 An ultrasound image depicting a large parotid pleomorphic adenoma (A). The accurate definition of the tumour margin is confirmed from the PET image of the same lesion (B). A   B

Nuclear medicine

Traditionally, technetium pertechnetate has been used to help in the diagnosis of Warthin's tumour and oncocytomas (Cogan *et al.* 1981; Brandwein and Huvos 1991). Both of these concentrate the injected tracer and produce hot spots on the resultant images. Anatomical structures are not demonstrated and only larger tumours can be resolved. It is not possible to distinguish confidently benign from malignant disease (Van Den Akker 1988); therefore, the use of these scans is very limited.

Positron emission tomography (PET) using fluoro-2-deoxy-D-glucose has been used successfully in evaluating tumours of the head and neck (Wong *et al.* 1997). The technique relies on the increased metabolic activity of tumours taking up the radioisotope. Its value lies in identifying recurrent disease, that would otherwise be

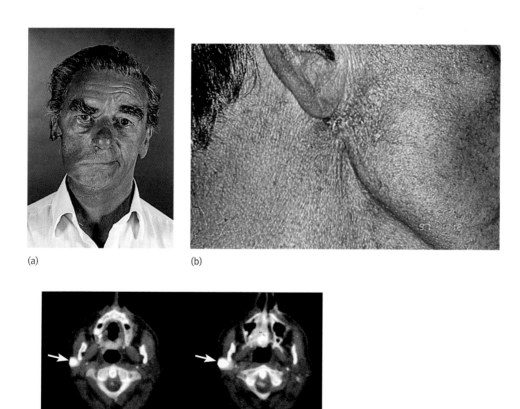

(a)　　　　　(b)

Fig. 4.2 Patient presented with facial palsy (a) and a small indurated mass below the right ear (b). A pleomorphic adenoma had been removed from the right parotid gland twenty years previously and the patient had received a course of adjuvant radiotherapy. The clinical concern was that a large diffuse cancer (adenocarcinoma) had disseminated through the infratemporal area. A co-localized PET scan demonstrated a localized and resectable cancer (c).

masked by scar tissue (Fig. 4.2), and it is useful in the search for the occult primary. It can be used in patients with atypical post-treatment symptoms as a form of intermittent surveillance to exclude early recurrence. It has little or no descriptive value unless the images are co-localized on CT or MR images. In this format, the tumour margin is shown more accurately compared with CT or MRI alone (Wong *et al.* 1996). Co-localized images have particular value in assessing the operability of large tumours that encroach on vital structures. It has no application for the evaluation of a discrete salivary lump.

Role of imaging in management

In the presence of a discrete, superficial clinically benign parotid lump, the routine use of imaging modalities has little impact on management. In practice, they represent a comfort factor for the surgeons. In benign tumours, their value lies in revealing the hidden neoplasm in the parapharyngeal space, ethmoid sinus, or maxillary antrum. They contribute to the assessment of advanced cancers (Fig. 4.3) which have evidence of frank malignancy, and when the full extent of the disease, including cervical nodal status, needs to be ascertained (Leverstein *et al.* 1995). Tumour margins are identified more easily on MRI compared with CT, and irregular tumour margins may suggest malignant disease (Mandebatt *et al.* 1987). Although a combination of clinical and radiological findings is claimed to distinguish benign from malignant disease in 90% of cases (Panush *et al.* 1993; Som and Shugar 1988), in practice, this is not the primary role of CT or MRI.

Imaging is especially valuable when a lesion is not suspected to be neoplastic, for example cystic, vascular, or bony lesions, and also in the submandibular area where it is important to distinguish whether the lesion is intra- or extraglandular.

Fine needle aspiration cytology (FNAC)

FNAC is a diagnostic test for which a clear role in the management of salivary gland lump has not yet been established. Reservations have generally arisen because of the

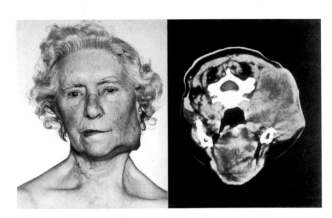

Fig. 4.3 CT or MR scans can make an important contribution to the management of salivary cancer and should be considered in most instances.

diverse microscopic appearance of salivary gland neoplasms. This is reflected in the WHO classification and also historically because these tumours pose a challenge to the pathologist even when the main specimen is available for histological evaluation (Chapter 3). The technique is operator dependent, and improved results are obtained if aspiration is performed by the cytologist directly (Cajulis *et al.* 1997). The theoretical risk of seeding has been now discredited as the overwhelming evidence indicates that FNAC is an oncologically safe procedure (see p. 47).

The role of FNAC in the management of salivary lumps

In order to establish the role of FNAC in management of a discrete salivary lump, in 1995 we undertook a review to determine the accuracy of the method for salivary tissue (McGurk and Hussain 1997). That review included 11 published series with comparable data. This has been updated for this chapter to include 15 studies, with a collective total of 4679 cases (Table 4.3). The original study was complimented by a worldwide survey of 30 head and neck centres to seek a consensus view. The results of these studies confirmed that the FNAC technique was operator sensitive but that, with experience, the technique produced reliable results. The ability to distinguish benign from malignant salivary gland neoplasm was generally good (range 81–98%), with sensitivities ranging from 64 to 100%, and specificities from 85 to 100%. However, the technique was much less effective in providing a correct histological diagnosis. This was estimated to be 77% (range 27–92%). To some extent, the technique is speciality driven as a Medline literature search (1991–1995) for articles with FNAC in the title ($n = 600$) showed that 61% were from departments of pathology and only 22% from clinical departments. The end-point used to assess FNAC in all these studies was invariably accuracy in distinguishing benign from malignant disease. Only one article investigated the value of the test result.

Use of this technique was tested by a questionnaire sent to 30 head and neck units. The question asked was 'What is the role of FNAC in the management of the discrete apparently benign parotid lump?'. All institutions replied but no consensus could be reached. Approximately a third did not use the method as it was thought not to influence management; a third used it routinely but not to distinguish benign from malignant disease, rather to provide as much information as possible to assist counselling the patient and, importantly, also to avoid unforeseen eventualities at surgery. A third used FNAC selectively and mainly in clinical situations where either it was thought the presence of a neoplasm was unlikely, or when the patient was old or infirm and so by confirmation of a benign lesion it meant that surgery could be *avoided*. This study, together with our own experience, led us to develop a selective approach to the use of FNAC with a list of selection criteria shown in Box 4.1.

In summary, parotid tumours can be separated on clinical grounds into the 'simple' discrete lump (the majority of cases as seen in Table 4.2), and the more 'complex' lump (defined by size >4 cm, hidden characteristics, and features of malignancy such as facial palsy and fixity). The policy adopted for the 'simple' lump is towards reliance on clinical judgement alone, whereas the 'complex' lump warrants further investigation through the selective use of the aforementioned investigative tools.

Table 4.3 Accuracy of FNAC in 15 published studies

Authors	No. of patients	Histology available	Accuracy benign versus malignant (%)	Cytohistological correlation (%)	Sensitivity (%)	Specificity (%)	Cytohistological correlation with histology (%)
Eneroth et al. (1967)	1000	690	89	64	64	95	54
Webb (1973)	66	50	98	92	100	96	92
Persson and Lettergren (1973)	362	216	95	86	86	99	70
Lindberg and Ackerman (1976)	860	461	81	63	67	85	50
Kline et al. (1981)	69	50	96	57	100	95	56
Sismanis et al. (1981)	51	51	91	74	85	96	60
Qizilbash et al. (1985)	160	101	98	88	88	100	79
O'Dwyer et al. (1986)	341	341	93	72	73	94	27
Layfield et al. (1987)	171	171	92	77	91	98	74
Kocjan et al. (1990)	52	29	86	79	89	94	83
MacLeod and Frable (1993)	582	21	98	96	93	99	90
Jayaram et al. (1994)	247	211	91	–	88	98	–
Atula et al. (1996)	438	218	–	–	70	87	–
Cajulis et al. (1997)	151	125	–	–	91	96	–
Filopoulos et al. (1998)	129	121	97	–	98	95	–
Total (ranges)	4679	2856	(81–98)	(63–96)	(64–100)	(85–100)	(27–92)

Box 4.1 Selective use of FNAC

- ◆ If lymphadenopathy is suspected, especially in a child, or benign lympho-epithelial disease, sarcoid, infections (i.e. Tuberculosis, histoplasmosis), and lymphoma

- ◆ In older and infirm patients, confirmation of a benign neoplasm will avoid the necessity for surgery

- ◆ To distinguish true parotid neoplasms from lymph nodes, branchial cysts, or submandibular gland lumps, when other tests are equivocal

- ◆ Metastasis either from skin or occult primary

- ◆ As a screening procedure, to select malignant neoplasms for referral to a tertiary centre

- ◆ In rare instances to help identify small malignant neoplasms that present only with pain and facial palsy

- ◆ Where there is risk of sacrifice to the facial nerve intra-operatively

Fine needle aspiration cytology: a 'surgical cytologist's' viewpoint   John Webb

Introduction

Writing as a general surgeon, it is necessary to outline my interest in clinical cytology. It commenced with bone marrow smears and continued with a research year (1963–1964), partly in Holland, studying FNAC. This knowledge I applied in my clinical practice in the management of salivary swellings (Webb 1973; Lewis *et al.* 1999) and other lesions (Webb 1967; Kissin *et al.* 1987; Anderson and Webb, 1987; Dunn *et al.* 1995).

The problem inherent to this disease is lack of experience. In a 29-year period at Bristol Health Trust (1967–1995), 1057 surgical salivary lesions (excluding mucoceles) were seen, of which 274 were 'mixed' tumours (pleomorphic adenomas). To compound the problem, in 1994, 33 epithelial neoplasms were treated by eight different surgeons (general, otolaryngological, and oro-maxillofacial). A similar experience was reported in other studies (Morgan and Mackenzie 1968; Poskitt *et al.* 1984; Gunn and Parrott 1988), and this limitation in experience inevitably contributes to clinical error or inappropriate surgery judged to occur in 15–33% of cases (Woods *et al.* 1975; Byrne and Spector 1988). This is in part because it is not possible to distinguish between benign and malignant neoplasms by clinical features alone; as approximately 55% of primary carcinomas appeared as an asymptomatic mass without demonstrable features of malignancy (Renehan *et al.* 1996). Hence the advantage of FNAC.

43

FNAC technique

FNAC is simple to perform but a technically demanding procedure. It has to be learned and regularly performed in order to ensure adequate smears.

The author's choice is a 21- or 23-gauge hypodermic needle (0.6–0.8 mm in diameter), coupled with a 10- or 20-ml disposable syringe using gentle constant suction by a 'braced thumb' technique (Webb 1982) (Fig. 4.4). This method is preferred to the syringe pistol invented by Franzen (1969). The aspirate is rapidly air-dried, methanol fixated, and stained with Giemsa alone or with May–Grünwald Giemsa. Wet fixation and Papanicolaou staining is also possible.

The puncture must be performed gently, and the number of 'needle passes' recommended varies from one to five (Shaha *et al.* 1990). The needle can be used as a tissue sensor, and puncture without the encumbrance of an attached syringe can be very precise, especially for small elusive lumps. The options of simple puncture and 'braced thumb' aspiration are an ideal, cheap, 'front line' combination (Nettle and Orell 1989).

With a sound technique, the incidence of inadequate smears for solid major salivary tumours should be less than 5%. Repeat procedures with a fine needle are acceptable practice, but a failure rate of around 15% is unacceptable (Wilson *et al.* 1985). CT, MRI, or US are not routinely required for parotid and submandibular masses. However, guided needle puncture may be required for deep lobe parotid parapharyngeal or recurrent tumours (Frable and Frable 1982).

The role of FNAC in the management of salivary lumps

Recent publications have elaborated the clinical utility of FNAC (for a review, see McGurk and Husain 1997). It should be used routinely but there are situations where there is a greater probability that the result will alter management. These are given in Box 4.2.

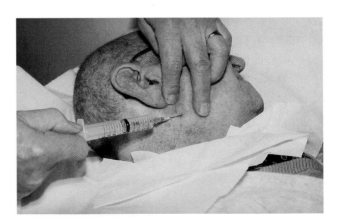

Fig. 4.4 Fine needle aspiration of a long-standing (15 years) cystic/infarcted parotid adenolymphoma; using the 'braced thumb' technique.

Box 4.2 **Optimizing the use of FNAC**

Shaha (1990):

♦ The patient and surgeon can plan an operation in the knowledge of the likely pathological diagnosis

♦ In human immunodeficiency virus (HIV) parotid disease where surgery can be avoided

♦ The unfit and elderly patients harbouring a benign tumour where again surgery may be avoided

♦ If Hodgkin's or non-Hodgkin's lymphoma is suspected

♦ Parotid lumps in children are seldom tumours and it is preferable to avoid surgery if a tumour can be excluded through FNAC

♦ Suspected inflammatory disease, Sjogren's syndrome, or a granulomatous condition

♦ Submandibular gland carcinoma—especially adenoid cystic—demands radical local excision and appropriate nodal clearance. Repeat operations are rarely successful

Palombini (1997):

♦ To determine the type and extent of surgery which is dictated in most cases

♦ To determine the urgency of surgery: this is particularly relevant to the current UK NHS setting where waiting lists are prevalent

♦ To improve the patient's and relatives' ability to give informed consent

♦ To render the patient psychologically prepared for the possibility of facial nerve impairment

♦ If it is suspected a lesion may be suited to radiotherapy or chemotherapy and not a major surgical intervention

The Bristol experience

Since 1967, the outcome of the author's personal series of FNAC diagnoses at the United Bristol Healthcare Trust from all organ sites has been subject to annual audit. For the purposes of this chapter, the total salivary gland entries were extracted from the pathology records. No mechanism was available to access the salivary patients who did not come to surgery.

Salivary gland series

Between 1967 and 1995, a total series of 440 epithelial tumours had accumulated. This section, which focuses on a series of 225 cases collected up to mid-1983 where the

Table 4.4 The Bristol Royal Infirmary salivary lesion series (1967–1983)

	n
Total salivary lesions	225
Children and adolescents under 16 years	23
Confirmed by histology:	
Primary 'mixed' tumour	59
Recurrent 'mixed' tumour	5
Adenolymphoma	36
Adenoid cystic carcinoma	5
Mucoepidermoid carcinoma	1
Acinic cell carcinoma	2
High-grade carcinoma	18
Lymphoma	17
Sensitivity of recognition of neoplasm	99%
Sensitivity of recognition of benign neoplasm	93%
Sensitivity of recognition of malignant neoplasm	90%
Sensitivity of recognition of adenolymphoma	90%
False negatives	1.3% (2/148)*
False suspicious	1.3% (2/148)†

* Two acinic cell carcinomas.

† Atypical pleomorphic adenomas versus adenoid cystic carcinoma.

author had performed FNAC, is illustrated in Table 4.4. A neoplasm was recognized in 99% of cases and the sensitivity for identifying benign, malignant, and Warthin's tumour was 93, 90, and 90% respectively. False-negative results occurred in 1.3% (2/148) cases, as did false-positives (1.3% or 2/148).

High-grade cancers

In the period 1966–1985, 34 high-grade parotid carcinomas of differing histological subtypes were selected for special study (Wyatt *et al.* 1989). Open incision biopsy was performed in 14, whereas FNAC was the diagnostic mode for 12. The cytological sensitivity was 100% (five adenocarcinomas and seven undifferentiated carcinomas). Surgery was performed in three and the cytological diagnosis was concordant with the histopathology; the remaining nine were treated by radiotherapy, and all died with clinical features totally consistent with the cytological diagnosis.

Adenolymphoma

The author has a longstanding interest in the adenolymphoma and preferred to remove these lesions by controlled enucleation (Ebbs and Webb 1986; Lewis *et al.* 1999). Pre-operative diagnosis was a real advantage by FNAC, but sensitivity was low (64%) because of tumour infarction and squamous metaplasia. The study was updated for

Table 4.5 Correlation of FNAC with adenolymphoma diagnosis

	n	% (95% CI)
Original report		
Diagnostic of adenolymphoma	21/32	66 (47–81)
Diagnosis and suggestive results combined	24/32	75 (57–89)
Suspicious cytology	3/32	9
Retrospective report (AJW)		
Diagnostic of adenolymphoma	25/32	78 (60–91)
Diagnostic and suggestive results combined	31/32	97 (84–100)

$\chi^2 = 5.14$, $P < 0.05$, McNemar Change Test, Yates correction.
CI = Confidence Interval.

1985–1995 (11 years) and in a series of 551 salivary lesions in 536 patients there were 222 salivary epithelial neoplasms, including 33 adenolymphomas (32 patients). The original cytological grading was 'suggestive' of adenolymphoma in 75% of cases (Table 4.5). A retrospective review of the cytology was undertaken by the author with a firm diagnosis or suggested features of adenolymphoma identified in 31/32 (97%).

Sensitivity for adenolymphoma recognition reached a mean of 82% in a subsequent blind retrospective review of cases with Kappa values (Lewis *et al.* 1999). In adenolymphoma, the acknowledged pitfalls of squamoid metaplasia and necrotic features leading to false-positive and suspicious readings of low-grade cystic mucoepidermoid carcinoma are significant and in some cases insuperable.

Tumour seeding and FNAC

The deterrent to FNAC is the possible risk of tumour seeding. The traditional view was that any form of biopsy seeded tumour cells. This concept received an authoritative boost from Ackerman and Wheat (1955), but core (2–3 mm diameter) and FNAC biopsy must be distinguished because there are rare but well documented examples of needle track seeding with 'core needle' size (Lambardini and Nesbit 1967), but not with FNAC.

During the past 30 years, careful studies from large series of FNACs have not identified track seeding (Eneroth and Zajicek 1965; Frable and Frable 1982; Klijanienko and Viehl 1997), and affirmed the overall safety of puncturing tumours. However, there are well recognized caveats. Zach (1972) advised against puncturing nodes possibly involved by metastatic melanoma or any rapidly growing neoplasm. Some organ sites, aside from subcutaneous tumours, are less favourable. Transperitoneal aspiration for pancreatic, ovarian, and retroperitoneal tumours carries the potential for seeding. However, the risk is low. McLoughlin and co-workers (1978) investigated 1275 FNACs from a variety of sites, including the parotid, followed for 5–10 years; there was no evidence of tumour implantation. Ferrucci and colleagues (1979) discovered one example of track tumour following percutaneous aspiration for pancreatic cancer within 5000 FNACs from a variety of organ sites. The Papanicolaou

Society (1997) issued authoritative guidelines for FNAC, identifying a seeding risk of 0.003–0.009 from many organ sites based upon needle sizes of 22–26 gauge.

In a personal experience of over 7000 FNACs from a range of sites, including salivary swellings, no seeding was identified but there were examples of subcutaneous tumour nodules following repeated paracentesis for carcinomatous ascites using 2–3 mm trocars. From the Bristol Royal Infirmary (Hughes and Lyons 1982), special review clinics were set up to study the outcome of 58 parotid pleomorphic adenomas and other lesions treated between 1968 and 1978. FNAC was performed in 26; 20 of which provided a precise diagnosis (79%). Two recurrences appeared after superficial parotidectomy preceded by FNAC. The first developed in a previously recurrent 'mixed' tumour after local excision; the second was a recurrent benign lymphoepithelial lesion (currently myoepithelial sialadenitis) which is naturally prone to recurrence. In neither case could recurrence be reasonably attributed to FNAC.

Pitfalls and problems in salivary cytology

It is not denied that FNAC is a testing area for cytological diagnosis. A cytological report should not 'go too far'. A report of benign or malignant is of great value to the surgeon: a precise histological label may not be possible. There are other difficulties, but the statement that FNAC may induce disruptive haemorrhage, infarction, squamoid metaplasia, and perversion of tumour histopathology (Hajdu and Melamed 1984) is not substantiated by a detailed study of adenolymphoma and mixed tumours (Lewis *et al.* 1999).

Some other specific problems that may be encountered in the cytological diagnosis of salivary tumours are illustrated by cases in Fig. 4.5.

Fig. 4.5 (A) Histological section of a 'mixed' parotid tumour, 24 h after FNAC, showing the track from a 21-gauge needle. The track measures ~0.7 mm in diameter and there is no significant damage to the neoplasm (original magnification ×50). (B) FNAC of a recurrent 'mixed' parotid tumour. The smear show atypical epithelial cells and a fibrillary mucopolysaccharide matrix contrasted with natural parotid acini (original magnification ×160). (C) FNAC of a parotid mass invading the angle of the mandible, producing trismus. The smear is typical of adenoid cystic carcinoma with a large 'mucoid globule' (original magnification ×160). (D) FNAC of a left parotid tumour in a 13-year-old black girl, revealing acinic cell carcinoma. The appearances differ little from natural acini. This was a false-negative reading (original magnification ×160). (E) FNAC of a left parotid mass from a 48-year-old woman. This cellular smear shows a low-grade non-Hodgkin lymphoma: classified in 1982 as a follicle centre cell lymphoma of cleaved cell type. The low-grade and nuclear cleavage is clear together with the intercellular cytoplasmic fragments known as lymph-glandular bodies. These are typical of lymphoid aspirates but not other 'round cell' neoplasms. (F) FNAC of a left parotid mass from a 60-year-old man, revealing a high-grade carcinoma of uncertain type. Radical parotidectomy and neck dissection (1968) was followed by death within 1 year. Current classification would regard this as a ductal carcinoma (original magnification ×40). (G) Cytological smear of a left parotid mass from an 18-month-old boy, outlining a malignant round cell tumour later revealed as a metastasis from a temporal bone Ewing's tumour. Intercellular lymphoglandular bodies are not seen (original magnification ×200). (H) A parotid mass in a 57-year-old male. The smear was misread as high-grade carcinoma but, on review, small amounts of pigment were found to be present. Superficial parotidectomy was performed with a histological verdict of secondary malignant melanoma. The patient died very rapidly (original magnification ×200).

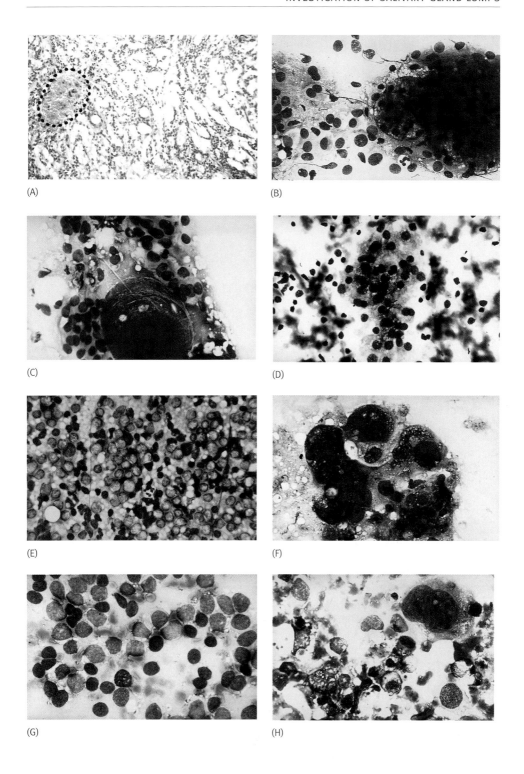

(A)

(B)

(C)

(D)

(E)

(F)

(G)

(H)

Acknowledgements

My colleague, Dr M.F. Lott, participated in the 'blinded', two-run cytology test, for which the slides were selected and numbered by Mrs B. Phillpotts, Chief Scientific Officer in Cytopathology. I am much indebted to them both. Dr S.T. Brooks kindly offered statistical advice and produced results derived from the adenolymphoma study. I am most grateful to Ms Marie Kingdon and Mrs Carol Bond for presentation of the manuscript. My special thanks are due to Professor J.R. Farndon. This research was made possible through his auspices, encouragement, and invaluable advice at all stages.

REFERENCES

Ackerman, L.V. and Wheat, M.W., Jr (1955) The implantation of cancer—an avoidable surgical risk? *Surgery*, **37**, 341–55.

Anderson, J.B. and Webb, A.J. (1987) Fine-needle aspiration biopsy and the diagnosis of thyroid cancer. *Br J Surg*, **74**, 292–6.

Atula, T., Greenman, R., Laippala, P., and Klemi, P.J. (1996) Fine-needle aspiration biopsy in the diagnosis of parotid gland lesions: evaluation of 438 biopsies. *Diagn Cytopathol*, **15**, 185–90.

Brandwein, M.S., Huros, A.G. (1991) Oncocytic tumors of major salivary glands: a study of 68 cases with follow-up of 44 patients. *Am J Surg Pathol*, **15**, 514–28.

Bryan, R.N., Miller, R.H., Ferreyro, R.I., and Sessions, R.B. (1982) Computed tomography of the major salivary glands. *AJR Am J Roentgenol*, **139**, 547–54.

Byrne, M.N. and Spector, J.G. (1988) Parotid masses: evaluation, analysis, and current management. *Laryngoscope*, **98**, 99–105.

Cajulis, R.S., Gokaslan, S.T., Yu, G.H., and Frias Hidvegi, D. (1997) Fine needle aspiration biopsy of the salivary glands. A five-year experience with emphasis on diagnostic pitfalls. *Acta Cytol*, **41**, 1412–20.

Cogan, M.I., Gill, P.S. (1981) Value of sialography and scintigraphy in diagnosis of salivary gland disorders. *Int J Oral Surg* (Supp 1), **10**, 216–22.

Da Xi, S., Hai Xiong, S., and Qiang, Y. (1987) The diagnostic value of ultrasonography and sialography in salivary gland masses. *Dentomaxillofac Radiol*, **16**, 37–45.

Dunn, J.M., Lucarotti, M.E., Wood, S.J., Mumford, A., and Webb, A.J. (1995) Exfoliative cytology in the diagnosis of breast disease. *Br J Surg*, **82**, 789–91.

Ebbs, S.R. and Webb, A.J. (1986) Adenolymphoma of the parotid: aetiology, diagnosis and treatment. *Br J Surg*, **73**, 627–30.

Eneroth, C.M. and Zajicek, J. (1965) Aspiration biopsy of salivary gland tumors. II. Morphologic studies on smears and histologic sections from oncocytic tumors (45 cases of papillary cystadenoma lymphomatosum and 4 cases of oncocytoma). *Acta Cytol*, **9**, 355–61.

Eneroth, C.M., Franzen, S., and Zajicek, J. (1967) Aspiration biopsy of salivary gland tumors. A critical review of 910 biopsies. *Acta Cytol*, **11**, 470–2.

Ferrucci, J.T., Wittenberg, J., Margolies, M.N., and Carey, R.W. (1979) Malignant seeding of the tract after thin-needle aspiration biopsy. *Radiology*, **130**, 345–6.

Filopoulos, E., Angeli, S., Daskalopoulou, D., Kelessis, N., and Vassilopoulos, P. (1998) Pre-operative evaluation of parotid tumours by fine needle biopsy. *Eur J Surg Oncol*, **24**, 180–3.

Frable, M.A. and Frable, W.J. (1982) Fine-needle aspiration biopsy revisited. *Laryngoscope*, **92**, 1414–8.

Franzén, S. Giertz, G., and Zajicek, J. (1969). Cytologic diagnosis of prostatic tumours by transrectal aspiration biopsy. *Br J Urol*, 7, 241–62.

Gritzmann, N. (1989) Sonography of the salivary glands. *AJR Am J Roentgenol*, **153**, 161–6.

Gunn, A. and Parrott, N.R. (1988) Parotid tumours: a review of parotid tumour surgery in the Northern Regional Health Authority of the United Kingdom 1978–1982. *Br J Surg*, **75**, 1144–6.

Hajdu, S.I. and Melamed, M.R. (1984) Limitations of aspiration cytology in the diagnosis of primary neoplasms. *Acta Cytol*, **28**, 337–45.

Hughes, R.G. and Lyons, T.J. (1982) Parotid tumours. *Lancet*, **1**, 1080.

Jayaram, G., Verma, A.K., Sood, N., and Khurana, N. (1994) Fine needle aspiration cytology of salivary gland lesions. *J Oral Pathol Med*, **23**, 256–61.

Kissin, M.W., Fisher, C., Webb, A.J., and Westbury, G. (1987) Value of fine needle aspiration cytology in the diagnosis of soft tissue tumours: a preliminary study on the excised specimen. *Br J Surg*, **74**, 479–80.

Klijanienko, J. and Vielh, P. (1997) Fine-needle sampling of salivary gland lesions. II. Cytology and histology correlation of 71 cases of Warthin's tumor (adenolymphoma). *Diagn Cytopathol*, **16**, 221–5.

Kline, T.S., Merriam, J.M., and Shapshay, S.M. (1981) Aspiration biopsy cytology of the salivary gland. *Am J Clin Pathol*, **76**, 263–9.

Kocjan, G., Nayagam, M., and Harris, M. (1990) Fine needle aspiration cytology of salivary gland lesions: advantages and pitfalls. *Cytopathology*, **1**, 269–75.

Lambardini, M.M. and Nesbit, R.M. (1967) Perineal extension of adenocarcinoma of the prostate gland after punch biopsy. *J Urol*, **97**, 891–3.

Layfield, L.J., Tan, P., and Glasgow, B.J. (1987) Fine-needle aspiration of salivary gland lesions. Comparison with frozen sections and histologic findings. *Arch Pathol Lab Med*, **111**, 346–53.

Leverstein, H., Castelijns, J.A., and Snow, G.B. (1995) The value of magnetic resonance imaging in the differential diagnosis of parapharyngeal space tumours. *Clin Otolaryngol*, **20**, 428–33.

Lewis, D.R., Webb, A.J., Lott, M.F., Brookes, S.T., and Farndon, J.R. (1999) Improving cytological diagnosis and surgical management of parotid adenolymphoma. *Br J Surg*, **86**, 1275–9.

Lindberg, L.G. and Akerman, M. (1976) Aspiration cytology of salivary gland tumors: diagnostic experience from six years of routine laboratory work. *Laryngoscope*, **86**, 584–94.

MacLeod, C.B. and Frable, W.J. (1993) Fine-needle aspiration biopsy of the salivary gland: problem cases. *Diagn Cytopathol*, **9**, 216–24.

Mandelblatt, S.M., Braun, I.F., Davis, P.C., Fry, S.M., Jacobs, L.H., Hoffman, J.C., Jr Parotid masses: MR imaging. *Radiology*, 1987; 163: 411–414.

McGhee, R.B., Jr, Chakeres, D.W., Schmalbrock, P., Brogan, M.A., and Negulesco, J.A. (1993) The extracranial facial nerve: high resolution three-dimensional Fourier transform MR imaging. *AJNR Am J Neuroradiol*, **14**, 465–72.

McGurk, M. and Hussain, K. (1997) Role of fine needle aspiration cytology in the management of the discrete parotid lump. *Ann R Coll Surg Engl*, **79**, 198–202.

McGurk, M., Renehan, A., Gleave, E.N., and Hancock, B.D. (1996) Clinical significance of the tumour capsule in the treatment of parotid pleomorphic adenomas. *Br J Surg*, **83**, 1747–9.

McLoughlin, M.J., Ho, C.S., Langer, B., McHattie, J., and Tao, L.C. (1978) Fine needle aspiration biopsy of malignant lesions in and around the pancreas. *Cancer*, **41**, 2413–9.

Morgan, M.N. and Mackenzie, D.H. (1968) Tumours of salivary glands. A review of 204 cases with 5-year follow-up. *Br J Surg*, **55**, 284–8.

Nettle, W.J. and Orell, S.R. (1989) Fine needle aspiration in the diagnosis of salivary gland lesions. *Aust N Z J Surg*, **59**, 47–51.

O'Dwyer, P., Farrar, W.B., James, A.G., Finkelmeier, W., and McCabe, D.P. (1986) Needle aspiration biopsy of major salivary gland tumors. Its value. *Cancer*, **57**, 554–7.

Palombini, L. (1997) Challenges in the interpretation of FNAs from the salivary glands. *Diagn Cytopathol*, **17**, 417–21.

Parush, D., Fulbright, R., Sze, G. *et al.* (1993) Inversion – recovery fast spin-echo imaging: efficacy in the evaluation of head and neck lesion. *Radiology*, **187**, 421–6.

The Papanicolaou Society (1997) Guidelines of the Papanicolaou Society of Cytopathology for fine-needle aspiration procedure and reporting. The Papanicolaou Society of Cytopathology Task Force on Standards of Practice. *Diagn Cytopathol*, **17**, 239–47.

Persson, P.S. and Zettergren, L. (1973) Cytologic diagnosis of salivary gland tumors by aspiration biopsy. *Acta Cytol*, **17**, 351–4.

Poskitt, K.R., Lambert, W.G., and Moore, P.J. (1984) Parotid tumours in a district general hospital. *Br J Clin Pract*, **38**, 384–7, 391.

Qizilbash, A.H., Sianos, J., Young, J.E., and Archibald, S.D. (1985) Fine needle aspiration biopsy cytology of major salivary glands. *Acta Cytol*, **29**, 503–12.

Renehan, A., Gleave, E.N., Hancock, B.D., Smith, P., and McGurk, M. (1996) Long-term follow-up of over 1000 patients with salivary gland tumours treated in a single centre. *Br J Surg*, **83**, 1750–4.

Rinast, E., Gmelin, E., and Hollands Thorn, B. (1989) Digital subtraction sialography, conventional sialography, high-resolution ultrasonography and computed tomography in the diagnosis of salivary gland diseases. *Eur J Radiol*, **9**, 224–30.

Schemelzeisen, R., Milbradt, H., Reimer, P., Gratz, P., and Wittekind, C. (1991) Sonography and scintigraphy in the diagnosis of diseases of the major salivary glands. *J Oral Maxillofac Surg*, **49**, 798–803.

Shaha, A.R., Webber, C., DiMaio, T., and Jaffe, B.M. (1990) Needle aspiration biopsy in salivary gland lesions. *Am J Surg*, **160**, 373–6.

Sismanis, A., Merriam, J.M., Kline, T.S., Davis, R.K., Shapshay, S.M., and Strong, M.S. (1981) Diagnosis of salivary gland tumors by fine needle aspiration biopsy. *Head Neck Surg*, **3**, 482–9.

Som, P.M. and Curtin, H.D. (1996) *Head and Neck Imaging*, Vol. 2, 3rd edn. pp. 834–5. Mosby, St Louis.

Som, P.M., Shugar, J.M., Sacher, M., Stollman, A.L., Biller, A.F. (1988) Benign and malignant parotid pleomorphic adenomas: CT and MR studies. *Journal of Computer Assisted Tomography*. **12**(1), 65–9, Jan–Feb.

Teresi, L.M., Lufkin, R.B., Wortham, D.G., Abemayor, E., and Hanafee, W.N. (1987) Parotid masses: MR imaging. *Radiology*, **163**, 405–9.

Thibault, F., Halimi, P., Bely, N., Chevallier, J.M., Bonfils, P., Lellouch Tubiana, A. *et al.* (1993). Internal architecture of the parotid gland at MR imaging: facial nerve or ductal system? *Radiology*, **188**, 701–4.

van der Akker, H.P. (1988) Diagnostic imaging in salivary gland disease. *Oral Surgery Oral Med Oral Path*, **66**, 625–37.

Webb, A.J. (1967) Cytological studies in retroperitoneal fibrosis. *Br J Surg*, **54**, 375–8.

Webb, A.J. (1973) Cytologic diagnosis of salivary gland lesions in adult and pediatric surgical patients. *Acta Cytol*, **17**, 51–8.

Webb, A.J. (1982) Surgical aspects of aspiration cytology. In: *Recent Advances in Surgery*. pp. 39–69. (ed. R.C. Russell) Churchill Livingstone, Edinburgh.

Wilson, J.A., McIntyre, M.A., Tan, J., and Maran, A.G. (1985) The diagnostic value of fine needle aspiration cytology in the head and neck. *J R Coll Surg Edinb*, **30**, 375–9.

Wittich, G.R., Scheible, W.F., Hajek, P.C. (1985) Ultrasonography of the salivary glands. *Radiol Clin North Am*, **231**, 29–37.

Wong, W.L., Hussain, K., Chevretton, E., Hawkes, D.J., Baddeley, H., Maisey, M. *et al.* (1996) Validation and clinical application of computer-combined computed tomography and positron emission tomography with 2-[18F]fluoro-2-deoxy-D-glucose head and neck images. *Am J Surg*, **172**, 628–32.

Wong, W.L., Chevretton, E.B., McGurk, M., Hussain, K., Davis, J., Beaney, R. *et al.* (1997) A prospective study of PET-FDG imaging for the assessment of head and neck squamous cell carcinoma. *Clin Otolaryngol*, **22**, 209–14.

Woods, J.E., Chong, G.C., and Beahrs, O.H. (1975) Experience with 1,630 primary parotid tumors. *Am J Surg*, **130**, 460–2.

Wyatt, M.G., Coleman, N., Eveson, J.W., and Webb, A.J. (1989) Management of high grade parotid carcinomas. *Br J Surg*, **76**, 1275–7.

Zach, J. (1972) *Praktische zytologie für internisten.* Thieme, Stuttgart.

Zhao, Y. and Zhang, R. (1990) [Differential diagnosis of parotid gland masses by gray scale real-time ultrasound]. *Hua Hsi I Ko Ta Hsueh Hsueh Pao*, **21**, 92–5.

Audience discussion

Profesor McGurk: Are there any comments on the proposal that an important indication for FNAC is when the lesion is not thought to be a tumour?

Professor van der Waal (Amsterdam, The Netherlands): I agree with Mr Webb, cytology is important and can make all the difference in determining the nature of a lump prior to surgery. But cytology is operator dependent and experience can make a tremendous difference to the result.

Dr Eveson (Bristol, UK): I believe that any information can be useful and I think the point has been made that the exclusion of things like lymphoma and non-neoplastic disease is as important as recognizing a malignancy or a benign tumour.

Mr Watkinson (Birmingham, UK): In Birmingham, we employ FNAC whenever possible when faced with lumps, particularly in the salivary glands. The surgeon should get as much information on the lesion to counsel the patient about the operation, and detail the probable course of surgery with its potential complication. You only have one chance to get it right. It also seems a little unfair to only refer the occasional difficult case to the cytologist and expect a correct answer on every occasion. Regular referral will provide the experience that must be drawn on to diagnose the difficult case.

Mr Bradley (Nottingham, UK): Having done a survey of benign salivary gland tumours in my Health Region, I would be embarrassed to undertake a similar survey of non-neoplastic lumps that have been removed surgically. Patients accept the risk of complications when the lesion is neoplastic but are less inclined to accept the morbidity when the lump is a lymph node, cyst, or sarcoidosis. I would definitely advocate fine needle aspiration cytology on the suspected non-neoplastic lesions in order to provide better informed consent.

Editorial comment

Two perspectives are adopted in this chapter. In the first, a general overview is given of diagnostic procedures available to the surgeon when managing a parotid lump. The strength of each test, and hence its most appropriate application, is emphasized. In the second, the application of FNAC to salivary gland lumps is described in detail. It is suggested that the battery of tests now available has tended to usurp the role of clinical judgement. A more discriminatory approach is advocated. This means there must be a critical appraisal of the relative value of investigations in elucidating diagnoses. It also importantly means that the role of clinical judgement has to be included as part of the diagnostic process.

SECTION TWO
Benign Neoplasms

CHAPTER 5

The surgical approaches to the treatment of parotid pleomorphic adenomas

Gordon Snow

Historical perspectives

Surgery for pleomorphic adenomas of the parotid gland underwent considerable change during the last century. Before the 1940s, the surgical management of pleomorphic adenomas of the parotid gland was unsatisfactory, mainly because of fear of damage to the facial nerve. The routine operation was enucleation and this was associated with a high recurrence rate (~35%) (McFarland 1936). In the 1940s, identification of the main trunk of the facial nerve followed by dissection was advocated (Bailey 1941; Janes 1940). Formal superficial parotidectomy became established as the appropriate treatment (Martin 1952; Patey and Thackray 1958). With this technique, recurrence rates declined dramatically to below 2%, while permanent facial nerve paralysis or paresis became rare (Woods *et al.* 1975; Stevens and Hobsley, 1982; Maynard 1988). With these favourable developments, in the last quarter of the last century attention gradually focused on other sequelae and complications of parotidectomy, such as Frey's syndrome, problems associated with transection of the greater auricular nerve, and cosmetic aspects. With the aim of reducing the morbidity of formal superficial parotidectomy and total parotidectomy, there is now a trend towards limited operations in the form of partial parotidectomy (with identification and dissection of the facial nerve first) and extracapsular dissection (without prior dissection of the facial nerve).

Surgical pathology

Standard surgical textbooks state that formal parotidectomy allows for the removal of benign tumours with an adequate margin of healthy parotid tissue. This statement would imply that the surgical specimen has the tumour in a central position totally surrounded by normal parenchyma. In many cases this is an illusion. In a consecutive series of 83 superficial parotidectomies for pleomorphic adenoma, Donovan and Conley (1984) reported that the surgical margins were considered adequate histologically in 35 cases (42%); the margins were considered close in 28 cases (34%). In those instances, there was only a thin rim of fibrous tissue separating the tumour from the margin of resection. In the remaining 20 cases, the tumour itself appeared to extend to the margin of the resection. The basis of this is the relationship of the tumour to the facial nerve or its branches, i.e. in 50–60% of the cases, the tumour is in close proximity to the nerve (Donovan and Conley 1984; McGurk *et al.* 1996), such that some modified type of limited extracapsular or capsular dissection must be carried out in order to preserve the nerve. Nevertheless, this operation is very successful in terms of very low recurrence rates, therefore it appears quite legitimate and appropriate to design and perform operations that *limit the amount of healthy parotid parenchyma to be removed as much as possible*. We describe the different approaches and examine whether this results in reduced morbidity without untoward effects on recurrence rates.

Classification of approaches

A proposed system of classification is shown in Box 5.1.

Partial parotidectomy

In partial parotidectomy, one adheres to the same principle as in formal superficial or total parotidectomy. First the main trunk or one (or more) of the peripheral branches of the facial nerve are identified and dissected, and subsequently the tumour is removed. For practical purposes, two main types of partial parotidectomy can be distinguished: partial superficial parotidectomy and selective deep lobe parotidectomy. The first operation is suitable for small tumours situated in the superficial lobe of the parotid gland, while the second operation is practicable for deep lobe tumours that are completely deep to the facial nerve and deep to the mandible. In both operations, the usual incision for parotidectomy is made starting just anterior to the tragus of the ear,

---

Box 5.1 Classification of approaches to parotid tumours

Formal parotidectomy
    superficial parotidectomy
    total parotidectomy
Limited operations
    Partial parotidectomy
        partial superficial parotidectomy
        selective deep lobe parotidectomy
    Extracapsular dissection

passing down in front of the lobule, thence curving posteriorly below the lobule and passing downward parallel to the posterior margin of the ascending ramus of the mandible, finally curving anteriorly below and parallel to the angle of the mandible. In all cases in which identification of the main trunk of the facial nerve is envisaged, the greater auricular nerve is identified running obliquely over the sternocleidomastoid muscle near the angle of the mandible. Unless precluded by the position of the tumour, the nerve is followed through the parotid gland to its posterior branch. This branch, which innervates the auricle and surrounding skin, is exposed completely after sacrificing the more anterior branches. Subsequently the nerve can be translocated posteriorly so as to avoid injury to it during identification of the main stem of the facial nerve.

Partial superficial parotidectomy

In partial superficial parotidectomy, identification and dissection of the nerve is limited to the part of the nerve that is in proximity to the tumour. The operation thus is very much determined by the position of the tumour and is rather a variant of the standard procedure. Depending on the location of the tumour, this operation can be started with exposure of the main trunk of the facial nerve, or with exposure of one (or more) of the

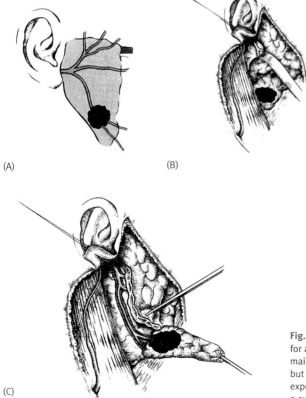

(A)   (B)

(C)

Fig. 5.1 Partial superficial parotidectomy for a posterior (lower pole) tumour (A). The main trunk of the facial nerve is identified but only relevant branches of the nerve exposed to allow removal of a tumour with a cull of normal salivary tissue.

59

peripheral branches of the nerve. The procedure is depicted for a tumour in the poste-rior/inferior part of the parotid gland in Fig. 5.1. After identification of the main stem and the main division of the facial nerve, dissection is continued along the cervicofacial trunk only, and the overlying parotid parenchyma is divided. The dissection is carried on to beyond the tumour and the tumour is then removed with a minimal amount of parotid parenchyma. The procedure, which starts with identification of the main trunk, is especially suitable for those patients in whom the tumour is located in the posterior part of the superficial lobe of the parotid gland. When the tumour is located in other parts of the superficial lobe, the dissection is started with exposure of one (or more) of the peripheral branches of the facial nerve just beyond the margin of the parotid gland. This procedure is described in great detail for the various tumour locations by Attie and Sciubba (1981).

In Fig. 5.2, the procedure is depicted for a tumour in the anterior part of the parotid gland near Stensen's duct. The skin flap is developed anteriorly to expose the parotid gland, Stensen's duct, and the peripheral buccal branches of the facial nerve anterior to the parotid gland. With the dissection starting at the duct anterior to the gland, the buccal branches are traced posteriorly. The anterior part of the parotid with the tumour is gradually lifted from the nerve in a posterior direction. When this has been continued to beyond the tumour, the tumour can be removed with a minimum of parotid parenchyma.

Selective deep lobe parotidectomy

This operation starts with identification of the main trunk and division of the facial nerve and dissection along both the temporofacial and cervicofacial trunks and their branches. Gradually the superficial lobe of the parotid is lifted from the nerve from behind forwards. This is continued to well beyond the posterior margin of the ascend-ing ramus of the mandible. However, the superficial lobe is not removed as it is in formal parotidectomy, but left attached anteriorly as a pedicle (Fig. 5.3). Subsequently

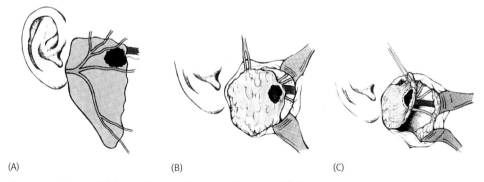

(A)   (B)   (C)

Fig. 5.2 Partial superficial parotidectomy for an anterior tumour (A). In order to limit unnecessary dissection of the gland, the relevant peripheral branches of the facial nerve are identified (B) and a retrograde dissection undertaken until the tumour can be removed with a minimum of parotid parenchyma.

60

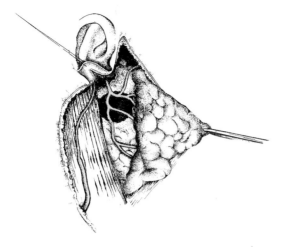

Fig. 5.3 Selective deep lobe parotidectomy.

the facial nerve and its branches are dissected off the deep lobe tumour, and the latter with the surrounding salivary tissue is delivered between the two major divisions of the nerve or by reflecting the entire nerve superiorly. The superficial lobe is replaced and sutured back in place with the intention of minimizing the incidence of Frey's syndrome, and maintaining the contour of the face.

Extracapsular dissection

This operation entails localized surgery done by careful dissection just outside or in the plane of the capsule of the tumour without prior dissection of the facial nerve and its branches. After the skin flaps have been raised, a cruciate incision is made over the lump and the glandular tissue is retracted with artery forceps as the plane is deepened by careful blunt dissection to the capsule of the tumour (Fig. 5.4). Care should be taken at all stages to look for and identify branches of the facial nerve which may be overlapping the tumour or lying in its bed. The lobular growth of pleomorphic

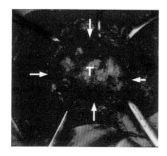
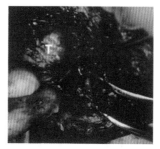
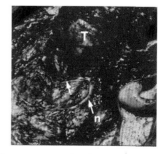

Fig. 5.4 Extracapsular dissection. T = Tumour; N = Facial Nerve. Arrows indicate extracapsular plane of dissection

adenomas should be remembered during resection in order to avoid rupture or out-growths of the tumour. The operation has been advocated in the USA by Anderson and Byars (1965), and in the UK by Gleave and colleagues (1979). The operation has been best described systematically by Gleave (1981, 1995). Gleave emphasizes in his publi-cation of 1981 that the decision as to the feasibility of this operation cannot be under-taken until the parotid gland has been fully explored. First the gland is exposed completely through an incision that is similar to the one used in formal parotidectomy. Subsequently the posterior border of the gland is separated from the mastoid process and the sternocleidomastoid muscle, and the main trunk of the facial nerve is identified. This allows palpation of the tumour from both superficial and deep aspects. The mobility of the tumour within the gland and its relationship to the plane of the facial nerve can thus be determined. In his later publication of 1995, Gleave states that he performed the operation latterly without full exploration of the parotid gland, needing only to raise the skin flap as far forward as to expose the tumour and so that the lobe of the ear and the posterior flap are mobilized as well. When adequate exposure has been obtained thus, careful assessment of the tumour is made in order to determine its mobility within the gland. The following factors favour a local approach to the tumour by (extra)capsular dissection: (i) mobility within the parotid gland; (ii) a thin covering of capsule and glandular tissue; and (iii) a tumour big enough to allow digital manipulation during dissection.

Comparison of limited versus formal operations

The principles of surgery for pleomorphic adenoma first of all are to ensure the intact removal of the tumour and to maintain the integrity of the facial nerve. Several reports bear evidence that recurrence rates after partial parotidectomy (Yamashita *et al.* 1993; Leverstein *et al.* 1997) and after extracapsular dissection (Anderson 1975; Martis 1983; McGurk *et al.* 1996) are equally low—both less than 2%—as those after formal superficial or total parotidectomy, while permanent facial nerve paralysis or paresis is equally rare. McGurk *et al.* (1996) found that extracapsular dissection was associated with a significantly reduced incidence of transient facial nerve damage compared with superficial parotidectomy. In partial superficial parotidectomy, there is also less risk of transient nerve injury, because less of the nerve is dissected than in formal superficial parotidectomy (Helmus 1997). There is overwhelming evidence that the incidence of Frey's syndrome is markedly reduced after partial parotidectomy (Leverstein *et al.* 1997; Helmus 1997) and after extracapsular dissection (Martis 1983; Prichard *et al.* 1992; McGurk *et al.* 1996) when compared with formal superficial parotidectomy, presumably because of the limited disruption of the parotid tissue.

Remarks

In experienced hands, limited operations such as partial parotidectomy and extra-capsular dissection are equally effective as formal superficial parotidectomy in eradi-cating pleomorphic adenoma without permanent facial nerve damage, and are

Table 5.1 Recurrence rates and morbidity for formal parotidectomy versus limited operations: comparative series

Study	Formal superficial parotidectomy	Partial superficial parotidectomy	Extracapsular dissection
Amsterdam series			
No. of patients	61	131	
Recurrence rate	0	0	
Facial palsy			
Permanent	0	0	
Transient	Overall 20%		
Frey's syndrome	8 (13)	9 (7)	
Manchester series			
No. of patients	95		380
Recurrence rate	2 (2)		7 (2)
Facial palsy			
Permanent	1 (1)		7 (2)
Transient	30 (32)		41 (11)
Frey's syndrome	36 (38)		18 (5)
Amputation neuroma	18 (19)		3 (1)

Amsterdam series (Leverstein *et al.* 1997); median follow-up = 95 months.

Manchester series (McGurk *et al.* 1996); median follow-up = 150 months.

Values in parentheses are percentages.

associated with considerably less morbidity such as Frey's syndrome (Table 5.1). However, this does not necessarily mean that partial parotidectomy and extracapsular dissection are to be recommended as standard techniques. Extracapsular dissection without prior dissection of the facial nerve is a technically demanding procedure and is not recommended as a standard technique. With partial superficial parotidectomy, the situation is more subtle. The majority of superficial pleomorphic adenomas are located in the posterior or inferior part of the superficial lobe of the parotid gland, and these lend themselves well to partial superficial parotidectomy with prior identification and dissection of the main trunk of the facial nerve. This procedure is not fundamentally different from formal superficial parotidectomy, but has considerable benefits for the patient and thus is recommended. For pleomorphic adenomas situated in the anterior part of the superficial lobe, partial parotidectomy would preferably entail initial dissection of one or more of the peripheral branches of the facial nerve from retrograde so as to minimize the amount of parotid parenchyma to be removed. However, the anterior approach is demanding and is not recommended as a standard operation. Furthermore, even when the parotidectomy in anteriorly situated tumours is done by initially dissecting the main trunk, a full superficial parotidectomy is rarely required. In deep lobe tumours that are completely deep to the facial nerve and the mandible, a selected deep lobe parotidectomy is recommended.

REFERENCES

Anderson, R. (1975) Benign mixed tumours of the parotid gland. In: *Cancer of the Head and Neck*. pp. 1555–8. (eds R.G. Chamvers, A.M.P. Janssen de Limpens, D.A. Jaques, and R.T. Routledge) Proceedings of an International Symposium 37, Excerpta Medica, Amsterdam.

Anderson, R. and Byars, L.T. (1965) *Surgery of the Parotid Gland*. pp 116–32. Mosby, St Louis.

Attie, J.N. and Sciubba, J.J. (1981) Tumors of major and minor salivary glands: clinical and pathologic features. *Curr Probl Surg*, **18**, 65–155.

Bailey, H. (1941) Treatment of tumours of the parotid gland with special reference to total parotidectomy. *Br J Surg*, **28**, 337–46.

Donovan, D.T. and Conley, J.J. (1984) Capsular significance in parotid tumor surgery: reality and myths of lateral lobectomy. *Laryngoscope*, **94**, 324–9.

Gleave, E.N. (1981) Tumours of the parotid gland. In: *Operative Surgery. Fundamental International Techniques. Head and Neck Part II*. pp. 848–61. (eds C. Rob and R. Smith) Butterworths, London.

Gleave, E.N. (1995) An alternative to superficial parotidectomy: extracapsular dissection. In: *Color Atlas and Text of the Salivary Glands. Diseases, Disorders and Surgery*. pp. 165–72. (eds J.E. de Burgh Norman and M. McGurk) Mosby-Wolfe, London.

Gleave, E.N., Whittaker, J.S., and Nicholson, A. (1979) Salivary tumours—experience over thirty years. *Clin Otolaryngol*, **4**, 247–57.

Helmus, C. (1997) Subtotal parotidectomy: a 10-year review (1985 to 1994). *Laryngoscope*, **107**, 1024–7.

Janes, R.M. (1940) The treatment of tumours of the salivary gland by radical excision. *Can Med Assoc J*, **43**, 554–9.

Leverstein, H., van der Wal, J.E., Tiwari, R.M., van der Waal, I., and Snow, G.B. (1997) Surgical management of 246 previously untreated pleomorphic adenomas of the parotid gland. *Br J Surg*, **84**, 399–403.

Martin, H. (1952) The operative removal of tumours of the parotid salivary gland. *Surgery*, **31**, 670–82.

Martis, C. (1983) Parotid benign tumors: comments on surgical treatment of 263 cases. *Int J Oral Surg*, **12**, 211–20.

Maynard, J.D. (1988) Management of pleomorphic adenoma of the parotid. *Br J Surg*, **75**, 305–8.

McFarland, J. (1936) Three hundred mixed tumours of the salivary glands, of which sixty-nine recurred. *Surg Gynecol Obstet*, **63**, 457–68.

McGurk, M., Renehan, A., Gleave, E.N., and Hancock, B.D. (1996) Clinical significance of the tumour capsule in the treatment of parotid pleomorphic adenomas. *Br J Surg*, **83**, 1747–9.

Patey, D.H. and Thackray, A.C. (1958) The treatment of parotid tumours in the light of a pathological study of parotidectomy material. *Br J Surg*, **55**, 477–87.

Prichard, A.J., Barton, R.P., and Narula, A.A. (1992) Complications of superficial parotidectomy versus extracapsular lumpectomy in the treatment of benign parotid lesions. *J R Coll Surg Edinb*, **37**, 155–8.

Stevens, K.L. and Hobsley, M. (1982) The treatment of pleomorphic adenomas by formal parotidectomy. *Br J Surg*, **69**, 1–3.

Woods, J.E., Chong, G.C., and Beahrs, O.H. (1975) Experience with 1,360 primary parotid tumors. *Am J Surg*, **130**, 460–2.

Yamashita, T., Tomoda, K., and Kumazawa, T. (1993) The usefulness of partial parotidectomy for benign parotid gland tumors. A retrospective study of 306 cases. *Acta Otolaryngol Suppl*, **500**, 113–6.

Audience discussion

Professor O'Brien (Sydney, Australia): Can Professor Snow tell us whether the technique of partial superficial parotidectomy (which is what I practice) is an operation only for pleomorphic adenoma, or in a previously untreated superficial, localized, and mobile tumour does it matter what the pathology is?

Professor Snow: I do this operation for every tumour where there are no clinical signs of malignancy because unless you have an expert cytologist the pathology is not known before the operation.

Mr Shaheen (London, UK): Would you expand on the advantage of saving the posterior branch of the greater auricular nerve? If the nerve is sacrificed, most of the sensation returns albeit in a slightly distorted form. How much more do you gain by preserving that posterior branch?

Professor Snow: This is a topic of debate. The sensitivity always recurs but it takes a long time. It is easy to preserve the nerve which I believe is possible in four out of five cases; there seems no logical reason to sacrifice it. The nerve suffers neuropraxia because of the dissection but in my experience the sensitivity comes back much earlier.

Professor Spiro (New York, USA): With respect to gustatory sweating (Frey's syndrome), in your series, were the patients tested or did you rely on patient symptoms? The second question is what do you think is adequate follow-up in terms of assessing recurrence of pleomorphic adenoma? My perception is that you really need something like 20 years in order to be sure.

Professor Snow: I summarized about 10 papers on this topic, and there is an enormous difference in incidence between studies depending on how detailed was the examination performed.

In answer to your second question. Recurrence can occur as late as 15 years after surgery. The average interval between the first operation and the first recurrence is about 7+ years. This leads me to another point, should you follow-up patients treated for pleomorphic adenoma? I have done so for 20–25 years and know my results (two recurrences in 250 cases). I now only follow-up patients if the case is abnormal (pathology or spillage).

Editorial comment

In his description of parotid procedures, Professor Snow raises two controversial issues. First, he reports a trend towards more conservative surgery for the benign lump and, secondly, a need for improved classification of parotid procedures. The two are inter-related because without a move to more limited procedures, there would only be the superficial and total parotidectomy.

The emerging evidence suggests that in appropriate surgical hands the extent of surgery has little impact on the risk of recurrent disease, but it does correlate with morbidity. Recurrence rates for pleomorphic adenoma in skilled hands have now been reduced to below 2%. Morbidity consequently has become the more dominant focus, particularly to the facial nerve. The risk to the nerve is directly proportional to the degree of nerve exposure at surgery.

A range of confusing terms has evolved to describe procedures less than the classic superficial or total parotidectomy (superficial parotidectomy, partial superficial parotidectomy, and lateral lobectomy and subtotal parotidectomy widely used in the USA). As the facial nerve is the principal cause of morbidity, perhaps a better approach would be to use the degree of facial nerve exposure as the discriminator in a revised classification of surgical techniques.

CHAPTER 6

The significance of the tumour capsule in pleomorphic adenoma

The changing face of conventional principles
John Langdon

The minimalist approach
Brian Hancock

The changing face of conventional principles   John Langdon

Historical perspectives

Prior to the 1940s, the surgical management of parotid tumours was unsatisfactory due to high rates of permanent facial nerve palsy and recurrence rates of between 20 and 45% (McFarland 1936). The poor results in the management of parotid tumours stemmed from inadequate resection through fear of injuring the facial nerve and lack of knowledge of facial nerve dissection technique (Martin 1952; Bearhs and Adsom 1958). This was the era of simple 'enucleation' for parotid tumours.

In an attempt to reduce high recurrence rates, Patey (1940), and later McEvedy and Ross (1976), advocated enucleation followed by irradiation either by implant/ brachytherapy or by external beam/teletherapy. Later, Patey (Patey and Thackray, 1958), still dissatisfied with outcomes, became one of the foremost advocates of formal parotidectomy following exposure of the facial nerve trunk. Until recently, this was the accepted surgical teaching for the treatment of benign parotid tumours; enucleation was considered 'bad' and formal parotidectomy should be the norm (Stevens and Hobsley 1982). Despite this, some surgeons continued to advocate 'enucleation' or, in most cases, extracapsular dissection, claiming low recurrence rates and a low incidence of facial nerve palsy (Stea 1975; Maimaris and Ball 1986; Hancock 1987; Prichard *et al.* 1992).

Mechanisms of recurrence

The two main theories explaining recurrence following treatment for the pleomorphic adenoma are the tumour bud concept and tumour rupture (Box 6.1). Multicentricity, as proposed by Redon (1953), has less proponents, but is still promulgated by some investigators (Aljamo *et al.* 1989).

> ## Box 6.1 Mechanisms of recurrence in pleomorphic adenomas
>
> ◆ Incomplete tumour capsule with protruding tumour—*tumour bud* concept
> ◆ Tumour rupture and spillage
> ◆ Multicentricity

The tumour bud concept

The proponents of formal parotidectomy base their arguments on the undisputed observation that although the pleomorphic adenoma is a benign neoplasm it is characterized by having a bosselated surface with an incomplete capsule and illusionary planes of cleavage (Stevens and Hobsley 1982). For these reasons, it is argued that superficial or total parotidectomy with preservation of the facial nerve is a procedure that ensures *en bloc* resection of the tumour with clear margins. However, those of us who practice parotid surgery are only too aware that the pleomorphic adenoma frequently is in intimate contact with the facial nerve which may be stretched over it. Peeling the nerve off the tumour cannot leave a cuff of normal parotid tissue.

The problem was quantified by Donovan and Conley (1984) who examined 100 consecutive superficial or total parotidectomies performed for benign tumours. They showed that in more than 60% of cases capsular dissection or limited enucleation occurs at some point in the procedure. Indeed, they stated 'it is an illusion to believe that the lateral lobe operation for resection of benign tumour of the superficial or deep lobe (of the parotid) produces a surgical specimen that has the neoplasm in a central position totally surrounded by normal parenchyma. True *en bloc* resection occurs in only approximately 40% of parotid tumours removed'.

Lam *et al.* (1990) confirmed these clinical suspicions in laboratory study using whole organ sectioning of 15 standard formal parotidectomy specimens. All tumours showed some exposed capsule or bare areas where the tumour had been dissected from the facial nerve. Indeed it was their conclusion based on this study that 'capsular incompleteness and tumour in-growth (into the capsule) make global capsular dissection unsafe. It is concluded that formal parotidectomy remains the operation of choice for pleomorphic adenoma of the parotid gland, although capsular dissection cannot be entirely avoided during the procedure'.

Tumour rupture

Tumour rupture and spillage are likely to be responsible for many recurrences. It appears certain that the rupture rate for enucleation is much higher than at formal parotidectomy. McEvedy and Ross (1976) reported 50% (using microscopic criteria), and Armistead *et al.* (1979) reported 21% based on operative observation. However,

Natvig and Soberg (1994) (Chapter 7) reviewed a series of 346 parotid operations for pleomorphic adenoma with an overall recurrence rate of 2.5%. Macroscopic tumour spillage occurred in 26 patients and only two of these (8%) developed recurrences. These authors questioned whether spillage of tumour cells played a significant role in the development of recurrent tumours.

Recurrence rates: formal parotidectomy versus limited resection

Without any doubt, in the early days of 'enucleation', recurrence rates were indeed high, ranging from 21 to 45% (Table 6.1). Lanier (1972) reported a 3.6% recurrence rate in 88 superficial parotidectomies compared with 20% recurrence in 20 enucleation procedures. Woods *et al.* (1975), in a large series of 436 enucleations, reported an 8%

Table 6.1 Rupture and recurrence rates after different treatment methods

Authors	No. of patients	Rupture rate	Recurrence rates	
			<10 year FU	**>10 year FU**
Enucleation only				
Wood (1904)	37		17 (45)	
Benedict and Meigs (1930)	40		17 (43)	
Stein and Geschickter (1934)	111		29 (26)	
McFarland (1936)	278		57 (21)	69 (35)
Rawson et al. (1950)	78			24 (31)
Enucleation plus RT				
Van Miert *et al.* (1968)	182		5 (2.7)	
Haw (1975)	57		2 (3.5)	
McEvedy and Ross (1976)	73	36 (50)	2 (2.7)	
Armistead *et al.* (1979)	76	16 (21)	1 (1.3)	
Formal parotidectomy				
Richardson *et al.* (1975)	90		1 (0.8)	
Woods *et al.* (1977)	360		8 (2)	
Gleave *et al.* (1979)	112	3 (2.5)		3 (2)
Chan and Gunn (1981)	20		0	
Steven and Hobsley (1982)	72	4 (6)	1 (0.8)	
Maynard (1988)	130		1 (0.8)	
Extracapsular dissection				
Anderson (1979)	131		2 (1.5)	
Prichard *et al.* (1992)	31		0	
McGurk *et al.* (1996)	380			9 (2)

FU, follow-up; RT, radiotherapy.

Values in parentheses are percentages.

recurrence rate compared with 2% in 388 formal superficial parotidectomies. Stevens and Hobsley (1982) claimed no recurrences in a series of 72 primary parotidectomies.

Advocates of extracapsular dissection claim that their tumour recurrence rates do not differ from those in formal parotidectomy. Gleave *et al.* (1979), in a series of 369 parotid pleomorphic adenomas from Manchester, reported a recurrence rate of 1.9% for extracapsular dissection and 1.8% when the facial nerve was formally exposed. Wennmo *et al.* (1988), in a smaller series of 57 superficial parotidectomies and 33 limited excisions, reported recurrence rates of 8.7 and 6%, respectively. McGurk *et al.* (1996) re-analysed the Manchester series and compared 380 extracapsular dissections with 95 superficial parotidectomies, and reported a 2% recurrence rate in both groups.

Are there differences in complication rates?

Facial nerve palsy

Tumour recurrence is not the only complication of parotid surgery. Temporary or permanent facial nerve weakness is an important cause of patient morbidity. If the facial nerve is not identified, it is put at greater risk because in the operation of enucleation

Tables 6.2 Facial nerve morbidity after different surgical approaches to parotid pleomorphic adenomas

Authors	No. of patients rate	Nerve damage Permanent	Transient rate
Formal parotidectomy			
Richardson *et al.* (1975)	90	0	(16)*
Woods *et al.* (1977)	360	9 (3)†	123 (41)†
Chan and Gunn (1981)	20	0	Not stated
Steven and Hobsley (1982)	72	0	Not stated
Maynard (1988)	130	1 (0.8)	19 (15)
Laccourreye *et al.* (1994)	229‡	9 (4)	161 (70)
McGurk *et al* (1996)	95	1 (1.1)	30 (32)
Moody *et al.* (1999)	111**	2 (1.8)	37 (33.3)
Extracapsular dissection			
Anderson (1979)	131	0	Not stated
Prichard *et al.* (1992)	31	0	1 (3)
Dallera *et al.* (1993)	71	1 (1.4)	8 (12)
McGurk *et al.* (1996)	380	7 (1.8)	41 (11)

Values in parentheses are percentages.

* Based on 467 total cases of parotidectomy.

† Based on 300 cases of superficial parotidectomy.

‡ All 229 patients had total parotidectomy.

** Number of cases for tumours treated by formal parotidectomy, not all pleomorphic adenomas.

the surgeon cannot know the exact position of the facial nerve and its branches (Touquet *et al.* 1990). This is demonstrated by the greater incidence of permanent (as opposed to temporary) facial nerve paralysis in the published series (Table 6.2).

Perhaps not surprisingly, Martis (1983) reported a higher incidence of temporary facial nerve paralysis with superficial parotidectomy compared with extracapsular dissection, and this observation has been confirmed by McGurk *et al.* (1996) who reported an incidence of 32 and 11%, respectively.

Frey's syndrome

A review of the historical aspects, incidence, diagnosis, and treatment of Frey's syndrome (gustatory sweating) has been covered comprehensively recently by Sood and colleagues (1998). The reported incidence of Frey's complication after parotid surgery is determined principally by the method of assessment and the extent of parotid surgery. With respect to the latter, rates decline from total parotidectomy (> 60%) to extracapsular dissection (<10%) (Table 6.3). In our series of parotidectomies for benign tumours at King's College Hospital, London, examined at two different time points, the incidences of Frey's were 13% (Langdon 1984) and 20% (Moody *et al.* 1999), respectively.

Tables 6.3 Frey's syndrome by extent of parotid surgery for pleomorphic adenomas

Authors	No. of patients	Rate
Total parotidectomy		
Laccourreye *et al.* (1994)	229	151 (66)
Superficial parotidectomy		
Richardson *et al.* (1975)	467	65 (14)
Woods *et al.* (1977)	360	86 (24)
Chan and Gunn (1981)	20	4 (20)
Steven and Hobsley (1982)	72	21 (30)
Maynard (1988)	130	22 (17)
Leverstein *et al.* (1997)	61	8 (13)
McGurk *et al.* (1996)	95	36 (38)
Partial superficial parotidectomy		
Leverstein *et al.* (1997)	131	9 (7)
Moody *et al.* (1999)*	111	22 (20)
Extracapsular dissection		
Prichard *et al.* (1992)	31	0
Dallera *et al.* (1993)	71	0
McGurk *et al.* (1996)	380	18 (5)

Values in parentheses are percentages.

* Number of cases for all tumours: partial superficial parotidectomty 92; total parotidectomy 19.

Implications for practice and training

The evidence outlined above shows that there are no differences in terms of recurrence rates between formal parotidectomy and extracapsular dissection. The author advocates an intermediate view as proposed by Lam and colleagues (1990), and believes that 'capsular incompleteness and tumour in-growth make capsular dissection unsafe'. Formal parotidectomy, therefore, remains the operation of choice (Fig. 6.1) although capsular dissection cannot be avoided entirely during the procedure. The author accepts that McGurk and colleagues (McGurk *et al.* 1996; McGurk 1997) provide con-

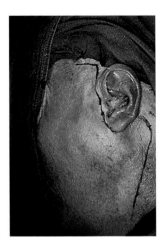
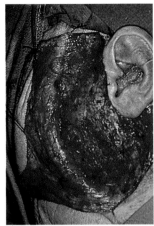
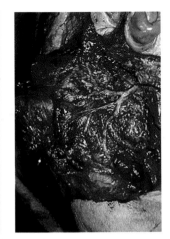

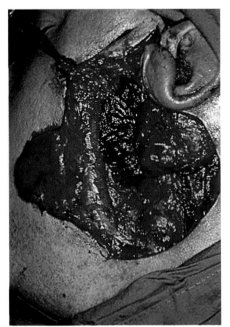

Fig. 6.1 A traditional superficial parotidectomy showing the dissection of the facial nerve. In this case, the soft tissue defect is repaired with a sternomastoid rotation flap.

vincing evidence that *in careful hands* extracapsular dissection may result in low recurrence rates and reduced morbidity. In accepting that their philosophy challenges conventional teaching, they do emphasize that surgery for pleomorphic adenomas is operator sensitive.

For these reasons, in training junior surgeons, it is difficult to justify capsular dissection as the operative procedure for parotid tumours. On the other hand, an excessively thick layer of overlying glandular tissue is not required. Wide local excision with a cuff of salivary tissue is adequate. The problem is that identification of a branch of the facial nerve in the middle of the parotid gland is more difficult than finding it at its trunk. Significantly, in his 1987 paper, Hancock (1987), who advocates extracapsular dissection, states that he uses a flexible approach and that in 78% of his cases the facial nerve trunk was identified at the start of the procedure. The bifurcation was exposed but only those branches passing towards the tumour were fully displayed.

The policy adopted by the author is supported by the work of Leverstein *et al.* (1997). They studied 245 patients who underwent parotid surgery for primary pleomorphic adenomas. For superficial lobe tumours, they performed *partial superficial parotidectomies* (Chapter 5). Two patients (both deep lobe tumours) developed recurrences. Tumour spillage occurred in 10 cases (4.1%); four of these received postoperative radiotherapy and none developed recurrences. There were no permanent facial nerve palsies although 20% had temporary weakness. The incidence of Frey's syndrome was 6.9%. The results of Yamashita *et al.* (1993) in their series of 112 patients with pleomorphic adenomas are comparable, with no tumour recurrences, 18% temporary facial nerve weakness, but a higher incidence of Frey's syndrome at 18%.

Submandibular gland and oral cavity

Pleomorphic adenomas are not confined to the parotid gland. When involving the submandibular gland they present no real surgical challenge. Although poorly encapsulated and bosselated, they are not invasive and do not extend beyond the capsule of the submandibular gland itself. Therefore, conventional excision of the submandibular gland should result in zero recurrence rates, unless the tumour is ruptured due to excessive retraction during surgery (Langdon 1998).

Within the oral cavity, the hard palate is the most frequent site of occurrence. Again although the tumour is poorly or incompletely encapsulated, it is not invasive and will not breach the periosteum. Therefore, simple excision in the subperiosteal plane is curative. Fenestration of the palate is not necessary and the periosteal attachment at the free end of the hard palate is continuous with the *aponeurosis* of the soft palate. This provides a plane of dissection when moving from bone to soft palate on which to remove the tumour safely.

Pleomorphic adenomas also occur more rarely in the submucosal tissues of the upper lip, cheeks, and floor of the mouth. As these areas are anatomically 'safe', extracapsular dissection is appropriate.

The minimalist approach   Brian Hancock

The philosophy of extracapsular dissection

The theories of the mechanisms underlying recurrence following surgery for pleomorphic adenoma have been outlined above. Of these, Alan Nicholson (Christie Hospital, Manchester, 1948–1973) was one of the first to recognize tumour rupture as the probable major cause of recidivism. He observed that many tumours were in close contact with the facial nerve branches so that performing a nerve dissection would not guarantee a complete covering of tumour by parotid tissue in every case. He reasoned that if the tumour was removed carefully without macroscopic rupture, recurrence should not occur, and that post-operative radiotherapy, which was still used routinely (in the 1950s), would be unnecessary. It was his practice to perform a local dissection for superficial and mobile parotid tumours. His successor, Neville Gleave (1973–1992), continued to practice this method and, having trained with both surgeons, I have used the same technique selectively in my practice at the South Manchester University Hospital (SMUH) (1976–1998). In previous publications (Gleave *et al.* 1979; Hancock 1987), we have called our method *local dissection*, but have latterly referred to it as *extracapsular dissection* (McGurk *et al.* 1996)—the terms should be considered as synonymous. The surgical techniques have been described in detail in Chapter 5, and in previous publications (Gleave 1979, 1995). I emphasize here that the decision to perform an extracapsular dissection is made after raising a standard preauricular flap, and is determined principally by mobility. If there is uncertainty about mobility or the lump is felt to extend deep to the main trunk of the facial nerve, the nerve is identified early and after dissecting the appropriate branches a partial superficial parotidectomy is completed (Chapter 5). In many of these cases, the capsule of the tumour was exposed because of close contact with branches of the nerve, so great care was taken to avoid rupture at this point.

The Manchester experience

The overview and demographics of the Christie series (1948–1992) have been described elsewhere (Renehan *et al.* 1996), and summarized in Chapter 1. To this, I add my personal series of patients with parotid tumours, which included 134 which were new pleomorphic adenomas (Hancock 1999). This experience is noteworthy on four counts: (i) large patient numbers; (ii) three surgeons operating with a uniform philosophy; (iii) careful prospective documentation; and (iv) long follow-up. The experience is also notable as pre-operative evaluation was clinically based (Chapter 4), and fine needle aspiration cytology was not used. The use of CT scan imaging was selective and limited to the last 10 years of the series.

The data and outcome for patients with new pleomorphic adenomas are presented in Table 6.4. The similarities between the Christie and SMUH series are striking. For the purpose of analysis, deep lobe tumours are excluded as they always required a nerve dissection and removal by a predominantly extracapsular dissection. In the Christie

Table 6.4 Comparison of results for formal parotidectomy versus extracapsular dissection in the Christie and South Manchester University Hospitals series

	Study period	FU duration (years) median (range)	No. of patients	Recurrence rates	Facial nerve injury		Frey's syndrome	Amputation neuroma
					Permanent	Transient		
Formal parotidectomy								
Christie*	1948–1992	12 (1–32)	95	2 (1.8)	1 (1)	30 (32)	36 (38)	18 (19)
SMUH†	1976–1998	8.5 (1–23)	61	0	0	20 (33)	15 (25)	–
Extracapsular dissection								
Christie			380	6 (1.6)	7 (2)	41 (11)	18 (5)	12 (3)
SMUH			56	0	0	2 (4)	0	–

* Christie series: overall new pleomorphic adenomas 551; analysis excluded 19 deep lobe tumours and 57 who received radiotherapy.

† SMUH (South Manchester University Hospital) series: overall new pleomorphioc adenoma 134; analysis excluded 17 deep lobe tumours, no patient had post-operative radiotherapy.

FU = Follow up

series, 57 patients who received radiotherapy were also excluded (36 patients with radium implants which were used routinely in the 1950s, and 21 who received post-operative radiotherapy for tumour spillage rupture. Post-operative radiotherapy was not used in the SMUH patients as no significant ruptures occurred.

In the Christie series, 80% of superficial tumours were removed by an elective extra capsular dissection compared with 45% in the SMUH series. With long-term follow-up in both series, the recurrence rate was similar for both surgical approaches (<2%). The patterns of morbidity were similar in both series, with three main messages: (i) permanent nerve injury is low (<2%) for both formal parotidectomy and extracapsular dissection; (ii) transient nerve injury occurs in approximately a third of patients following formal parotidectomy, but in only (approximately) 10% of patients undergoing extracapsular dissection; and (iii) Frey's syndrome occurs in approximately a third of patients following formal parotidectomy but in less than 5% of those undergoing extracapsular dissection.

Practical implications

Extracapsular dissection has been shown to be safe in the hands of three Manchester surgeons. Numbers are large and follow-up is long and complete. It is most important that this operation is not associated with the discredited operation termed *enucleation* which is the rapid shelling out of the lump through a limited incision and is associated with a high risk of tumour rupture. Enucleation has been used by other authors to refer to any form of local removal, but this term should be relegated to history. It must be clearly understood that the method currently described is a painstaking meticulous dissection every bit as demanding as a nerve dissection aiming for absolutely no tumour rupture (Fig. 6.2).

Accepting that extracapsular dissection can be done with minimal long-term recurrence, what are the implications for parotid surgery? First, it shows us that the microscopic projections of tumour into and through the capsule are of no practical significance to the surgeon. Secondly, it supports the concept that macroscopic rupture of the tumour is the main cause of recurrence and is therefore avoidable. This message is relevant whether performing an extracapsular dissection or a nerve dissection.

These results from Manchester show clearly that the outcome of surgery for pleomorphic adenoma is surgeon dependent and raise doubt as to the clinical relevance of the tumour bud concept.

REFERENCES

Aljamo, E., Polli, G., and De Meester, W. (1989) Total parotidectomy—a routine treatment for parotid gland swellings? *J Laryngol Otol*, **103**, 181–6.

Anderson, R. (1975) Benign mixed tumours of the parotid gland. In: *Cancer of the Head and Neck*. Pp. 1555–8. (eds. R.G. Chamvers, A.M.P. Janssen de Limpens, D.A. Jacques, and R.T. Routledge) Proceedings of an International Symposium 37, Encerpta Medica, Amsterdam.

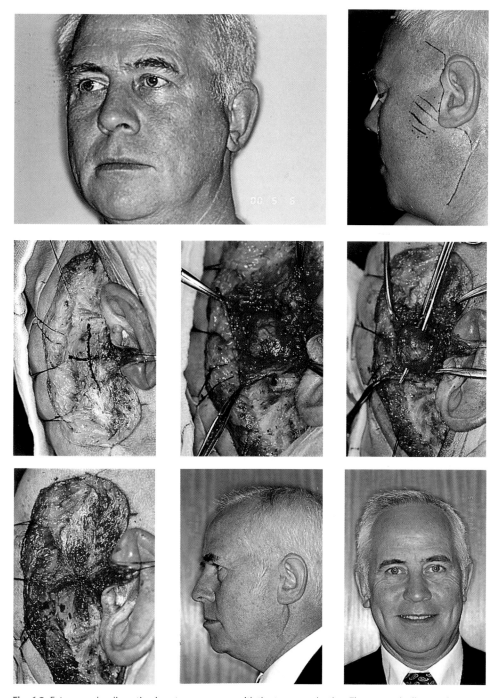

Fig. 6.2 Extracapsular dissection is not synonymous with the term enucleation. The tumour is dissected carefully in an extracapsular plain, rolling the tumour from side to side as it is dissected free from the bed of the parotid. The parotid capsule closes easily after the tumour is removed, leaving a normal contour and reducing the risk of Frey's syndrome.

Armistead, P.R., Smiddy, F.G., and Frank, H.G. (1979) Simple enucleation and radiotherapy in the treatment of the pleomorphic salivary adenoma of the parotid gland. *Br J Surg*, **66**, 716–7.

Bearhs, O.H. and Adsom, M.A. (1958) The surgical anatomy and technique of parotidectomy. *Am J Surg*, **95**, 885–96.

Benedict, E.G. and Meigs, J.V. (1930) Tumours of the parotid gland. A study of 225 cases with complete end results in 80 cases. *Surg Gynaecol Obsts*, **51**, 626–47.

Chan, S. and Gunn, A. (1981) Conservative parotidectomy by the peripheral approach. *Br J Surg*, **68**, 405–7.

Dallera, P., Marchetti, C., and Campobassi, A. (1993) Local capsular dissection of parotid pleomorphic adenomas. *Int J Oral Maxillofac Surg*, **22**, 154–7.

Donovan, D.T. and Conley, J.J. (1984) Capsular significance in parotid tumor surgery: reality and myths of lateral lobectomy. *Laryngoscope*, **94**, 324–9.

Gleave, E.N. (1979) Tumours of the parotid gland in operative surgery. pp. 848–54 (eds, C. Rob and R. Smith) 3rd edition. Butterworth, London.

Gleave, E.N. (1995) An alternative to superficial parotidectomy: extra-capsular dissection. In: *Color Atlas and Text of the Salivary Glands. Diseases, Disorders and Surgery*. pp. 165–72. (eds, J. de Burgh Norman and M. McGurk) Mosby-Wolfe, London.

Gleave, E.N., Whittaker, J.S., and Nicholson, A. (1979) Salivary tumours—experience over thirty years. *Clin Otolaryngol*, **4**, 247–57.

Hancock, B.D. (1987) Pleomorphic adenomas of the parotid: removal without rupture. *Ann R Coll Surg Engl*, **69**, 293–5.

Hancock, B.D. (1999) Clinically benign parotid tumours: local dissection as an alternative to superficial parotidectomy in selected cases. *Ann R Coll Surg Engl*, **81**, 299–301.

Haw, C.S. (1975) Pleomorphic adenoma of the parotid gland. A review of results of treatment. *J R Coll Surg Edinb*, **20**, 25–9.

Laccourreye, H., Laccourreye, O., Cauchois, R., Jouffre, V., Menard, M., and Brasnu, D. (1994) Total conservative parotidectomy for primary benign pleomorphic adenoma of the parotid gland: a 25-year experience with 229 patients. *Laryngoscope*, **104**, 1487–94.

Lam, K.H., Wei, W.I., Ho, H.C., and Ho, C.M. (1990) Whole organ sectioning of mixed parotid tumors. *Am J Surg*, **160**, 377–81.

Langdon, J.D. (1984) Complications of parotid gland surgery. *J Maxillofac Surg*, **12**, 225–9.

Langdon, J.D. (1998) Submandibular gland surgery. In: *Operative Maxillofacial Surgery*. (eds J.D. Langdon and M.F. Patel) Chapman and Hall, London.

Lanier, V.C., Jr., McSwain, B., and Rosenfeld, L. (1972) Mixed tumors of salivary glands: a 44 year study. *South Med J*, **65**, 1485–8.

Leverstein, H., van der Wal, J.E., Tiwari, R.M., van der Waal, I., and Snow, G.B. (1997) Surgical management of 246 previously untreated pleomorphic adenomas of the parotid gland. *Br J Surg*, **84**, 399–403.

Maimaris, C.V. and Ball, M.J. (1986) Treatment of parotid gland tumours by conservative parotidectomy. *Br J Surg*, **73**, 897.

Martin, H. (1952) The operative removal of tumours of the parotid salivary gland. *Surg*, **31**, 670–82.

Martis, C. (1983) Parotid benign tumors: comments on surgical treatment of 263 cases. *Int J Oral Surg*, **12**, 211–20.

Maynard, J.D. (1988) Management of pleomorphic adenoma of the parotid. *Br J Surg*, **75**, 305–8.

McEvedy, M.V. and Ross, W.M. (1976) The treatment of mixed parotid tumours by enucleation and radiotherapy. *Br J Surg*, **63**, 341–2.

McFarland, J. (1936) Three hundred tumours of the salivary glands of which 69 recurred. *Surg Gynaecol Obstet*, **63**, 457–68.

McGurk, M. (1997) Parotid pleomorphic adenoma. *Br J Surg*, **84**, 1491–2.

McGurk, M., Renehan, A., Gleave, E.N., and Hancock, B.D. (1996) Clinical significance of the tumour capsule in the treatment of parotid pleomorphic adenomas. *Br J Surg*, **83**, 1747–9.

Moody, A.B., Avery, C.M., Taylor, J., and Langdon, J.D. (1999) A comparison of one hundred and fifty consecutive parotidectomies for tumours and inflammatory disease. *Int J Oral Maxillofac Surg*, **28**, 211–5.

Natvig, K. and Soberg, R. (1994) Relationship of intraoperative rupture of pleomorphic adenomas to recurrence: an 11–25 year follow-up study. *Head Neck*, **16**, 213–7.

Patey, D.H. (1940) The treatment of mixed tumours of the parotid gland. *Br J Surg*, **28**, 29–38.

Patey, D.H. and Thackray, A.C. (1958) The treatment of parotid tumours in the light of a pathological study of parotidectomy material. *Br J Surg*, **55**, 477–87.

Prichard, A.J., Barton, R.P., and Narula, A.A. (1992) Complications of superficial parotidectomy versus extracapsular lumpectomy in the treatment of benign parotid lesions. *J R Coll Surg Edinb*, **37**, 155–8.

Rawson, A.J., Howard, J.M., Royster, H.P., and Horn, R.C. (1950) Tumours of the salivary glands. A clinicopathological study of 160 cases. *Cancer*, **3**, 445–58.

Redon, H. (1953) Discussion of the surgical treatment of parotid tumours. *Proc R Soc Med*, **46**, 1013–20.

Renehan, A., Gleave, E.N., Hancock, B.D., Smith, P., and McGurk, M. (1996) Long-term follow-up of over 1000 patients with salivary gland tumours treated in a single centre. *Br J Surg*, **83**, 1750–4.

Richardson, G.S., Dickason, W.L., Gaisford, J.C., and Hanna, D.C. (1975) Tumors of salivary glands. An analysis of 752 cases. *Plast Reconstr Surg*, **55**, 131–8.

Sood, S., Quraishi, M.S., and Bradley, P.J. (1998) Frey's syndrome and parotid surgery. *Clin Otolaryngol*, **23**, 291–301.

Stea, G. (1975) Conservative surgical treatment of mixed tumours of the parotid gland. *J Maxillofac Surg*, **3**, 135–7.

Stein, I. and Geschickter, C.F. (1934) Tumours of the parotid gland. *Arch Surg*, **28**, 482–526.

Stevens, K.L. and Hobsley, M. (1982) The treatment of pleomorphic adenomas by formal parotidectomy. *Br J Surg*, **69**, 1–3.

Touquet, R., Mackenzie, I.J., and Carruth, J.A. (1990) Management of the parotid pleomorphic adenoma, the problem of exposing tumour tissue at operation. The logical pursuit of treatment policies. *Br J Oral Maxillofac Surg*, **28**, 404–8.

Van Miert, P.J., Dawes, J.D., and Harkness, D.G. (1968) The treatment of mixed parotid tumours. A report of 183 cases. *J Laryngol Otol*, **82**, 459–68.

Wennmo, C., Spandow, O., Emgard, P., and Krouthen, B. (1988) Pleomorphic adenomas of the parotid gland: superficial parotidectomy or limited excision? *J Laryngol Otol*, **102**, 603–5.

Wood, F.C. (1904) Mixed tumours of the salivary glands. *Ann Surg*, **39**, 57.

Woods, J.E., Chong, G.C., and Beahrs, O.H. (1975) Experience with 1,360 primary parotid tumors. *Am J Surg*, **130**, 460–2.

Woods, J.E., Weiland, L.H., Chong, G.C., and Irons, G.B. (1977) Pathology and surgery of primary tumors of the parotid. *Surg Clin North Am*, **57**, 565–73.

Yamashita, T., Tomoda, K., and Kumazawa, T. (1993) The usefulness of partial parotidectomy for benign parotid gland tumors. A retrospective study of 306 cases. *Acta Otolaryngol Suppl*, **500**, 113–6.

Audience discussion

Professor Snow (Amsterdam, The Netherlands): In partial parotidectomy, you leave a large area of functioning parotid tissue, has this resulted in an increased incidences of sialocoeles?

Mr Hancock: When people started to do   .rtial superficial parotidectomy, this was cited as the main risk. But it does not happen, there is no increased incidence of sialocoeles or fistulae.

Mr Shaheen (London, UK): I support these comments, I think I have had two in 35–40 years but they always stopped in the end.

Mr Webb (Bristol, UK): If you look at the histopathology of these lesions as I have done recently in 130 tumours, the so-called space around them which Mr Hancock says he can find is very minimal in most of the cases. If you use special stains, there is mucus together with pleomorphic cells right up to the edge I doubt if the average person has a patron saint like Mr Hancock.

Dr Morgan (London, UK): Can I continue on the histopathology of the capsule. If you cut into an unfixed specimen there is a very quick retraction of what little capsule exists, leaving naked surface of tumour. In a fixed specimen, the dehydration processing with alcohol presses down the delicate collagen capsule on to the tumour. What intrigues me is how pathologists can distinguish between proximity to the excision margin, penetration of the capsule, and direct contact with the excision margin.

Mr Webb: If you do not use fine needle aspiration (FNAC), do you use frozen section and how often is a second operation required because of unsuspected cancer?

Professor Snow: We use FNAC in every case but I lack confidence in the test. There are cases of a completely clinically benign tumour which is reported as an adenoid cystic carcinoma. You take that into account when you do the operation but even then it does not change my operation very much. May I elaborate. The subdigastric area is always palpated, particularly in suspicious cases, which leads me on to your second question. I never use frozen section on the primary tumour but I do use it on the subdigastric nodes. Once or twice a year I encounter a patient where there is very little suspicion of malignancy yet the subdigastric node contains metastasis. You also asked whether a partial parotidectomy was appropriate with this senario in mind. I recommend it as standard surgery because it is no different from a formal total superficial parotidectomy except you are restricting the surgery to the lower portion of the gland. You identify the main trunk but just follow the division and the branches that have a close relationship to the tumour. There is nothing magic about it.

But I agree entirely with Mr Hancock that the care with which the surgery is undertaken is all-important. It really does not matter on the choice of the procedure but how it is done. Carefulness, that is very important.

Mr Thomas (London, UK): I suspect that most people now perform a partial superficial parotidectomy although they may describe it as a superficial parotidectomy. It is not uncommon when operating on recurrent pleomorphic adenomas to find rather a healthy portion of superficial lobe left after an apparently superficial parotidectomy.

With regards to recurrent tumours, every time a patient is referred to me with a recurrent pleomorphic adenoma the first question I ask them is did you have weakness of the face, in other words neuropraxia, after the first operation. If the answer is that they had perfect facial function after the first operation then almost certainly the operation for the recurrent pleomorphic adenoma will be easy because the surgeon almost certainly has not dissected the facial nerve fully. Whereas if they had a severe neuropraxia after the first operation those are the patients I think that one can expect to see multifocal recurrent tumour sitting on the stem and divisions of the facial nerve.

Mr Carter (London, UK): I would like to ask from the panel if they use facial nerve monitors or stimulators, when they do parotidectomies? Should we use them with the medical climate as it is?

Mr Hancock: I use neither.

Professor Snow: I do not use it routinely but in some very difficult cases of recurrent tumour. In our country (The Netherlands) it is not required for medico-legal purposes but it may arise in the future.

Mr Carter: Do you use magnifying glasses or microscope?

Mr Hancock: I use spectacles as I get older, but no I do not use magnification, just good illumination with a headlight.

Professor Natvig (Oslo, Norway): Mr Hancock, in your series of extracapsular dissection for the cases of pleomorphic adenoma, were there any cases that turned out to be malignant and what happened to those patients?

Mr Hancock: I am very pleased you asked that question because it does worry people a lot and it worries me. Yes, I have. I have had three cases now that were reported as malignant tumours but they looked exactly like a pleomorphic adenoma when I removed them. One was a low-grade mucoepidermoid carcinoma, and the patient is well without disease at 9 years post-operatively. The other two were reported as adenoid cystic carcinomas and this was confirmed by a second pathology opinion. I went back and did a superficial parotidectomy to cover my operative field. There was no residual tumour found in the specimen and they are 5 years post-surgery without evidence of disease. So the answer is yes, I have encountered low-grade malignant tumours but I think if they look like a benign tumour when you are operating they will be cured. I think the editors have further data on this and will discuss it later (Chapter 14).

Professor O'Brien (Sydney, Australia): Do you treat palatal tumour without a previous biopsy? If you knew it was an adenoid cystic carcinoma, would it alter your treatment?

Professor Langdon (London, UK): We always do an incisional biopsy on palatal tumours pre-operatively. There is no evidence that supraradical surgery for adenoid cystic carcinomas makes any difference to long-term outcome. So I would do a partial maxillectomy based on the dimensions and locations of the particular tumour and I would always have pre-op imaging, preferably MRI, and all patients would have post-operative radiotherapy going up to the base of skull. I disagree with Brian Hancock in that I would have used adjuvant radiotherapy.

Mr Shaheen: How serious do you regard the problem of spillage when operating on pleomorphic adenomas; what do you do about it?

Professor Snow: First of all it is extremely important to prevent spillage. The high risk case is a large tumour wedged between the mandible and the mastoid. Do not try to identify the main trunk but undertake a retrograde dissection from peripheral branches. If spillage occurs, you should try to contain it immediately; the tear is over-sewed and the area irrigated. I always irrigate the wound after every parotidectomy; I think this is important.

Mr Hancock: There are varying degrees of capsular rupture. In my series, I have had two splits. I do not think macroscopically any tumour escaped but there was technically a breach of the capsule. So there is a whole range of rupture from tiny splits in the capsule to major ruptures and they represent different risks for recurrence. Major ruptures are the cause of the multifocal recurrences.

Professor Langdon: We have had three ruptures of parotid pleomorphic adenomas and one in the submandibular gland. They have all had post-operative radiotherapy regardless of age and there have been no recurrences over a 16 years follow-up.

Mr Renehan (Manchester, UK): If I could add a final comment with regards to Frey's syndrome. We have heard that the incidence of this complication is heavily dependent on the vigour with which it is pursued. The factor of time is often forgotten. When we looked at the Manchester Christie series, in the hands of two consecutive parotid surgeons reviewing their patients with long-term follow-up, the incidence of post-operative Frey's syndrome was determined not only by extent of surgery but also length of follow-up (Fig. 6.3).

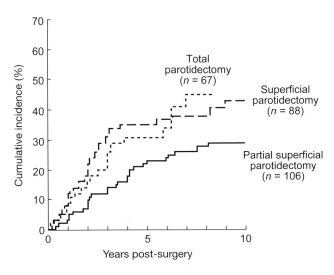

Fig. 6.3 Cumulative incidence (using Kaplan-Meier life-table estimates) of post-operative Frey's syndrome after different levels of parotidectomy in 261 patients at the Christie Hospital, Manchester (1956–1992, surgeons: Mr WAB Nicholson, Mr EN Gleave). Various histologies including: pleomorphic adenoma, 105: Warthin's, 43: chronic sialadenitis, 46. Frey's syndrome was defined on clinical criteria. Median follow-up was 8.5 (range 1–30) years.

Editorial comment

Pleomorphic adenoma has a long-held reputation for recurrence and this has clouded our intellectual perspective towards the emerging scientific facts. Based on the work of Patey and Thakery, the superficial parotidectomy became the procedure of choice for pleomorphic adenoma. However, the logical basis of this operation is open to sceptical scrutiny because in 60% of cases the dissection is in close proximity to the capsule (the bare area) which in theory carries a risk of recurrent disease. Such recurrences have not occurred, so a number of surgeons are adopting a more conservative surgical approach to parotid pleomorphic adenoma.

What is the limit of conservatism in this context? We think that this question has been settled decisively by Mr Hancock's data, i.e the limit of safe surgery is extra-capsular dissection. This procedure contravenes present accepted precepts and the results are understandably difficult to accept, and there is concern that extra-capsular dissection is an excessively demanding technique. Moreover, the results presented by the Manchester surgeons create an intellectual problem, as they defy the conventional wisdom, vigorously supported by pathologists, that pleomorphic adenomas have tumour buds and are incompletely enclosed by tumour capsule, and thus explains the tumour's reputation for recurrence. It is interesting to hear in the discussion from Dr Morgan (Oral Pathologist) that the microscopic appearance of tumour buds may in fact be an artefact of fixation. With over 350 cases treated by extracapsular dissection and with long-term follow-up, the Christie results are a confirmed fact. The clinical and pathological findings appear to be contradictory.

CHAPTER 7

The treatment of spillage and residual pleomorphic adenoma

The argument for post-operative radiotherapy
Nicholas Slevin

Pursuing a conservative policy
Ketil Natvig

The argument for post-operative radiotherapy
Nicholas Slevin

The propensity for pleomorphic adenoma to recur is well recognized and has already been highlighted (Chapter 6). Recurrence rates from contemporary series are typically quoted at less than 2% following parotid surgery. These figures are selective, being generally from large centres with corresponding surgical expertise, sometimes with exclusion of those patients referred for post-operative radiotherapy, and in others there is limited follow-up. In practice, with multioperators, rates may be as high as 4–8%. Professor Langdon has already demonstrated that tumour rupture and/or spillage occurs in approximately 5% of cases, and these patients are at increased risk of recurrence (Chapter 6). The optimum method of treatment in these circumstances remains unclear.

The clinical dilemma is whether it is better to wait for recurrent tumour to appear before attempting treatment, or use prophylactic radiotherapy to reduce the risk of recurrent disease. The whole debate revolves around the issue of morbidity. A second parotid operation, especially when a comprehensive nerve dissection was undertaken at the primary procedure, presents a significant risk to the facial nerve, a point highlighted in Chapter 8.

The Manchester experience

The role of post-operative radiotherapy was evaluated in a retrospective study of 187 patients with residual pleomorphic adenoma treated with radiotherapy between 1951 and 1984 (Barton *et al.* 1992). In that series, 115 of 187 cases (61%) were given radiotherapy immediately after their first operation because either tumour was spilled at operation or the surgeon was suspicious that residual tumour remained in the tumour bed (group I). A second group of 72 cases (39%) were referred for radiotherapy after one or more excisions for tumour recurrence (group II). Radiotherapy

> ## Box 7.1 Techniques of radiotherapy
>
> ◆ Needle implant (radium or caesium) as a single plane or V-plane with the posterior needles deep to the ascending ramus of the mandible. The intended dose was 60 Gy at 0.5 cm in 7 days. The last implant was done in 1976.
>
> ◆ External beam megavoltage photon radiotherapy using a beam-directed lateralized two- or three-field technique with an inclined plane to avoid the eyes. The dose was 50 Gy in 15–16 daily fractions over 20 days.

was given by one of the two techniques shown in Box 7.1. Median follow-up was 14 years in this study.

The results are highlighted in Table 7.1. In the 115 cases given immediate post-operative radiotherapy after initial surgery, there was only one local recurrence (0.9%). This case of local recurrence had initial surgery (local excision only) at a peripheral hospital and then treatment by a V-plane radioactive needle implant, and after further surgery the patient was clinically disease-free 27 years following his initial treatment. Within this group was a smaller subgroup of 41 patients with new pleomorphic adenoma whose primary surgery had been performed at the Christie Hospital and referred for immediate post-operative radiotherapy because of perceived risk of recurrence. There were no recurrent tumours in this subgroup of patients.

Of the 72 cases given radiotherapy for recurrent disease, nine patients (12.5%) had a subsequent recurrence of their pleomorphic adenoma. These recurrences had no relationship to either the previous number of recurrences or to radiotherapy modality.

Clinical implications

In experienced hands, the rate of recurrence following surgery for pleomorphic adenoma is low and, therefore, the role of radiotherapy in primary tumours is small.

Table 7.1 Results of two treatment approaches to cases at risk of recurrent tumour. Group I – immediate (prophylactic) radiotherapy; Group II – wait for current disease and treat by surgery and adjuvant radiotherapy

	Description	No. of patients	Recurrence rates
Group I	Immediate radiotherapy	115*	1 (0.9)
Group II	Delayed radiotherapy	72†	9 (13)

Values in parentheses are percentages.

* Forty-one had initial surgery at the Christie, 74 were referred from a large number of District General Hospitals (~20) throughout the North West of England; many of these 74 cases had local excision only.

† Of the recurrent cases, 44 had further surgery at the Christie Hospital, 28 were surgically managed at peripheral hospitals. The number of episodes of recurrences encountered by the 72 patients before radiotherapy were as follows: one recurrence in 41 patients (57%), two recurrences in 20 (28%), three recurrences in six (8%), and four recurrences in five patients (7%). The time to first recurrence was from 0 to 5 years in 24 patients, 5 to 10 years in 29 patients, 10 to 20 years in 16 patients and more than 20 years in three patients.

However, the experience at the Christie Hospital suggests that for patients who are suspected of having inadequate clearance of tumour or spillage at surgery, post-operative radiotherapy reduces the recurrence rate to almost zero.

This decision must be weighed against potential complications of radiotherapy which can be a problem in this area, and include persistent xerostomia, ear problems, and occasional bone necrosis (see below). There is no simple rule or formula that can resolve the issue. Patient, tumour, and treatment factors all have to be taken into consideration when making a decision for or against prophylactic radiotherapy. A history of a slow growing tumour over many years, young age, potential for salvage surgery without sacrifice of the facial nerve, and a capsule tear/spillage (as opposed to macroscopic evidence of residual tumour) residuum are factors that favour the adoption of a wait and see approach. This is one situation where experience is of inestimable value and underlines the importance of centralization of head and neck tumour management and the need for multidisciplinary discussion.

Potential long-term radiotherapy-related complications

The list of potential complications is shown in Box 7.2.

Skin stigmata

Unlike oral cancer, the patients with salivary tumours are relatively young and often female. Consequently, there is obviously a concern about skin stigmata but, with the use of moderate doses (~85% of the definitive dose for squamous carcinoma) and avoiding excessive skin bolus, unsightly skin changes are uncommon. However, this does not apply to multinodular recurrence. In this situation, a skin bolus should be

---

Box 7.2 Potential long-term radiotherapy-related sequelae

Skin stigmata and telangectasia

Xerostomia and dental problems

◆ Dental caries

◆ Periodontitis

Osteoradionecrosis

Neural dysfunction

Ear problems

◆ Sensorineural damage

◆ Otitis externa

Risk of malignant change

considered to ensure that the subcutaneous tissue over the whole parotid bed is within the high-dose volume of radiation.

Xerostomia

Xerostomia and consequent dental problems (caries and periodontitis) can be limited by minimizing the dose of radiation to the contralateral parotid gland. This can be achieved either by mixing electrons with photons or by using a lateral oblique pair of fields which exit on either side of the contralateral parotid.

Osteoradionecrosis

We previously reported two cases (one major and one minor) of osteoradionecrosis in a series of 52 patients receiving radiotherapy using older techniques. With modern computer planning techniques which help ensure dose homogeneity, osteoradionecrosis of the mandible is almost never seen.

Neural dysfunction

Facial nerve palsy does not occur with radiotherapy of salivary tumours. Occasionally patients experience an unpleasant hypersensitivity within the treatment field which can be difficult to ameliorate.

Ear problems

Complications of radiotherapy relate to both dose fractionation and treatment technique. This is illustrated in the case of sensorineural damage from radiotherapy to the inner ear. A study of 28 patients treated at the Christie Hospital showed that 15 had significant audiometric hearing deficit on the irradiated side and that this was predominantly *sensorineural* in type (Singh and Slevin 1991). The likely explanation is the high biological effective dose and large daily fraction size of 3.3 Gy when a regimen of 50 Gy in 3 weeks is utilized. A similar study using the conventional 2 Gy per day fractionation up to 60 Gy revealed no evidence of significant hearing loss (Evans *et al.* 1988). Consequently, the Christie schedule has been modified over the last 10 years to 45–47.5 Gy in 20 fractions over 4 weeks, which brings us into line with other UK centres which do not use conventional fractionation (50–60 Gy, 2 Gy daily) Clinical problems with the ear are now restricted to *otitis externa* in some patients (with wax plugging), but audiovestibular problems are not reported.

Malignant change

There are two concerns here. First is the case of a second tumour arising in a radiation field. Since the commencement of the prospective collection of data on salivary tumours at the Christie Hospital in 1948, there have been only two well-documented cases of this event. One case was a squamous carcinoma related to radioactive implant treatment 35 years previously, the other a fibrosarcoma also following a radium implant with a latent period of 15 years. Secondly is the concern of malignant transformation within recurrent pleomorphic adenomas, and the possibly stimulatory effects of radiotherapy. This has perhaps been overestimated in some series (Gnepp 1993). A review of 311 pleomorphic adenoma patients treated with radiotherapy found only four malignancies (1–2%) within the treatment field 14–20 years after treatment (Watkin and Hobsley 1986). In the Christie series of 187 patients with recurrent pleomorphic adenomas of the parotid, there were four malignancies; all transformations occurred after at least four recurrences, and all had received radiotherapy (Renehan *et al.* 1996). These data suggest that the risks of malignant changes are very small.

Pursuing a conservative policy   Ketil Natvig

Rather than apply different treatment strategies to minimize the risk of recurrent disease, an alternative approach or question is simply to quantify the actual risk that accompanies tumour rupture to see if remedial treatment is in fact necessary. Not surprisingly, this question is addressed infrequently as surgeons are reluctant to publish results following 'surgical errors' in their treatment.

The present author was impressed by the apparent low incidence of recurrent disease in his department (Department of Otolaryngology, Oslo) after rupture of the tumour capsule during surgery, and this was the stimulus to undertaking the study described in detail in this chapter (Natvig and Soberg 1994). A second Scandinavian study (Henriksson *et al.* 1998) was published shortly after ours with similar findings, and this is also discussed.

The Oslo experience

Medical records of 346 patients who were operated on between 1965 and 1981 at the Department of Otolaryngology, National Hospital, Norway, were reviewed. All patients had a histologically verified pleomorphic adenoma of the parotid gland, and all the pathology notes were studied in detail. After excluding recurrent cases, adequate information and follow-up were available in 238 patients with primary tumours.

Patients with malignant degeneration of their adenoma or with parapharyngeal tumours are not included in this material. The patients were operated on by many different surgeons, either experienced staff surgeons or residents in training. The specimens were examined as a matter of routine by different staff members from the Department of Pathology. No histological reassessment has been performed. The mean observation time was 18 (range 11–25) years. None of our patients received postoperative irradiation.

Operation notes were assessed carefully with particular reference to tumour spillage and the tumour being visible during removal. There were three categories: rupture of the capsule ($n = 26$ or 11%); the capsule being visible ($n = 87$ or 36%); and the capsule not being visible ($n = 121$ or 51%). In four cases, the relationship was not known.

Six (2.5%) patients had a recurrence, 7–18 years following initial surgery (mean 11.8 years). Of the 26 patients with macroscopic spillage of tumour cells, only two (8%) developed recurrent tumours (Table 7.2). Of the 87 patients in whom surgical dissection was close to the capsule, there was only one recurrence (1.1%). In the

Table 7.2 Recurrences compared with macroscopic relationship of capsule and visualization of tumour—Oslo series

Category	No. of patients	Recurrence rates
Rupture of capsule	26	2 (8)
Capsule visible	87	1 (1.0)
Capsule not visible	121	3 (2.5)

Information was incomplete in four cases.

Values in parentheses are percentages.

Table 7.3 Recurrences compared with microscopic surgical resection margins—Oslo series

Category	No. of patients	Recurrence rates
Positive and/or close margins	87	2 (2.0)
Tumour cells growing through capsule	48	1 (2.0)
Negative margins	100	2 (2.0)
Surgical margins not described	3	1

Values in parentheses are percentages.

remaining patients, there were three (2.5%) patients who developed recurrences despite the consideration that the surgical procedure was oncologically sound in that the capsule was not exposed or seen.

The study also examined the rate of recurrence according to the microscopic status of the surgical margins. There was a positive margin in 24 cases (10%), tumour cells growing through the capsule in 48 (20%), and negative margins in the remainder (70%). Despite these histological differences, the recurrence rates were similar in all three groups (Table 7.3).

The Swedish study

The Swedish study comprised 255 patients operated on for pleomorphic adenomas from all three major anatomic salivary sites. A total of 213 patients (parotid, 197; submandibular and minor glands, 16) had long-term follow-up (median 8.3 years) and were the focus for the analysis.

There were a number of similarities to the Oslo study: (i) the review involved multiple surgeons; (ii) there was long-term follow-up; and (iii) 28 patients (12%) were noted to have macroscopic capsular rupture (all in the parotid gland). The results were also similar. In the capsular rupture group, the recurrence rate was 7% (2/28). For the remaining 'uncomplicated tumours', the recurrence rate was 4% (7/185). The authors observed that in five out of the nine primary tumours which subsequently recurred, pseudopodia extended through the pseudocapsule, but the statistics were inadequate to distinguish whether this finding alone was predictive of recurrence above that for those without pseudopodia.

Remarks

Despite a number of methodological impurities in these two retrospective analyses, nonetheless, there are a number of pertinent and common observations. First, both studies were multioperator series with overall recurrence rates of 3–5%. These rates are higher than those of many contemporary series (Chapter 6), and may be representative of surgical practice across a general population (i.e. includes both specialized and non-specialized practice). Secondly, the Oslo series corresponds to the observations of others (Donovan and Conley 1984; McGurk *et al.* 1996) that the tumour capsule is visible in approximately 60% of parotid pleomorphic adenomas during formal parotidectomy, but without inevitable recurrence. Thirdly, both studies have shown that capsular rupture and/or spillage may occur in up to 12% of cases but that overall recurrence rates are less than half this figure. Recurrence following tumour rupture is therefore not an inevitability. Fourthly, both studies show that even where the capsule is not visible (i.e. an uncomplicated surgical procedure), there is still a recognized (albeit small) rate of recidivism.

Taken together, these two studies raise questions about the traditional ways in which we explain the development of recurrence following surgery for pleomorphic adenomas (the tumour bud concept and tumour rupture). The theory of multicentricity proposed by the French surgeon Redon (1953) over four decades ago has been dismissed by many authorities (Eneroth 1965). The finding of 2% muliticentricity in an Italian series (Alajmo *et al.* 1989) of 239 parotid pleomorphic adenomas stands alone as a unique observation which has not been replicated by others.

In conclusion, the importance of tumour rupture with or without spillage has been re-appraised. In terms of clinical practice, none of the patients in these series received post-operative radiotherapy. Nevertheless, the recurrence rates among patients with tumour rupture were modest and, as a consequence, I question the justification for and benefit of the automatic use of post-operative radiotherapy in patients with spilled benign disease.

REFERENCES

Alajmo, E., Polli, G., and De Meester, W. (1989) Total parotidectomy—a routine treatment for parotid gland swellings? *J Laryngol Otol*, **103**, 181–6.

Barton, J., Slevin, N.J., and Gleave, E.N. (1992) Radiotherapy for pleomorphic adenoma of the parotid gland. *Int J Radiat Oncol Biol Phys*, **22**, 925–8.

Donovan, D.T. and Conley, J.J. (1984) Capsular significance in parotid tumor surgery: reality and myths of lateral lobectomy. *Laryngoscope*, **94**, 324–9.

Eneroth, C.M. (1965) Mixed tumors of major salivary glands: prognostic role of capsular structure. *Ann Otol Rhinol Laryngol*, **74**, 944–53.

Evans, R.A., Liu, K.C., Azhar, T., and Symonds, R.P. (1988) Assessment of permanent hearing impairment following radical megavoltage radiotherapy. *J Laryngol Otol*, **102**, 588–9.

Gnepp, D.R. (1993) Malignant mixed tumors of the salivary glands: a review. *Pathol Annu*, **28**, 279–328.

Henriksson, G., Westrin, K.M., Carlsoo, B., and Silfversward, C. (1998) Recurrent primary pleomorphic adenomas of salivary gland origin: intrasurgical rupture, histopathologic features, and pseudopodia. *Cancer*, **82**, 617–20.

McGurk, M., Renehan, A., Gleave, E.N., and Hancock, B.D. (1996) Clinical significance of the tumour capsule in the treatment of parotid pleomorphic adenomas. *Br J Surg*, **83**, 1747–9.

Natvig, K. and Soberg, R. (1994) Relationship of intraoperative rupture of pleomorphic adenomas to recurrence: an 11–25 year follow-up study. *Head Neck*, **16**, 213–7.

Redon, H. (1953) Discussion of the surgical treatment of parotid tumours. *Proc R Soc Med*, **46**, 1013–20

Renehan, A., Gleave, E.N., and McGurk, M. (1996) An analysis of the treatment of 114 patients with recurrent pleomorphic adenomas of the parotid gland. *Am J Surg*, **172**, 710–4.

Singh, I.P. and Slevin, N.J. (1991) Late audiovestibular consequences of radical radiotherapy to the parotid. *Clin Oncol R Coll Radiol*, **3**, 217–9.

Watkin, G.T. and Hobsley, M. (1986) Influence of local surgery and radiotherapy on the natural history of pleomorphic adenomas. *Br J Surg*, **73**, 74–6.

Audience discussion

Professor Spiro (New York, USA): We have data that I will be showing you that supports Dr Natvig's point about the questionable impact of tumour spillage contrary to what logic would dictate.

Mr Hancock (Manchester, UK): If rupture of the capsule is not an important cause of recurrence, what do you believe is the cause of recurrence?

Professor Spiro: We have a paradigm for this same phenomenon with cancer in general. We know that cancer cells can be found in the marrow and peripheral blood in a variety of neoplastic disorders without subsequent growth of tumour.

Mr Danford (London, UK): I would like to ask Dr Slevin what morbidity he is aware of from radiotherapy to the parotid area?

Dr Slevin: When I arrived at the Christie, the dose used for benign and malignant disease was identical. Over the last 10–15 years, we have substantially reduced the dose so that, anecdotally, I believe serious problems are uncommon. But, using the old techniques, patients had skin stigmata, problems with otitis externa, and occasionally audiovestibular problems. A priority in benign disease is to avoid serious morbidity from radiotherapy.

Professor Spiro: Dr Slevin, I am struck by two settings in which the radiation issue comes up. One which is hard to justify namely because of concern about spillage. The second which I believe you alluded to is the treatment of recurrent disease. If the patient develops a second recurrence and is lucky enough to still have some functioning nerves, the pressure is then to avoid the third recurrence when the nerve is almost certain to go. Do you have a comment?

Dr Slevin: We have looked at 72 cases of recurrent disease where radiotherapy was given post-operatively. The overall local control was 88%, that means that 12% recurred despite the radiotherapy. There is no doubt that radiotherapy is less effective for recurrent disease than when given after the first operation.

Professor Spiro: In our experience, the recurrence rate after one operation for resection is at least 30%, which is probably a low estimate.

Professor McGurk (London, UK): The use of adjuvant radiotherapy should have a logical basis. If a tumour is spilled, the recurrence rate is approximately 8%; if adjuvant radiotherapy is used, the recurrence rate is 1%. Would it be logical to consider another relevant factor, i.e. magnitude of the original operation? After a conventional superficial parotidectomy, the risk of permanent damage to the facial nerve at a subsequent operation is about 50%. Now, if this situation pertains in a young person at risk of recurrence would you favour adjuvant radiotherapy? In an older age group (65+) it may not be as important; a recurrent tumour may not need to be treated. This option is not available in a 40-year-old. In which age group would you use adjuvant radiotherapy?

Dr Slevin: If the initial operation has been done by an experienced surgeon and if there is spillage, I think we can adopt a wait and see approach. However, if I am referred a patient who has had an enucleation in an outside hospital and histologically these have a high recurrence rate, do we advise a second operation, wait and see, or give radiotherapy?

Professor McGurk: Could I take the contrary view? As long as the original surgery has been minimal, you have a good chance of going back and doing a total parotidectomy or a superficial parotidectomy with minimal damage to that nerve. So in fact I would reverse your criteria for radiotherapy. If an experienced surgeon has undertaken a full nerve dissection and is worried about possible risk of recurrence, I think serious consideration should be given to adjuvant radiotherapy.

Professor Spiro: It is my perception that capsular disruption and tumour spillage is primarily a retraction problem. I do not think that you regularly rupture the capsule during the course of a nerve dissection but rather an overzealous assistant.

Mr Hancock: I agree. In my own series, I have had two splits in tumours pressed hard against the mastoid process. I was working down a very narrow angle and had to retract the tumour to get to the nerve. Excessive retraction is a danger point.

Editorial comment

The management options for tumour spillage have been discussed in this chapter. There is still a general reluctance to use radiotherapy in the management of benign disease because of the potential long-term sequelae, and the theoretical risk of radiation-induced second neoplasia.

Within the literature, the term 'contamination' is often used without clarification but, where it is defined, it appears that a simple rupture without gross wound contamination seems to have only a moderate rate of recurrence (8%), and so radiotherapy does not need to be used routinely for this type of spillage. On the other hand, the argument is stronger for using post-operative radiation if there has been gross contamination or where the degree of contamination is not known, for example a referred case. Ultimately, each case has to be addressed according to the particular problems, and management tailored to the individual patient.

CHAPTER 8

Treatment of recurrent pleomorphic adenomas

Andrew Renehan

Introduction

Historically, the propensity for salivary pleomorphic adenomas to recur has been well recognized and the possible mechanisms underlying these occurrences have been debated in the last two chapters. With modern surgical techniques, recurrence rates are less that 5% and, in experienced hands, probably less than 2%. Experience in the re-treatment of pleomorphic adenomas is uncommon and limited to all but a few institutes. This chapter is based on the large experience at the Christie Hospital Manchester.

Clinical features

The typical time period from initial treatment to recurrence was 5–10 years. Interestingly, a number of studies point out that the median age of patients with recurrent tumour is on average younger than that of patients at first presentation with new pleomorphic adenomas (Malone and Baker 1984; Maran *et al.* 1984). McGregor *et al.* (1988) implied that tumours occurring in young patients are inherently more aggressive, but this supposition was not supported by analyses correlating age with subsequent recurrences (see below). An alternative explanation provided by Norman (1995) would appear more plausible—a surgeon may be reluctant to undertake a comprehensive approach in a young person with a small lump and prefer a lesser procedure with the inevitable risk of recurrence.

From the clinical viewpoint, two forms of recurrent tumour are recognized; uninodular or solitary, and multinodular. The latter account for 47–67% of cases, depending on referral patterns (Maran *et al.* 1984; Fleming, 1987; Phillips and Olsen 1987). Solitary recurrences are thought to arise from dislocation of a tumour bud as it protrudes through the tumour pseudocapsule; multinodular recurrences, on the other hand, are assumed to occur following rupture of the tumour during primary surgery and consequent seeding of the surgical bed.

Treatment philosophies

The treatment approaches to recurrent pleomorphic adenomas fall into three broad categories (Table 8.1). One is radical excision with sacrifice of the facial nerve and acceptance of a consequent high post-operative morbidity. Others have questioned whether the integrity of the facial nerve should be forfeited in the presence of benign disease, and have advocated dissection and preservation of the nerve. However, nerve-preserving surgery alone in the context of *recurrent* tumour has been associated with a high rate of further recurrence. Consequently, adjuvant radiotherapy has been advocated, and some authors recommend this modality as routine (Dawson 1989).

At the Christie Hospital, adjuvant radiotherapy was used in approximately half the recurrent pleomorphic adenoma cases. To clarify the approach to radiotherapy selection, we undertook a retrospective review of our patients focusing in particular on the outcome of treatment by modality (surgery alone versus surgery with radiation) sub-analysed by type of recurrence (solitary versus multinodular). We have published these results (Renehan *et al.* 1996), and present updated data for this chapter.

Table 8.1 Results of treatment of recurrent parotid pleomorphic adenomas

Treatment groups	No. of patients	Further recurrence (%)	Permanent nerve injury (%)
Aggressive surgical approach			
Hanna *et al.* (1976)	47	23	Not stated
Conley and Clairmont (1979)	42	5	57
Niparko *et al.* (1986)	30	47	29
Routine post-operative RT			
Dawson (1989)	20	10	Not stated
Samson *et al.* (1991)	21	19	5
Jackson *et al.* (1993)	38	Not stated	Not stated
Nerve-preserving surgery with selective use of RT			
Fee *et al.* (1978)	26	35	29
Piorkowski and Guillamondegui (1981)	58	14	Not stated
Maran *et al.* (1984)	19	11	16
Watkin and Hobsley (1984)	65	18	Not stated
O'Dwyer *et al.* (1986)	32	31	26
Fleming (1987)	19	10.5	Not stated
Phillips and Olsen (1995)	126	33	19
Renehan *et al.* (1996)	114	15	15
Liverstein *et. al.* (1997)	40	5	3
Laskawi *et al.* (1998)	94	21	14

RT, radiotherapy.

The beneficial effect of adjuvant radiotherapy in multinodular recurrences

During the period 1952–1992 there were 170 patients with pleomorphic adenomas of the parotid gland referred with recurrences. The analysis focused on 114 patients who had first-time recurrences, defined as a disease-free interval greater than 6 months. All but nine of these patients had their initial operation at another institute. The demographic characteristics of the patients with recurrences compared with data of 551 patients with primary pleomorphic adenomas treated at the Christie over the same period are shown in Table 8.2.

Recurrences were multinodular in 52 patients (46%) and uninodular in 62 patients (54%), the distinction being made at the time of surgery. The type of salvage surgery was determined by the extent and location of recurrent disease. Adjuvant radiotherapy (Chapter 7) was administered in 51 (45%) patients; 32 out of 52 patients with multinodular recurrence and 19 out of 62 with solitary recurrence.

The overall rate of second recurrence was 15% (17/114). This compared with a recurrence rate of 1.6% (9/551) for patients primarily treated at the Christie (Chapter 6). The

Table 8.2 Characteristics of primary referred patients versus patients at first recurrence, Christie Hospital 1952–1992

	Primary treatment	First recurrences
No. of patients	551	114†
Male:female	1:1.6	1:2.1
First treatment		
Median age (range)	47 (5–87)	32 (9–76)*
Second treatment		
Median age (range)	–	45 (13–87)

† Details of previous treatment were available in 77 cases. Local excision or enucleation was reported in 67 (87%) cases. Five patients developed recurrent tumours following superficial parotidectomy or total parotidectomy. An additional five patients had been treated by local excision and radiotherapy prior to referral. The median time from initial surgery to first recurrence was 96 (range 6–383) months.

* The difference in median ages between recurrent and primary groups was significant (Mann–Whitney, two-tailed P <0.0001).

Table 8.3 The effect of surgery on the rate of second recurrence

Type of re-operation	No. of patients	Rate of second recurrence
Extracapsular dissection	33	4 (13)
Superficial parotidectomy	54	8 (15)
Total parotidectomy	21	4 (19)
Parotidectomy with sacrifice of VII*	6	1

Values in parentheses are percentages.

* Nerve sacrifice: partial in four, total in two patients. Two patients also had a downfracture of the mastoid bone for access purposes; another patient had an extended radical parotidectomy and primary reconstruction with a pectoralis major myocutaneous flap.

median time to second recurrence was 73 (range 5–283) months. The rate of *second* recurrences was not influenced by gender ($P = 0.16$), age at initial treatment ($P = 0.76$), time to first recurrence ($P = 0.9$), and type of prior treatment ($P = 0.67$). There was no significant difference in control rates between the surgical categories (Table 8.3).

Direct comparison between treatment modalities showed that adjuvant radiotherapy significantly improved the rate of subsequent or *second* recurrence from 24% to 8% at 15 years ($P = 0.01$). Subanalysis revealed that this advantage in tumour control was confined to the multinodular recurrent tumour group (surgery versus surgery + radiotherapy; 43% versus 4% at 15 years, $P = 0.008$; Fig. 8.1) On the other hand, there was no difference between treatment modalities in the uninodular recurrent tumour group (surgery versus surgery + radiotherapy; 15% versus 13% at 15 years, $P = 0.9$; Fig. 8.2)

Multinodular recurrence implies that at primary surgery the wound was contaminated with neoplastic cells, and that subsequent surgical resection cannot reliably encompass all disease. Radiotherapy appears to eradicate this microscopic residuum. In contrast, radiation made no difference to the outcome of treating isolated or isolated recurrences, suggesting that this subgroup may be dealt with satisfactorily by surgery alone. Similar findings, albeit with smaller numbers of patients, have been observed in a more recent study (Carew *et al.* 1999).

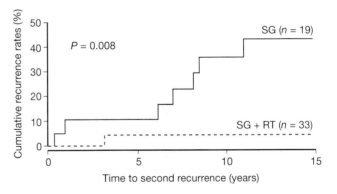

Fig. 8.1 Cumulative incidence (using Kaplan–Meier life-table estimates) of recurrence after the first re-operation according to treatment modality in patients with multinodular recurrence (SG, surgery alone; SG + RT, surgery plus radiotherapy).

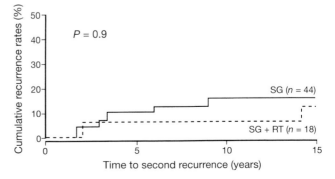

Fig. 8.2 Cumulative incidence (using Kaplan–Meier life-table estimates) of recurrence after the first re-operation according to treatment modality in patients with uninodular recurrence (SG, surgery alone; SG + RT, surgery plus radiotherapy).

Complications associated with re-treatment

The overall incidence of permanent facial nerve injury was 15% (17/114). This compared with 2.5% (14/551) for primary tumours (Table 8.4). With a *second* recurrence, five patients (30%) had a permanent facial palsy (intentional sacrifice, four; unintentional, one). Irradiation appeared to protect against the development of Frey's syndrome and amputation neuroma of the great auricular nerve stump. Radiation-related complications (in the 51 patients who received radiotherapy) included acute skin and mucosal reactions in 35% of patients. Long-term radiation side effects included persistent otitis externa ($n = 7$ or 14%), troublesome xerostomia ($n = 3$ or 6%), and hearing and vestibular disturbances (two patients each or 4%). Radionecrosis of the skin was seen in one patient.

Permanent facial nerve injury is the principal risk when treating recurrent parotid pleomorphic adenomas. The incidence in this series was 15% which compared favourably with other published reports of 16–29% (see Table 8.1). In practice, the risk to the facial nerve depends on the extent of previous surgery and the resultant scarring, with dense scar predisposing to nerve injury. If the first operation was only a minor procedure, then second treatment by a standard parotidectomy may be low risk to the nerve. However, three out five patients in this series initially treated by parotidectomy developed a permanent facial nerve injury following re-operation. Management without further surgery may be a prudent option in this subgroup.

Malignant degeneration in recurrent tumours

The literature reports varying rates from 0 to 16% for malignant degeneration occurring in recurrent pleomorphic adenomas (Fee *et al.* 1978; Fleming 1987; Myssiorek *et al.* 1990; Phillips and Olsen 1995). These must be considered in the light of the

Table 8.4 Comparison of complications following surgery for primary and first recurrent tumours

	Primary (n = 51)	First recurrence SG (n = 63)	SG + RT (n = 51)
Facial nerve damage			
Deliberate nerve division*	6 (1)	2 (3)	4 (8)
Accidental damage			
Permanent	8 (1.5)	6 (9)	5 (10)
Transient	71 (13)	22 (35)	15 (29)
Frey's syndrome	54 (11)	22 (35)	6 (12)†
Amputation neuroma	36 (7)	10 (16)	0
Fistula		3	1

Values in parentheses are percentages.

SG, surgery; RT, radiotherapy.

* All resulted in a permanent facial nerve palsy.

† $P < 0.001$, χ^2 test.

number and types of previous treatments. Thus, there were no malignant transformations in our series in those patients who developed one recurrence only, but three patients did develop malignant disease over the total study period who each had three or more recurrences. All three had also received radiation therapy, and the implication is that repeated intervention is partly responsible for the malignant degeneration seen. These observations agree with the comments of Myssiorek *et al.* (1990) that 'there is little proof that recurrent pleomorphic adenomas are (inherently) malignant' and, indeed, malignant transformation is rare.

Indications for surgical intervention: a shift in perspective

Three aspects of management of recurrent pleomorphic salivary adenoma are highlighted in this series. First, a surgical policy aimed principally at preserving nerve integrity yields recurrence rates of the order of 15%. Adjuvant radiotherapy is useful in this setting especially in the presence of multinodular disease. Secondly, the risk of permanent nerve damage is approximately 15% for first re-operation but rises to 30% for second re-operation. Thirdly, the risk of malignant degeneration is in practice very small, and indeed its development may be associated with repeated surgical and radiotherapy intervention.

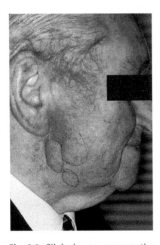

Fig. 8.3 Clinical case: conservative treatment of recurrent pleomorphic adenoma. This patient, now 83 underwent a superficial parotidectomy for a pleomorphic adenoma during the 1960s by Mr Patey. The patient presented 30 years later with multinodular recurrence. The patient suffered from cardiac failure. Taking this together with the recognized increased risk of permanent facial nerve injury, the patient and clinician decided to treat conservatively. Five years later, there has been no change in the size of these recurrences.

These findings have brought about a re-evaluation of the management of both primary and recurrent pleomorphic adenomas. The main reason for surgical removal of a primary parotid tumour (which are mostly pleomorphic adenoma) is to establish a histological diagnosis. In the past, the principal motive for treating recurrent disease had been driven by fear of malignant degeneration. This now appears a questionable reason. As there is a significant risk of permanent facial nerve damage following surgery for recurrent pleomorphic adenoma, there is a case for a 'wait and see' policy (Fig. 8.3). This ethos represents a shift in the approach to these tumours, as a whole brought about through better understanding of the natural history of this tumour.

REFERENCES

Carew, J.F., Spiro, R.H., Singh, B., and Shah, J.P. (1999) Treatment of recurrent pleomorphic adenomas of the parotid gland. *Otolaryngol Head Neck Surg*, **121**, 539–42.

Conley, J. and Clairmont, A.A. (1979) Facial nerve in recurrent benign pleomorphic adenoma. *Arch Otolaryngol*, **105**, 247–51.

Dawson, A.K. (1989) Radiation therapy in recurrent pleomorphic adenoma of the parotid. *Int J Radiat Oncol Biol Phys*, **16**, 819–21.

Norman, J.E. de B (1995) Recurrent mixed tumours of the major and minor salivary glands. In: *Color Atlas and Text of the Salivary Glands. Disease, Disorders and Surgery.* pp. 234–44. (eds J.E.de Burgh Norman and M. McGurk) Mosby-Wolfe, London.

Fee, W.E., Jr, Goffinet, D.R., and Calcaterra, T.C. (1978) Recurrent mixed tumors of the parotid gland—results of surgical therapy. *Laryngoscope*, **88**, 265–73.

Fleming, W.B. (1987) Recurrent pleomorphic adenoma of the parotid. *Aust NZ J Surg*, **57**, 173–6.

Hanna, D.C., Dickason, W.L., Richardson, G.S., and Gaisford, J.C. (1976) Management of recurrent salivary gland tumors. *Am J Surg*, **132**, 453–8.

Jackson, S.R., Roland, N.J., Clarke, R.W., and Jones, A.S. (1993) Recurrent pleomorphic adenoma. *J Laryngol Otol*, **107**, 546–9.

Laskawi, R., Schott, T., and Schroder, M. (1998) Recurrent pleomorphic adenomas of the parotid gland: clinical evaluation and long-term follow-up. *Br J Oral Maxillofac Surg*, **36**, 48–51.

Leverstein, H., Tiwari, R.M., Snow, G.B., van der Wal, J.E., and van der Waal, I. (1997) The surgical management of recurrent or residual pleomorphic adenomas of the parotid gland. Analysis and results in 40 patients. *Eur Arch Otorhinolaryngol*, **254**, 313–7.

Malone, B. and Baker, S.R. (1984) Benign pleomorphic adenomas in children. *Ann Otol Rhinol Laryngol*, **93**, 210–4.

Maran, A.G., Mackenzie, I.J., and Stanley, R.E. (1984) Recurrent pleomorphic adenomas of the parotid gland. *Arch Otolaryngol*, **110**, 167–71.

McGregor, A.D., Burgoyne, M., and Tan, K.C. (1988) Recurrent pleomorphic salivary adenoma—the relevance of age at first presentation. *Br J Plast Surg*, **41**, 177–81.

Myssiorek, D., Ruah, C.B., and Hybels, R.L. (1990) Recurrent pleomorphic adenomas of the parotid gland. *Head Neck*, **12**, 332–6.

Niparko, J.K., Beauchamp, M.L., Krause, C.J., Baker, S.R., and Work, W.P. (1986) Surgical treatment of recurrent pleomorphic adenoma of the parotid gland. *Arch Otolaryngol Head Neck Surg*, **112**, 1180–4.

O' Dwyer, P.J., Farrar, W.B., Finkelmeier, W.R., McCabe, D.P., and James, A.G. (1986) Facial nerve sacrifice and tumor recurrence in primary and recurrent benign parotid tumors. *Am J Surg*, **152**, 442–5.

Phillips, P.P. and Olsen, K.D. (1995) Recurrent pleomorphic adenoma of the parotid gland: report of 126 cases and a review of the literature. *Ann Otol Rhinol Laryngol*, **104**, 100–4.

Piorkowski, R.J. and Guillamondegui, O.M. (1981) Is aggressive surgical treatment indicated for recurrent benign mixed tumors of the parotid gland? *Am J Surg*, **142**, 434–6.

Renehan, A., Gleave, E.N., and McGurk, M. (1996) An analysis of the treatment of 114 patients with recurrent pleomorphic adenomas of the parotid gland. *Am J Surg*, **172**, 710–4.

Samson, M.J., Metson, R., Wang, C.C., and Montgomery, W.W. (1991) Preservation of the facial nerve in the management of recurrent pleomorphic adenoma. *Laryngoscope*, **101**, 1060–2.

Watkin, G.T. and Hobsley, M. (1986) Influence of local surgery and radiotherapy on the natural history of pleomorphic adenomas. *Br J Surg*, **73**, 74–6.

Audience discussion

Professor McGurk (London, UK): Given the very high rate of permanent facial nerve palsy in those patients who have had a full superficial parotidectomy, and also the findings that malignant transformation is rare, in recurrent disease is there any role for radiotherapy alone with no surgery?

Mr Renehan: No. There is no direct evidence for the efficacy of radiotherapy in the treatment of macroscopic disease. There is indirect evidence to support its use in the post-operative situation.

Dr Slevin (Manchester, UK): I note that for multinodular recurrence, adjuvant radiotherapy reduces subsequent recurrence from 43 to 4%, but yet recurrence rates were approximately 15% for uninodular disease, with or without post-operative radiotherapy?

Mr Renehan: We looked at this at the time we were writing this, and we too were initially puzzled. The answer probably lies in the statistics. Despite the fact that we have the largest series of recurrent tumours, the number of cases available for analysis at 15 years is small, and small changes have a disproportionate effect on the log-rank statistical model. If you do not censor the data for patients lost, etc., the crude re-recurrence rates for uninodular recurrences were about 10%, which is closer to 4%.

Professor Langdon (London, UK): May I ask the unspeakable? If I followed Mr Renehan's argument correctly, he is saying that for recurrent pleomorphic adenoma, a wait and see policy is reasonable if the tumour presents no cosmetic problem. If that is so, why do we advocate surgery for the primary tumour? The strongest argument for surgery is a risk of subsequent malignancy. But we are now beginning to question the validity of this risk. Should we be advising patients with small parotid pleomorphic adenomas to have surgery?

Professor Spiro (New York, US): If I may answer this question. Even if I am 90% confident that a lump is benign, the only way we know for sure is to remove it. The difference in recurrent disease is that you are fairly confident of the histology, i.e. that it is a pleomorphic adenoma, as malignant transformation for the first recurrence is a very rare event. I have a photograph of a chap who for 12 years had absolutely no change in what was a pleomorphic adenoma on needle aspiration biopsy and who adamantly refused intervention.

Mr Watkinson (Birmingham, UK): Do we not still teach that if a pleomorphic adenoma recurs the first thing to do is look at the original histology? Andrew (Renehan) has mentioned a number of patients that when the tumour recurred, and the original specimen was examined, it proved to be a mucoepidermoid carcinoma, etc. Therefore, is there not still an obligation to get a new biopsy on your recurrent tumour?

Editorial comment

Mr Renehan's paper is distinctive in that he analysed first-time recurrence only. He has been able to conduct a long (10–14 years) follow-up which is essential in the assessment of recurrent pleomorphic salivary adenomas. Its second feature has been the presence of a uniform treatment philosophy for a large number of cases and for a long period of time. Since the study was neither prospective nor randomized, the groups are not directly comparable, but they represent the best material currently available for evaluation. Recurrent disease is now much less common than 40 years ago and so a similar series (>100 cases) will be difficult to acquire today, so in this sense the study may prove to be unique.

The study has two clear conclusions. First, recurrent pleomorphic adenomas present in two forms: uninodular and multinodular. Surgical removal of the uninodular recurrent lump has a 10–15% risk of a second recurrence; a multinodular recurrence treated by surgery alone has a much higher risk of second recurrence approaching 45% at 15 years. Post-operative radiotherapy significantly reduces this risk. Secondly, malignant transformation is rare in first and even second recurrences. As malignant transformation is held to be one of the main reasons for repeat surgery, the automatic need for re-operation is questioned in the elderly or infirm patient.

CHAPTER 9

What is the evidence for the progression from benign to malignant pleomorphic adenoma?

John Eveson and Andrew Yeudall

Introduction

As late as 1970, the very concept of carcinoma arising in pleomorphic adenoma (malignant mixed tumour) was still being questioned by some (Evans and Cruikshank 1970). In addition, it was also recognized that many of the tumours described in the previous literature as carcinoma in pleomorphic adenoma were misdiagnoses of other tumour types. Until that time, there had been a prevailing concept that pleomorphic adenomas were 'semi-malignant' tumours, and some pathologists described a spectrum of pleomorphic adenomas including: 'benign', 'semi-malignant', and 'malignant'. The picture was confused further when such terms as 'primary malignant mixed tumour' were used to describe what was considered to be a carcinoma in pleomorphic adenoma arising *de novo* (Kleinsasser and Klien 1968). In addition, there were scattered reports of histologically benign pleomorphic adenomas that had undergone distant metastasis.

Carcinoma arising in pleomorphic adenoma is now a well-established diagnosis. It is defined as a 'tumour showing definitive evidence of malignancy, such as cytological and histological characteristics of anaplasia, abnormal mitoses, progressive course, and infiltrative growth, and in which evidence of pleomorphic adenoma can still be found' (Seifert and Sobin 1991). Within this category, there is a spectrum of tumours that includes: carcinoma in pleomorphic adenoma, non-invasive (*in situ* or intra-capsular carcinoma), carcinosarcoma, and metastasizing benign pleomorphic adenoma (Figs 9.1–9.6)

A diagnosis of carcinoma arising in pleomorphic adenoma can only be made with certainty if a focus of benign pleomorphic adenoma can be identified or if there is a history of a benign pleomorphic adenoma having been removed from the site of a malignant recurrence. However, this strict definition probably underestimates the true frequency of carcinoma arising in pleomorphic adenoma as many appear to arise in an old, scarred pleomorphic adenoma with little if any of the original tumour remaining, and in other cases the original tumour is probably replaced by the malignant elements.

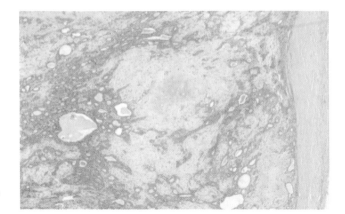

Fig. 9.1 Typical pleomorphic adenoma with cartilaginous and epithelial elements and a discrete fibrous capsule.

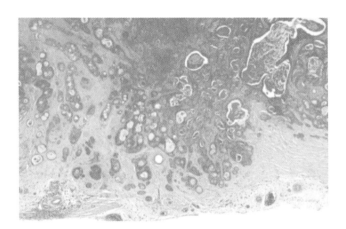

Fig. 9.2 A pleomorphic adenoma with extensive invasion of the capsule. This does not constitute malignant change.

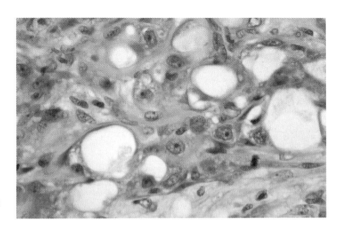

Fig. 9.3 High power showing dysplastic changes in pleomorphic adenoma ('non-invasive carcinoma in pleomorphic adenoma').

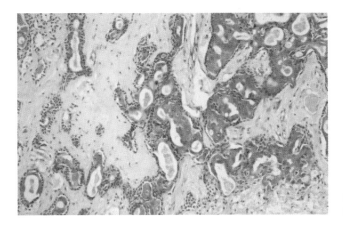

Fig. 9.4 Carcinoma (right) arising within a pleomorphic adenoma.

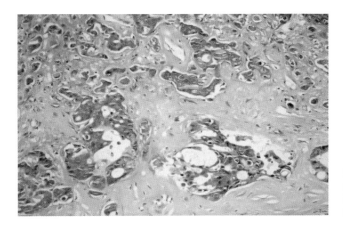

Fig. 9.5 Carcinoma arising in the scarred fibrous remnant of a long-standing pleomorphic adenoma.

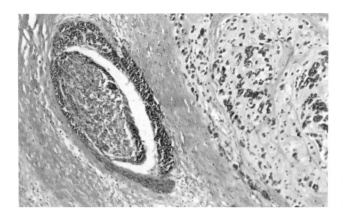

Fig. 9.6 Carcinosarcoma (left) showing perineural invasion and chondrosarcoma (right)

107

Carcinoma in pleomorphic adenoma accounted for 3.6% of all salivary gland tumours in a review of a series of 60 papers on this tumour published after 1950 (Gnepp 1993). In the Armed Forces Institute of Pathology (AFIP) series, carcinoma in pleomorphic adenoma formed 6.5% of the total malignant salivary gland tumours and was the sixth most common salivary gland malignancy (Gnepp and Wenig 1991). The evidence for the development of malignancy in pleomorphic adenoma is clinical, pathological, and molecular.

Clinical evidence

There is an increasing likelihood of malignant change in pleomorphic adenoma with time. Eneroth and Zetterberg (1974) reported a rate of malignant change in pleomorphic adenoma of 1.6% in 0–4 years, 5.9% in 10–14 years, and 9.4% in tumours present for more than 15 years. In other series of carcinoma in pleomorphic adenoma, most patients were aware of a mass in the salivary gland for many years that frequently had undergone a sudden increase in size or ulcerated. However, LiVolsi and Perzin (1977) state that in 45% of cases of carcinoma in pleomorphic adenoma, a mass had been present for less than 3 years. In the series reported by Spiro and colleagues (1977), a swelling had been present for less than 2 years in about half of their cases. However, some of the cases in Spiro's series had arisen in the deep lobe of the parotid and this may have masked their presence for some time.

There is an increased frequency of carcinoma in pleomorphic adenoma in patients who have had one or more operations for pleomorphic adenoma before the diagnosis of malignancy. For example, in the series reported by LiVolsi and Perzin (1977), nine out of their 47 cases (20%) of carcinoma in pleomorphic adenoma followed previous surgery for pleomorphic adenoma. However, post-operative radiation had been given in two cases. In the AFIP series (Gnepp and Wenig 1991), 86% of cases arose in the major glands, even though they only accounted for 71% of all cases of pleomorphic adenoma. It was thought that this related to the much higher rate of recurrence of pleomorphic adenoma in the major as opposed to the minor glands.

There is a strong relationship between carcinoma in pleomorphic adenoma and the age of the patient. Most series show that the average age at presentation for patients with carcinoma in pleomorphic adenoma is 10–20 years later than patients with pleomorphic adenoma. In the AFIP series (Gnepp and Wenig 1991), the average age was 46.9 years for pleomorphic adenoma and 60.1 years for carcinoma in pleomorphic adenoma. In the British Salivary Gland Tumour Panel series (Eveson and Cawson 1985), the equivalent ages were 46 and 63.3 years. In addition, carcinoma in pleomorphic adenoma is very uncommon in younger patients and there were no cases in two major series of salivary gland tumours in children (Krolls *et al.* 1972; Lack and Upton 1988).

There appears to be an association between the size of the tumour and the likelihood of malignancy in pleomorphic adenoma, particularly in tumours over 5 cm in diameter (Nagao *et al.* 1981).

Pathological evidence

Within the spectrum of carcinoma in pleomorphic adenoma, there is a grouping of non-invasive (intracapsular or *in situ*) carcinoma and, in addition, some recognize minimally invasive mixed tumour (Brandwein *et al.* 1996). These tumours show dysplastic features without invasion of the surrounding structures. The presence of aneuploid cell populations in 70% of tumours examined (Brandwein *et al.* 1996), suggested that these tumours are a histological category distinct from benign pleomorphic adenoma. However, a further study of 16 benign pleomorphic adenomas showed that only 25% were aneuploid (Martin *et al.* 1994). Dysplastic pleomorphic adenomas appear to have a similar prognosis to benign pleomorphic adenoma but probably represent part of a spectrum that ultimately would lead to frankly invasive carcinoma (Clark *et al.* 1993).

Molecular evidence

The progression from dysplastic epithelium and/or adenoma through to carcinoma is well recognized in colorectal and oesophageal carcinogenesis, and is related to the accumulation of genetic mutations (Fig. 9.7A and B). It is tempting to postulate a similar situation for salivary glands and, in particular, from pleomorphic adenoma to carcinoma (Fig. 9.7C).

During the development of pleomorphic adenomas, chromosomal rearrangements occur at 8q12–15 and 12q13–15. The former results in promoter swapping between the pleomorphic adenoma gene (*PLAG1*) which encodes a zinc finger protein, and the gene encoding β-catenin (*CTNNB1*) (Kas *et al.* 1997; Aström *et al.* 1999). The latter leads to abnormalities of the gene encoding a high mobility group protein (*HMGIC*) (Geurts *et al.* 1997).

Activation of c-*myc*, $p21^{RAS}$, and *p53* mutations may also be important (Rosa *et al.* 1996). Loss of heterozygosity (LOH) of the *p53* gene was detected in 57% of pleomorphic adenomas and 86% of carcinomas in pleomorphic adenomas (Yamamoto *et al.* 1998). In a small series of four pleomorphic adenomas with documented malignant transformation, Righi and colleagues (1994) found identical *p53* mutations in both pleomorphic adenomatous tissue and transformed malignant specimens. In addition, overexpression of p53 was detected immunohistochemically in 13% of adenomas, in 50% of transitional areas, and in 75% of carcinomas in pleomorphic adenomas. All of the tumours with immunoreactivity for p53 showed LOH. These findings strongly suggest that mutation of the *p53* gene is an early event in the progression of benign to malignant pleomorphic adenoma.

It has also been suggested that inactivation of the *p16* gene (a putative tumour suppressor gene) and genetic instability are a feature of malignant transformation in carcinoma in pleomorphic adenoma (Suzuki and Fujioka, 1998).

During conversion of pleomorphic adenoma to carcinoma, LOH occurs at multiple chromosomal loci. LOH at loci on 8q has been widely reported in pleomorphic adenoma (el Naggar *et al.* 1997). The incidence is not increased in areas of focal carcinoma, which suggests that LOH at 8q is an early event in tumorigenesis (Gillenwater

(a)   **Colorectal adenoma-carcinoma sequence**

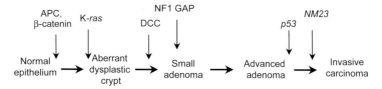

(b)   **Oesophageal metaplasia-carcinoma sequence**

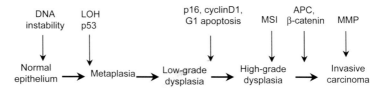

(c)   **Proposed salivary carcinogenesis**

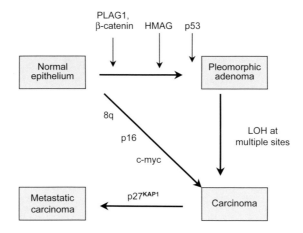

Fig. 9.7 Similarities between the multistep genetic processes during carcinogenesis of colorectal cancer (A), oesophageal cancer (B), and proposed model for salivary carcinoma in-pleomorphic adenoma (C). See text for explanation of terms.

et al. 1997). It has been shown that there may be loss of chromosome 17 in pleomorphic adenoma before the development of carcinoma and, in addition, polysomy 17 was found to be more frequent in carcinoma in pleomorphic adenoma than pleomorphic adenoma and was associated with mutation of *p53* (Li *et al.* 1997). In addition, loss of the short arm of chromosome 17 may also be related to tumour progression (el Naggar *et al.* 1997).

Taken together, the molecular changes underlying the development of the pleomorphic adenoma are beginning to be unravelled, but detailed molecular knowledge of the progression to carcinoma is still limited.

REFERENCES

Astrom, A.K., Voz, M.L., Kas, K., Roijer, E., Wedell, B., Mandahl, N. *et al.* (1999) Conserved mechanism of PLAG1 activation in salivary gland tumors with and without chromosome 8q12 abnormalities: identification of SII as a new fusion partner gene. *Cancer Res*, **59**, 918–23.

Brandwein, M., Huvos, A.G., Dardick, I., Thomas, M.J., and Theise, N.D. (1996) Noninvasive and minimally invasive carcinoma ex mixed tumor: a clinicopathologic and ploidy study of 12 patients with major salivary tumors of low (or no?) malignant potential. *Oral Surg, Oral Med, Oral Pathol Oral Radiol Endod*, **81**, 655–64.

Clark, J., Bailey, B.M., and Eveson, J.W. (1993) Dysplastic pleomorphic adenoma of the sublingual salivary gland. *Br J Oral Maxillofac Surg*, **31**, 394–5.

el Naggar, A.K., Dinh, M., Tucker, S.L., Gillenwater, A., Luna, M.A., and Batsakis, J.G. (1997) Chromosomal and DNA ploidy characterization of salivary gland neoplasms by combined FISH and flow cytometry. *Hum Pathol*, **28**, 881–6.

Eneroth, C.M. and Zetterberg, A. (1974) Malignancy in pleomorphic adenoma. A clinical and microspectrophotometric study. *Acta Otolaryngol*, **77**, 426–32.

Evans, R.W. and Cruikshank, A.H. (1970) *Epithelial Tumours of the Salivary Glands*. W.B.Saunders Co., Philadelphia.

Eveson, J.W. and Cawson, R.A. (1985) Salivary gland tumours. A review of 2410 cases with particular reference to histological types, site, age and sex distribution. *J Pathol*, **146**, 51–8.

Geurts, J.M., Schoenmakers, E.F., Roijer, E., Stenman, G., and Van de Ven, W.J. (1997) Expression of reciprocal hybrid transcripts of HMGIC and FHIT in a pleomorphic adenoma of the parotid gland. *Cancer Res*, **57**, 13–7.

Gillenwater, A., Hurr, K., Wolf, P., Batsakis, J.G., Goepfert, H., and El Naggar, A.K. (1997) Microsatellite alterations at chromosome 8q loci in pleomorphic adenoma. *Otolaryngol Head Neck Surg*, **117**, 448–52.

Gnepp, D.R. (1993) Malignant mixed tumors of the salivary glands: a review. *Pathol Annu*, **28** 1, 279–328.

Gnepp, D.R. and Wenig, B.M. (1991) Malignant mixed tumors. In: *Surgical Pathology of the Salivary Glands*. pp. 1350–1368. (eds G.L. Ellis, P.L. Auclair, and D.R. Gnepp) W.B.Saunders Co., Philadelphia.

Kas, K., Voz, M.L., Roijer, E., Astrom, A.K., Meyen, E., Stenman, G. *et al.* (1997) Promoter swapping between the genes for a novel zinc finger protein and beta-catenin in pleiomorphic adenomas with t(3;8)(p21;q12) translocations. *Nat Genet*, **15**, 170–4.

Kleinsasser, O. and Klein, H.J. (1968) [Secondary carcinoma in primary non-malignant mixed tumors of the salivary glands]. *Arch Klin Exp Ohren Nasen Kehlkopfheilkd*, **190**, 272–85.

Krolls, S.O., Trodahl, J.N., and Boyers, R.C. (1972) Salivary gland lesions in children. A survey of 430 cases. *Cancer*, **30**, 459–69.

Lack, E.E. and Upton, M.P. (1988) Histopathologic review of salivary gland tumors in childhood. *Arch Otolaryngol Head Neck Surg*, **114**, 898–906.

Li, X., Tsuji, T., Wen, S., Mimura, Y., Sasaki, K., and Shinozaki, F. (1997) Detection of numeric abnormalities of chromosome 17 and p53 deletions by fluorescence *in situ* hybridization in pleomorphic adenomas and carcinomas in pleomorphic adenoma. Correlation with p53 expression. *Cancer*, **79**, 2314–9.

LiVolsi, V.A. and Perzin, K.H. (1977) Malignant mixed tumors arising in salivary glands. I. Carcinomas arising in benign mixed tumors: a clinicopathologic study. *Cancer*, **39**, 2209–30.

Martin, A.R., Mantravadi, J., Kotylo, P.K., Mullins, R., Walker, S., and Roth, L.M. (1994) Proliferative activity and aneuploidy in pleomorphic adenomas of the salivary glands. *Arch Pathol Lab Med*, **118**, 252–9.

Nagao, K., Matsuzaki, O., Saiga, H., Sugano, I., Shigematsu, H., Kaneko, T. *et al.* (1981) Histopathologic studies on carcinoma in pleomorphic adenoma of the parotid gland. *Cancer*, **48**, 113–21.

Righi, P.D., Li, Y.Q., Deutsch, M., McDonald, J.S., Wilson, K.M., Bejarano, P. *et al.* (1994) The role of the p53 gene in the malignant transformation of pleomorphic adenomas of the parotid gland. *Anticancer Res*, **14**, 2253–7.

Rosa, J.C., Fonseca, I., Felix, A., and Soares, J. (1996) Immunohistochemical study of c-erbB-2 expression in carcinoma ex-pleomorphic adenoma. *Histopathology*, **28**, 247–52.

Seifert, G. and Sobin, L.H. (1991) *WHO International Histological Classification of Tumours. Histological Typing of Salivary Gland Tumours*, 2nd edn. Springer-Verlag, Berlin.

Spiro, R.H., Huvos, A.G., and Strong, E.W. (1977) Malignant mixed tumor of salivary origin: a clinicopathologic study of 146 cases. *Cancer*, **39**, 388–96.

Suzuki, H. and Fujioka, Y. (1998) Deletion of the p16 gene and microsatellite instability in carcinoma arising in pleomorphic adenoma of the parotid gland. *Diagn Mol Pathol*, **7**, 224–31.

Yamamoto, Y., Kishimoto, Y., Wistuba, II, Virmani, A.K., Vuitch, F., Gazdar, A.F. *et al.* (1998) DNA analysis at p53 locus in carcinomas arising from pleomorphic adenomas of salivary glands: comparison of molecular study and p53 immunostaining. *Pathol Int*, **48**, 265–72.

Audience discussion

Mr Renehan (Manchester, UK): The proposed progression of pleomorphic adenoma into a carcinoma might reasonably be compared with the well-established model for progression of adenoma to carcinoma in the gut. But it is very clear in the gastro-intestinal tract that an adenoma is always dysplasic. Is there always a degree of dysplasia in the pleomorphic adenoma? The second point is that you mentioned Eneroth's paper. This paper has been very influential in supporting the progression from benign pleomorphic adenoma to its malignant counterpart. But, of course, it is based on retrospective recollection by patients reporting the duration of symptoms (i.e. presence of a lump)—this evidence is indirect and weak.

Dr Eveson: It is difficult to envisage a malignant tumour going on for 15 years before someone does something about it. So even as indirect evidence it is useful. If the cancer has not arisen in a pleomorphic adenoma, where has it come from? The WHO classification of carcinoma ex-pleomorphic adenoma requires histological evidence of pre-existing pleomorphic adenoma but I take a more liberal view and include scarring or multiple differentiation as supportive evidence. To complicate matters further, a lot of papers now refer to de-differentiated tumours so you can have a de-differentiated acinic cell carcinoma or adenoidcystic carcinoma.

Mr Hancock (Manchester, UK): I clearly remember that Alan Nicholson told me that 50% of all his patients with high-grade carcinomas gave a history of a lump in the parotid for more than 10 years. He always argued that we should remove all parotid tumours because then we can reduce the high-grade parotid carcinoma by 50%. The reason we see relatively few high-grade tumours today could be because we are removing all benign tumours and not leaving them.

Dr Eveson: I do not think there is any evidence the high-grade tumours were more common in the 1940s and 1950s than they are now. But there is circumstantial evidence that pleomorphic adenomas will change to a high-grade tumour. In some cases, you cannot even recognize histologically any elements of pleomorphic adenoma in these often undifferentiated cancers.

Professor Spiro (New York, USA): If that were so, then when the incidence of carcinoma mixed pleomorphic adenoma is examined in two different time frames it should decline. We were unable to show that in our experience. When we looked at our malignant mixed tumours, there seemed to be two clinical categories: a carcinoma ex-pleomorphic adenoma which arose after a history of multiple recurrence, and another that just appeared *de novo* and had the same histological appearance.

Dr Eveson: I do not understand what it is meant by the term *de novo*. I cannot visualize a benign and malignant tumour arising simultaneously, so logically you would have thought one would precede the other and that the benign will precede the malignant. This is biological common sense.

Professor Spiro: Also, it seems that the variety that appear *de novo* behave more aggressively so the basic evolutionary process of pleomorphic adenoma to something else must have happened with much greater rapidity.

Editorial comment

The perplexing nature of carcinoma ex-pleomorphic adenoma is due mainly to the fact that pathologists have been unable to reach a clear consensus on what constitutes the histological criteria for making the diagnosis. This is illustrated by Dr Eveson's's comments on the WHO definition which can be interpreted liberally. If there is no firm histological basis, then it is very difficult to establish a correlation between pathological findings and clinical data.

However, happily there is one area in this problem-ridden field that is tolerably clear—that is the existence of two separate clinical entities that can be differentiated from each other. It is a well established fact that repeated interference with a benign lesion (presumably due to release of growth promotion substances) leads to the development of overt malignant disease. This phenomenon has been observed widely and is well documented in the specific case of pleomorphic adenoma. The second clinical entity is more controversial—that a pleomorphic *de novo* adenoma can degenerate into a carcinoma. This proposition is based on explanation of 'de-differentiation' or anecdotal clinical histories; all evidence which is uncertain. An analogy is drawn with adenomas of the large bowel but this concept is not really tenable because the large bowel adenomas invariably have histological dysplastic features which make the concept of malignant change comprehensible. However, with salivary adenomas, there is seldom evidence of earlier histological dysplasia. In other words, the concept of malignant change in a pleomorphic adenoma is rather like thunder out of a blue sky; it might occur but it seems very improbable that it is an inevitable event. In medicine it is accepted that anything can happen but in the present context of salivary tumours one is looking for regular occurrences that permit predictions to be made.

CHAPTER 10

The influence of multicentricity in the treatment of Warthin's tumour

The Amsterdam experience

Isaac van der Waal and Gordon Snow

The Manchester experience

Brian Hancock

Warthin's tumour is a somewhat controversial lesion which is almost exclusively restricted to the parotid gland. [The World Health Organization stated that the term Warthin's tumour is preferred to other terms such as adenolymphoma and papillary cystadenoma lyphomatosum (Seifert 1992).] The controversy is multifaceted and relates to aspects of both pathogenesis and treatment. Extensive reviews of this tumour by Chapnik (1983) and Lamelas and colleagues (1987) alluded to the frequent observation of multicentricity and raised questions as to whether this characteristic may affect the approach to treatment. In the present chapter, studies from two centres specifically address this issue.

The Amsterdam experience
Isaac van der Waal and Gordon Snow

Background
In a series of 278 cases from the files of the British Salivary Gland Tumour Panel (Eveson and Cawson 1986), multicentric disease was evident on clinical examination of the surgical specimens in 10% of cases; no mention was made of microscopic multi-centricity. Subsequent studies found similar rates for multiple tumours identified marcoscopically at the time of operative removal (Table 10.1). Second tumours occurring in the other parotid gland are also well recognized and may present at the time of initial diagnosis (bilateral synchronous tumours) or at a later time (bilateral meta-chronous tumours). Following routine histological examination, the proportion of resections demonstrating multiple tumours rises to approximately 20% (Fig. 10.1). In contrast, following a thorough microscopic examination by a serial section technique, the rate of multicentricity may rise to greater than half (Lam et al. 1994).

Table 10.1 Studies of multicentricity in Warthin's tumour

Study	No. of resections	Multicentricity rate	
		Macroscopic	Microscopic
Per-operative assessment			
Eveson and Cawson (1984)	278	28 (10)	
Heller and Attie (1988)	162	15 (9)	31 (19)
Leverstein et al. (1997)	88	9 (10)	17 (19)
Serial section techniques			
Lam et al. (1994)	24		13 (54)

Values in parentheses are percentages.

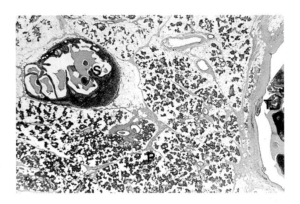

Fig. 10.1 Macroscopic focus (labelled S) of Warthin's tumour at some distance from the main tumour (labelled T). Parenchymal salivary tissue is labelled by P (H & E stain; original magnification ×10).

Warthin's tumour and other salivary gland tumours

In addition to the development of multiple Warthin's tumours in the same individual, Warthin's is not infrequently associated with other salivary pathologies, for instance pleomorphic adenomas (Lefor and Ord 1993; Seifert and Donath 1996). Of all salivary tumours, Warthin's is the most frequent to become complicated by infection or infarction, and may thus present as pain or facial nerve weakness (Newman et al. 1993).

Multicentricity and recurrence rate

We reviewed a number of studies examining specifically the rate of second tumours in cases of Warthin's tumour (Table 10.2). For both second ipsilateral and second contralateral Warthin's tumours, the prevalences were between 3 and 13%. We specifically examined for the rates of 'true' recurrences, i.e. the occurrence of a second Warthin's tumour within the surgical bed of an operated gland. While this was not defined uniformly, the values shown in Table 10.2 suggest that this is less than 2%.

In our own series from Amsterdam (Leverstein et al. 1997), we looked for the influence of different surgical techniques on the recurrence rate in 88 resection cases of Warthin's tumours in 85 patients. In each procedure, after resecting the tumour,

Table 10.2 Second tumours and 'true' recurrences following treatment for Warthin's tumour

Study	No. of resections	Second tumours		'True' recurrence
		Ipsilateral	Contralateral	
Local resection				
Heller and Attie (1988)	113	15 (13)	12 (11)	2 (1.7)
Christie series*	92	5 (5)	5 (5)	1
Nerve identification				
Leverstein et al. (1997)†	88	3 (3)	5 (6)	0
Christie series*	43	1	2 (5)	2 (1.5)

Values in parentheses are percentages.

* Unpublished data (courtesy of Mr A. Renehan).

† One surgeon: 52 'partial' superficial parotidectomies; 22 'standard' superficial parotidectomies; 12 'partial' superficial/deep lobe parotidectomies; and two 'selective' deep lobe parotidectomies.

careful examination of the remainder of the gland was performed to exclude other simultaneous lesions. In seven of the 22 patients who underwent a standard superficial parotidectomy, there was gross or microscopic evidence of multicentricity; it was also observed in 13 out of 66 patients whom underwent a 'partial' parotidectomy. None of the patients developed recurrent disease in either group, with a median follow-up of 93 months. We stressed the need for careful per-operative inspection of the remaining gland for additional lesions.

Clinical recommendations

Reported 'recurrence rates' following surgical removal of Warthin's tumours range from 5 to 12%; these figures probably reflect second tumour rates rather than 'true' recurrences, which probably occur in less than 2% of cases. Most importantly, the microscopic multicentricity rates of approximately 20% do not translate into a significant clinical problem. Nonetheless, since it is estimated that at least one out of 10 patients with Warthin's tumour will have gross multicentric disease, meticulous per-operative inspection and palpation to avoid overlooked synchronous tumour foci and subsequent recurrence is recommended. Partial superficial parotidectomy and careful extracapsular dissection seem to be adequate methods of treating the majority of Warthin's tumours.

The Manchester experience   Brian Hancock

The multicentric nature of Warthin's tumour at a macroscopic level has long been appreciated (as shown by Professor van der Waal above), but that the extent of this may be significantly greater, as observed at a microscopic level, is relatively recent. These issues have raised questions about the oncological principles underlying the surgical approach to this tumour and, consequently, some authors have advocated total parotidectomy as routine (Alajmo et al. 1989).

For many decades, the Christie Hospital, Manchester, has followed a practice of *extracapsular dissection* for mobile superficial lumps (Chapter 7). This included many Warthin's tumours. The aspect addressed here is if microscopic multicentricity was important, one would expect a high rate of recurrences following the use of an *ultra-conservative* operation, i.e. extracapsular dissection. We explored this in our series comparing long-term outcome in patients with Warthin's tumour treated surgically by extracapsular dissection versus superficial parotidectomy.

Study cohort

During the period 1948–1992, there were a total of 825 new epithelial parotid neoplasms treated by one surgical unit (Renehan *et al.* 1996). Of these, 140 (17%) patients had a histological diagnosis of a Warthin's tumour. Seven patients were lost early to follow-up. Thus, 133 patients formed the basis of this analysis; three had bilateral tumours at presentation, i.e. 136 surgical resections. The median follow-up was 6.5 (range 1–27) years. Tumours were designated multicentric if: (i) multiple foci were found on histological examination; (ii) two or more tumours were removed individually from one gland at the same operation; and (iii) bilateral synchronous tumours if bilateral tumours were present at initial presentation. Over the 40-year study period, surgery was performed by three surgeons, Mr W.A.B. Nicholson (1952–1972), B.D. Hancock (1973–1975), and E.N. Gleave (1975–1992), ensuring a consistent surgical approach.

Counted as 136 operative cases, extracapsular dissection was employed in 92 cases (68%) and a partial or standard superficial parotidectomy with nerve identification in 39 (29%). A deep lobe parotidectomy was performed in four, and one patient required a parotidectomy with sacrifice of some branches of the facial nerve.

Of the 133 patients, 17 (14%) had multicentric tumours, i.e meeting any three of the above criteria (Table 10.3). Six patients developed a second tumour in the ipsilateral gland with a median time of 5.4 (range 2.6–11.7) years. A careful examination of the operation notes and pathology reports suggested that only two were 'true' recurrences (i.e. a recurrence rate of 1.5%) with the others probably representing metachronous Warthin's tumours. Two of these patients with second tumour were in the group of 17 patients with multicentric tumours, and four in the group of 116 patients with solitary tumours (Table 10.3). Five second ipsilateral tumours (5%) occurred following 92 extracapsular dissections, and one (3%) occurred after 44 partial or superficial

Table 10.3 Second Warthin's tumours by nature of initial tumour—Christie Hospital series, 1948–1992

Nature of tumour	No. of resections	Second ipsilateral	Second contralateral
Solitary	116	4 (3)	5 (4)
Multicentric	17	2 (12)*	2 (12)*

Values in parentheses are percentages.

* Not significant by χ^2 test.

Table 10.4 Complications following treatment for Warthin's tumours at the Christie Hospital, 1948–1992

Complications	Extracapsular dissection (n = 92)	Superficial parotidectomy (n = 43)	P-value*
Permanent facial weakness	1	0	
Transient facial weakness	7 (8)	12 (30)	<0.001
Frey's syndrome	7 (8)	9 (23)	<0.001

Values in parentheses are percentages.

* χ^2 test.

parotidectomies. Seven patients (5%) developed a second tumour in the contralateral gland in a median time of 3.7 (1.3–12) years. Collectively these data demonstrate that between 5 and 10% of patients with Warthin's tumour develop second tumours in either the ipsilateral gland or contralateral gland, and their development was uninfluenced by the extent of surgery.

The complication rates by type of surgery are shown in Table 10.4. Similarly to the comparison of complications for extracapsular dissection versus superficial parotidectomy in pleomorphic adenomas (Chapter 6), there were no differences in rates of permanent facial nerve weakness. However, the complications of transient facial weakness and Frey's syndrome were significantly decreased in the extracapulsar dissection group.

Remarks

With long-term follow-up, the principal findings in this study were threefold. First, consistent with the earlier comments of Professors van der Waal and Snow, the rate of 'true' recurrences following the treatment of Warthin's tumour was low (<2%). Secondly, there was a 5–10% rate of second tumours (both ipsilateral and contralateral). Thirdly, these rates were uninfluenced by the extent of the initial operation, and a conservative approach to the surgical treatment of Warthin's can prevail.

To our knowledge, this is the first study of Warthin's tumour in which outcome has been evaluated comparing multicentric verses solitary lesions. The incidence of 17% multicentricity is comparable with other series (Table 10.1). Nonetheless, the results do not support the hypothesis that multicentricity of Warthin's tumour at the initial operation may later be associated with a high rate of ipsilateral and contralateral tumours, and that minimal surgery does not result in unacceptable problems of recidivism after treatment for Warthin's tumours. This is supported further by a recent publication (Yu et al. 1998).

The use of extracapsular dissection in the Christie series was associated with significantly reduced morbidity. The conservative policy can be extended to two further situations: (i) a second salivary tumour in an individual with a previous Warthin's; and (ii) an elderly individual with a parotid lump where the suspicion is that of a Warthin's [e.g. supplemental evidence from fine needle aspiration cytology, sonography (partly cystic), or technesium scan (increased uptake)]. In the former, a non-surgical approach is an option, and indeed was the case for six out of the 13 second tumours in the Christie series. For the primary lump, the foremost reason for surgery is to determine its pathological nature, with cosmetic considerations secondary. In the main, an untreated Warthin's tumour will probably remain static, or at worst fluctuate in size due to infection. A small number may become painful through infarction, and malignant transformation is extremely rare (Warnock 1991). In patients with significant co-morbidity, a watchful policy may be prudent.

REFERENCES

Alajmo, E., Polli, G., and De Meester, W. (1989) Total parotidectomy—a routine treatment for parotid gland swellings? *J Laryngol Otol*, **103**, 181–6.

Chapnik, J.S. (1983) The controversy of Warthin's tumor. *Laryngoscope*, **93**, 695–716.

Eveson, J.W. and Cawson, R.A. (1986) Warthin's tumor (cystadenolymphoma) of salivary glands. A clinicopathologic investigation of 278 cases. *Oral Surg, Oral Med Oral Pathol*, **61**, 256–62.

Heller, K.S. and Attie, J.N. (1988) Treatment of Warthin's tumor by enucleation. *Am J Surg*, **156**, 294–6.

Lam, K.H., Ho, H.C., Ho, C.M., and Wei, W.I. (1994) Multifocal nature of adenolymphoma of the parotid. *Br J Surg*, **81**, 1612–4.

Lamelas, J., Terry, J.H., Jr, and Alfonso, A.E. (1987) Warthin's tumor: multicentricity and increasing incidence in women. *Am J Surg*, **154**, 347–51.

Lefor, A.T. and Ord, R.A. (1993) Multiple synchronous bilateral Warthin's tumors of the parotid glands with pleomorphic adenoma. Case report and review of the literature. *Oral Surg, Oral Med Oral Pathol*, **76**, 319–24.

Leverstein, H., Van der Wal, J.E., Tiwari, R.M., Van der Waal, I., and Snow, G.B. (1997) Results of the surgical management and histopathological evaluation of 88 parotid gland Warthin's tumours. *Clin Otolaryngol*, **22**, 500–3.

Newman, L., Loukota, R.A., and Bradley, P.F. (1993) An infarcted Warthin's tumour presenting with facial weakness. *Br J Oral Maxillofac Surg*, **31**, 311–2.

Renehan, A., Gleave, E.N., Hancock, B.D., Smith, P., and McGurk, M. (1996) Long-term follow-up of over 1000 patients with salivary gland tumours treated in a single centre. *Br J Surg*, **83**, 1750–4.

Seifert, G. (1992) [New pathohistologic WHO classification of salivary gland adenomas]. *Pathologe*, **13**, 322–35.

Seifert, G. and Donath, K. (1996) Multiple tumours of the salivary glands—terminology and nomenclature. *Eur J Cancer B Oral Oncol*, **32**, 3–7.

Warnock, G.R. (1991) Papillary cystadenoma lymphomatosum (Warthin's tumor). In: *Surgical Pathology of the Salivary Glands*. pp. 192. (eds G.L. Ellis, P.L. Auclair, and D.R. Gnepp) W.B. Saunders Co., Philadelphia. pp. 192–201.

Yu, G.Y., Ma, D.Q., Liu, X.B., Zhang, M.Y., and Zhang, Q. (1998) Local excision of the parotid gland in the treatment of Warthin's tumour. *Br J Oral Maxillofac Surg*, **36**, 186–9.

Audience discussion

Mr Webb (Bristol, UK): At Bristol, we have used the operation termed 'controlled enucleation' for Warthin's—I must explain this as it has been denigrated. The method has been described by Steve Ebbs and myself (1986), and in our cases we know the diagnosis before surgery (from FNAC). We used the facial nerve stimulator at all stages. The surgery was undertaken very carefully and the only time the Warthin's tumour was ruptured was when it was both thin and very large. I am sure many people carry adenolymphomas around and they do not progress. Yet suddenly one may undergo dramatic enlargement due to infarction. One of my patients had an adeno-lymphoma for 16 years, the only treatment was aspiration when it filled up, in order to be sure it was not becoming malignant.

Mr Bradley (Nottingham, UK): Have we any evidence that Warthin's tumours will become malignant?

Dr Eveson (Bristol, UK): Yes. There have been isolated cases of carcinomas arising in Warthin's tumours including squamous cell carcinomas, and there have prob-ably been a number of misdiagnoses as well because they can often show either squamous metaplasia or mucous metaplasia, and some of the so-called *mucopedermoid carcinomas arising in Warthin's tumour* have probably been misdiagnosed (Seifert 1997).

Professor O'Brien (Sydney, Australia): Why don't you call those deposits in the related lymph nodes metastases?

Professor van der Waal: Good question; they do not behave like metastases, they do not spread outside the neck but stay in the intra-parotid lymph nodes.

Mr Baraka (Lancaster, UK): How would you explain the 8% incidences of Frey's in extracapsular cases where parotid tissue is not removed?

Mr Webb: I think the answer must be that Mr Nicholson and Mr Gleave (Manchester) did an extracapsular dissection for really large tumours and they did expose the nerve to some extent in the bed of the tumour. My impression is that the risk of Frey's increases in proportion to the degree of dissection in the parotid gland.

Mr Bradley: Both presenters seem to identify smoking as an aetiology factor for Warthin's tumour. Is that really true?

Mr Webb: I think it was Ebbs and myself who first described the association with smoking and the idea was supported by Professor Hobsley (Cadier *et al.* 1992). I think on balance it does fit and there are subsequent publications to back it up (Yoo *et al.* 1994; Yu *et al.* 1998).

REFERENCES

Cadier, M., Watkin, G., and Hobsley, M. (1992) Smoking predisposes to parotid adenolymphoma. *Br J Surg*, **79**, 928–30.

Ebbs, S.R. and Webb, A.J. (1986) Adenolymphoma of the parotid: aetiology, diagnosis and treatment. *Br J Surg*, **73**, 627–30.

Seifert, G. (1997) [Carcinoma in pre-existing Warthin tumors (cystadenolymphoma) of the parotid gland. Classification, pathogenesis and differential diagnosis]. *Pathologe*, **18**, 359–67.

Yoo, G.H., Eisele, D.W., Askin, F.B., Driben, J.S., and Johns, M.E. (1994) Warthin's tumor: a 40-year experience at The Johns Hopkins Hospital. *Laryngoscope*, **104**, 799–803.

Yu, G.Y., Liu, X.B., Li, Z.L., and Peng, X. (1998) Smoking and the development of Warthin's tumour of the parotid gland. *Br J Oral Maxillofac Surg*, **36**, 183–5.

Editorial comment

Two questions are raised by the observation that microscopic multicentric disease is present in over half of the cases of Warthin's. The first is whether this leads to a higher recurrence rate. The second is whether Warthin's is a neoplasm in the true sense of the word. If it is a true tumour, one would expect all these foci to grow inexorably over time and with it would come a powerful argument for superficial or total parotidectomy.

Thankfully, we have the answer. By chance and before anyone was aware of the multicentric nature of the disease, a relatively large number of these tumours were treated by what would have been considered 'inadequate' surgery, i.e. extracapsular dissection. The results show that recurrence with this very conservative approach is rare.

So from a surgical perspective, these histological features of multifoci disease can be ignored although the advice to palpate the gland for additional nodules is appropriate in the circumstances. Multicentricity should not alter the approach to surgery: local dissection is adequate. The problem which remains is whether a disease that is multicentric but does not recur, and which also is present in local lymph nodes but does not disseminate, can be considered a true neoplasm?

CHAPTER 11

Childhood parotid tumours

A surgeon's perspective
Robert Frankenthaler

A paediatric oncologist's perspective
Bernadette Brennan

A surgeon's perspective Robert Frankenthaler

Epidemiology

Epithelial neoplasms in children, neonates, and young adults are rare. It has been estimated that 1–5% of all salivary tumours occur in this population (Kauffman and Stout 1963; Galich 1969; Castro *et al.* 1972; Jacques *et al.* 1976; Bianchi and Cudmore 1978; Shikhani and Johns 1988; Fonseca *et al.* 1991). They comprise 10% of all paediatric head and neck tumours. Primary salivary neoplasms must be differentiated from the more common benign inflammatory processes of mumps, lymphadenopathy, and cysts of branchial, sebaceous, or parotid origin (Krolls *et al.* 1972; Wright *et al.* 1985). In neonates and children under 10 years of age, vascular lesions such as lymphangiomas and haemangiomas are the most common causes of parotid enlargement (Shikhani and Johns 1988). It is in the setting of a young healthy child presenting with salivary gland enlargement with anxious parents that the pediatrician and oncologist must decipher the life-threatening from the self-limited reactive process. An appropriate history, physical exam, viral titres (Epstein–Barr virus human immunodeficiency virus, cytomegalovirus, and mumps), toxoplasmosis titre, and tuberculosis testing will considerably narrow the differential diagnosis. A history of recent viral symptoms, the presence of a cystic lesion, or multiple nodules all point more to the inflammatory and benign aetiologies (Byers *et al.* 1984; Baker and Malone 1985).

Clinical presentation

The heightened concern comes in the setting of an otherwise asymptomatic child presenting with an isolated salivary gland nodule or mass. The nodule may come up quickly or may have been present for several years. Knowledge of the most likely sites, age group, and gender helps to define further the likelihood of a neoplasm. By far the most common site of presentation in young patients is the parotid gland (90%) followed by the submandibular gland (Krolls *et al.* 1972; Schuller and McCabe 1977). There are rare reports of sublingual and minor salivary gland neoplasms comprising less than 1% of all paediatric salivary gland tumours (Hendrick 1964; Danziger 1964). Although there have been isolated reports of neonates and children presenting with salivary neoplasms, they are quite rare. Two-thirds of paediatric salivary tumours occur between the ages of 10 and 16 years (Chong *et al.* 1975; Luna *et al.* 1991). There is a slightly higher incidence in females, comprising 60% of all tumours (Callender *et al.* 1992).

The pathology of childhood salivary tumours

Once an epithelial tumour has been suspected in a child, it is important to consider the fact that the majority of these are malignant (49–70%). Fortunately, most of these tumours are low and intermediate grade, rarely demonstrating negative prognostic findings (Lack and Upton 1988). Mucoepidermoid carcinomas are followed most frequently by adenoid cystic carcinoma and undifferentiated carcinomas, each accounting for 5–10% each (Shikhani and Johns 1988). Acinic cell cancers are slightly more common in this group, which may account for some of the higher incidence of salivary gland cancer in girls. For the benign tumours, the pleomorphic adenoma reigns supreme as the most common benign epithelial neoplasm. Other benign tumours such as monomorphic adenomas, Warthin's tumours, myoepithelial epitheliomas, and the unusual embryoma (sialoblastoma) are rare but have been reported (Batsakis and Frankenthaler 1992).

As with their adult counterparts, most paediatric salivary tumours are, therefore, low- to intermediate-grade mucoepidermoid carcinomas, or pleomorphic adenomas involving the superficial lobe of the parotid gland. For these tumours, I do not routinely obtain a fine needle aspiration (FNAC) or an imaging study. For the rare minor salivary gland tumour, sublingual tumour, deep lobe parotid tumour, undifferentiated lesion, or unresectable tumour, I would obtain imaging.

Treatment

The treatment of any salivary gland tumour begins and ends with a carefully thought out and executed surgical plan. Radiation treatment in this population carries additional long-term risks and only highlights the need for a very skilled oncological surgeon. With the establishment of the efficacy of post-operative radiation's ability to decrease the incidence of local–regional recurrence, perhaps some surgeons have tried to perform mere enucleations and to be less concerned about microscopic residual disease. The need to perform a complete tumour resection is paramount whether the patient is young or old. As paediatric tumours more frequently involve the superficial lobe of the parotid or submandibular gland and are more often of low grade, an *en bloc* resection should be more possible. Leaving disease not only complicates a patient's prognosis but it necessitates the need for radiation. For children, the risks of epiphyseal damage, facial deformity, long-term risk of osteoradionecrosis, and post-radiation sarcomas cannot be minimized by any current treatment protocol. Simply stated, the treatment plan is the same for the young or old. The cost of leaving disease and needing adjunctive radiation treatment to clean up residual disease is greater for children and adolescents. For most of the paediatric salivary gland tumours, complete removal of the tumour with nerve preservation should be curative without the need for radiation. A neck dissection is indicated only in the rare patient who presents with clinical or radiological evidence of regional disease.

Aggressive disease is the exception

Infrequently, there are tumours occurring in children that may require more aggressive therapy. It used to be thought that as long as a surgeon could find a larger area to remove, surgery could cure all solid tumours of the salivary gland. Unfortunately, this premise resulted in higher rates of recurrence. Clearly, there are tumour properties that do not lend themselves to cure by surgery alone.

Similarly to their adult counterparts, tumours demonstrating perineural invasion, soft tissue invasions, intralymphatic invasion, or significant extracapsular lymph node involvement will require combined treatment. Fortunately for the children, the need for radiation should be rare. The indiscriminate use of radiation for all salivary neoplasms, and particularly in children, should be stopped.

Outcome

Given our knowledge of the histological location and malignant potential of most child-hood salivary gland tumours, survival should be excellent. Callender and colleagues (1992), from the M.D. Anderson Hospital, reported 2- and 5-year survival rates of 100 and 90%, respectively. The factors most commonly associated with poor survival are high-grade, perineural invasion, intravascular or lymphatic invasion, extraglandular parotid extension, and lymph node metastasis. The survival rates for these tumours (20–30%) mirror those of the adult tumours. Distant metastases in this high-risk population and lack of adequate treatment for this greatly contribute to the overall poor outcomes.

For these reasons, I propose nothing radical other than that the surgeon be gifted with good surgical technique and judgement so that he will remove the disease completely and with minimal lasting deformity.

A paediatric oncologist's perspective Bernadette Brennan

The proportion of malignant salivary tumours of childhood

In common with the epidemiology of salivary gland tumours in general (Chapter 1), accurate population-based descriptive statistics for childhood salivary neoplasms are also lacking. Problems frequently are encountered with the definition of childhood

Table 11.1 Childhood salivary tumours

	Total	Children	Remark	Site			Epithelial tumours	
				Parotid	Submandibular	Minor	Benign	Malignant
Population-based								
Bianchi and Cudmore (1978)	937	12 (1.3)	≤16 years	12	0	0	10	2 (17)
North West Region UK*		25	≤16 years	21	3	1	17	8 (32)
Surgical series								
Castro et al. (1972)	2135	38 (1.8)	≤16 years	33	5	0	19	19 (50)
Krolls et al. (1972)	9993	430 (4.3)	<15 years	Not stated	Not stated	Not stated	60	35 (37)
Callender et al. (1992)	1822	29 (1.6)	≤16 years	21	Not included	Not included	8	21 (72)
Christie series†	1194	23 (1.9)	≤16 years	22	1	0	18	5 (22)
Pathology series								
Lack and Upton (1988)		80	<18 years	79	1		10	15 (60)
AFIP (1991)	13263	422 (3.2)	≤16 years	Not stated	Not stated	Not stated	210	212 (50)

Values in parentheses are percentages.

* Unpublished data. Period 1956–1996 (Courtesy of Professor J. Birch).

† Unpublished data. Period 1952–1992 (Courtesy of Mr A. Renehan).

(which should be 16 years and under) and also the range of pathology. There is general agreement in adult salivary tumours that the denominator is epithelial neoplasms but, as numbers are often small in childhood series, there is a temptation to include mesenchymal and other neoplasms.

Against this background, a review of the larger published series of childhood salivary gland tumours was undertaken and analysed (Table 11.1). To these data were added figures from the North West Childhood Tumour Registry (1956–1996) which covers a North West population of 12 million people (courtesy of Professor J. Birch, Manchester). This is a comprehensive Cancer Research Campaign-supported database which is inclusive of all childhood tumours, and is updated every 2 years. In particular, the author addressed the perception in the literature that there is an increased proportion (>50%) of malignant salivary tumours in childhood, compared with adults. The summary data suggest that this is indeed true for surgical and pathology series, but that this is probably a misrepresentation due to referral biases. In a retrospective review of the Merseyside population, Bianchi and Cudmore (1978) found 12 childhood tumours over a two-decade period (1951–1973), but only two of these were malignant. In the North West of England series of 25 cases, the proportion of malignant tumours was only 32%. This suggests that the reported 50% of malignant salivary tumours in childhood is probably an overestimate, and that the figure is closer to 20–30%.

In common with adult salivary tumours, the majority of childhood tumours are in the parotid gland. The 10:1 ratio rule for parotid to submandibular tumours (Chapter 1) seems to hold, but minor salivary gland tumours are reported infrequently, and the assumption is that they are very rare.

Clinical presentation and initial management

In a paediatric oncology practice, the most common cause of parotid swelling is leukaemic infiltration, which typically is bilateral (Fig. 11.1). This is included here as it is seldom referred to in the surgical literature.

The differential diagnosis of a unilateral salivary swelling (principally parotid gland) is that of a 'lump in the neck'. Inflammatory processes of mumps and other viruses, juvenile recurrent parotitis, tuberculosis, lymphadenopathy and Goodman's syndrome, and branchial cysts form the differential diagnosis. For childhood salivary tumours, the relative proportions for different diagnoses differ by age. This is illustrated for the cumulative data from six different studies shown in Fig. 11.2. There is a peak of haemangiomas and vascular anomalies in the first 3 years of life, when other neoplasms are very rare. After 5 years of age, primary epithelial neoplasm are encountered with the above caveat; malignant epithelial

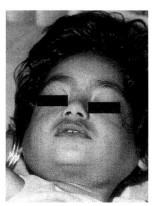

Fig. 11.1 A 6-year-old boy with bilateral parotid swelling secondary to leukaemic infiltrates. The diagnosis is obvious from the clinical history, blood count, and bone marrow examination. This is a common observation in paediatric oncology practice. The parotid swelling resolves within days following commencement of chemotherapy.

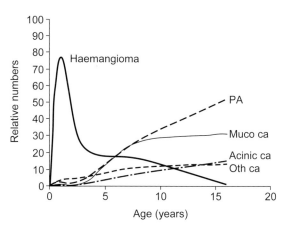

Fig. 11.2 Relative number of cases of different salivary gland tumours by age categories in childhood. Haem, haemangioma; PA, pleomorphic adenoma; Muco ca, mucoepidermoid carcinoma; Acinic ca, acinic cell carcinoma; oth Ca, other carcinomas. Cumulative data from six studies [Castro 1972; Krolls *et al.* 1972; AFIP 1991; Callender *et al.* 1992; Christie Hospital unpublished data (1952–1992) (Mr A. Renehan); North West Childhood Tumour Registry (1956–96) (Professor J. Birch)].

tumours account for 20–30%. Most carcinomas are either mucoepidermoid or acinic cell carcinomas, and are low grade. For the benign tumours, almost all are pleomorphic adenomas.

As the treatment of rare tumours should be centralized, salivary gland childhood tumours should not be an exception. There is considerable evidence that one of the main reasons underlying the large improvements in childhood cancer survival (in general) over the last 3 years has been attributable to centralization. While there is no direct evidence for this in salivary tumours (because they are rare), basic principles would dictate so. The centralized team includes head and neck surgeons familiar with childhood tumours and surgery, paediatric and radiation oncologists, paediatric anaesthetists, radiologists, and pathologists.

Solitary superficial lumps in the parotid gland may be treated adequately by surgery alone with no untoward consequences, because in the majority of cases the histology will be a pleomorphic adenoma or a low-grade carcinoma. We stress that anything else 'a bit unusual' should be evaluated thoroughly pre-operatively. In this regard, we find cross-sectional imaging very helpful in planning the extent of surgery. In my paediatric oncology practice, I still see head and neck lumps where surgeons 'had a go' without really thinking about the diagnosis—the consequences can be unnecessary morbidity, and can even be fatal. We do not find FNAC useful, as it: (i) requires a general anaesthetic to perform in young children; (ii) is generally not accurate enough conclusively to diagnose 'the unusual' tumour; and (iii) is equally not accurate enough to diagnosis the benign inflammatory processes.

The late-effects clinic

The complications following radiotherapy for salivary gland tumours have been alluded to in Chapter 7. In children, there are additional problems or 'late effects' (Box 11.1). For almost two decades, the long-term effects of cancer therapy in survivors of childhood malignancies in the Greater Manchester area have been monitored in late-effects clinics. The psychological, cardio-respiratory, and endocrine effects in

Box 11.1 Potential late effects from radiotherapy for childhood salivary tumours

Second tumours

◆ second primary tumour

◆ radiation-induced second tumour

Retarded facial skeletal growth

◆ cosmetic deformities

◆ dental malocclusion

◆ psychological problems

Anterior pituitary hormone deficiencies

(oropharyngeal and nasopharyngeal cancers only)

Others (detailed in Chapter 6)

◆ xerostomia

◆ osteoradionecrosis

◆ otitis externa

◆ sensorineural damage to the cochlea

this cohort have been described for the more common cancers such a leukaemia (Brennan *et al.* 1998; Murray *et al.* 1999). Childhood salivary gland tumours are rare and what is said here is based not on quantifiable data but experience gained in related areas.

Radiation-induced tumour and second primary tumours

From the outset, a distinction should be drawn between second tumours occurring in a field of radiation therapy in which the radiation received may have contributed to the development of that tumour, and a second primary tumour (SPT) developing *de novo* and not necessarily within the same site of origin. In the absence of radiotherapy, the risk of SPT represents a form of genetic predisposition. After all first childhood tumours (except retinoblastoma), the inherent risk of a SPT is fourfold (Hawkins 1990). Among a cohort of almost 10 000 survivors of childhood cancers (excluding retinoblastoma) treated in Britain before 1980, there were no SPTs of salivary gland origin.

Several studies from survivors of the Hiroshima and Nagasaki atomic bombs have shown an association between radiation exposure and the subsequent development of salivary gland neoplasia (Chapter 2). In particular, these studies demonstrate: (i) a dose–response relationship; (ii) a relatively long latency period; and (iii) a stronger yield of malignant neoplasia that that of benign tumours. Experience from other childhood tumours has demonstrated a real but moderate increase in risk of radiation-induced second tumours within a radiation field (Bhatia *et al.* 1996). However, the evidence for salivary gland tumours is lacking. Specifically, a distinction should be made between true radiation-induced second tumours and carcinoma arising within recurrent pleomorphic adenomas. To date, there are no cohorts large enough to detect discernibly an increased risk of radiation-induced malignancy following radiation for childhood salivary tumours.

Mandibular growth retardation

The growth centre in the mandibular condyle is responsible for the majority of lengthening and forward growth of the lower jaw during puberty and post-pubertal modelling of the facial skeleton. This area is directly within the radiation field for parotid gland tumours. Experience from other anatomical sites shows that chondrocytes are very sensitive to radiation and, therefore, unilateral retardation of mandibular growth is a real potential problem following radiotherapy. The results are facial asymmetry, dental malocclusion, and temporomandibular joint dysfunction. The cosmetic deformity may predispose to a variety of psychological anxieties. However, we are unaware of any data which have quantified the incidence or severity of these problems, though we have seen a small number of severe cases in our clinic.

Radiation and pituitary dysfunction

Deficiency of one or more anterior pituitary hormones may follow treatment with external radiation when the hypothalmic–pituitary axis falls within the fields of radiation. This is a distinct possibility for rare salivary gland malignancies of the naso- and oropharynx. In general, the pituitary falls outside the radiation fields for parotid tumours, though there are no studies which have searched for hitherto unrecognized hormone deficiencies.

There is a well recognized pattern of loss of anterior pituitary hormones following radiation—growth hormone (GH) > gonadotropin or cortiotropin > thyroid-stimulating hormone (TSH)—that are dose and latency dependent. The threshold for damage is lower in children compared with adults (Shalet 1993; Shalet and Brennan 1998). For most patients, these deficiencies are subclinical, but the importance of detecting them is borne out by the benefits in quality of life and mortality gained from replacement therapy of the appropriate hormone.

REFERENCES

Baker, S.R. and Malone, B. (1985) Salivary gland malignancies in children. *Cancer*, **55**, 1730–6.

Batsakis, J.G. and Frankenthaler, R. (1992) Embryoma (sialoblastoma) of salivary glands. *Ann Otol Rhinol Laryngol*, **101**, 958–60.

Bhatia, S., Robison, L.L., Oberlin, O., Greenberg, M., Bunin, G., Fossati Bellani, F. *et al.* (1996) Breast cancer and other second neoplasms after childhood Hodgkin's disease. *N Engl J Med*, **334**, 745–51.

Bianchi, A. and Cudmore, R.E. (1978) Salivary gland tumors in children. *J Pediatr Surg*, **13**, 519–21.

Brennan, B.M., Rahim, A., Mackie, E.M., Eden, O.B., and Shalet, S.M. (1998) Growth hormone status in adults treated for acute lymphoblastic leukaemia in childhood. *Clin Endocrinol Oxf*, **48**, 777–83.

Byers, R.M., Piorkowski, R., and Luna, M.A. (1984) Malignant parotid tumors in patients under 20 years of age. *Arch Otolaryngol*, **110**, 232–5.

Callender, D.L., Frankenthaler, R.A., Luna, M.A., Lee, S.S., and Goepfert, H. (1992) Salivary gland neoplasms in children. *Arch Otolaryngol Head Neck Surg*, **118**, 472–6.

Castro, E.B., Huvos, A.G., Strong, E.W., and Foote, F.W., Jr (1972) Tumors of the major salivary glands in children. *Cancer*, **29**, 312–7.

Chong, G.C., Beahrs, O.H., Chen, M.L., and Hayles, A.B. (1975) Management of parotid gland tumors in infants and children. *Mayo Clin Proc*, **50**, 279–83.

Danziger, H. (1964) Adenoid cystic carcinoma of the submaxillary gland in an 8-month-old infant. *Can Med Assoc J* **91**, 759–61.

Fonseca, I., Martins, A.G., and Soares, J. (1991) Epithelial salivary gland tumors of children and adolescents in southern Portugal. A clinicopathologic study of twenty-four cases. *Oral Surg, Oral Med Oral Pathol*, **72**, 696–701.

Galich, R. (1969) Salivary gland neoplasms in childhood. *Arch Otolaryngol*, **89**, 878–82.

Hawkins, M.M. (1990) Second primary tumors following radiotherapy for childhood cancer. *Int J Radiat Oncol Biol Phys*, **19**, 1297–301.

Hendrick, J.W. (1964) Mucoepidermoid cancer of the parotid gland in a one-year-old child. *Am J Surg*, **108**, 907–909.

Jaques, D.A., Krolls, S.O., and Chambers, R.G. (1976) Parotid tumors in children. *Am J Surg*, **132**, 469–71.

Kauffman, S.I. and Stout, A.P. (1963) Tumours of the major salivary glands in children. *Cancer*, **16**, 1317–31.

Krolls, S.O., Trodahl, J.N., and Boyers, R.C. (1972) Salivary gland lesions in children. A survey of 430 cases. *Cancer*, **30**, 459–69.

Lack, E.E. and Upton, M.P. (1988) Histopathologic review of salivary gland tumors in childhood. *Arch Otolaryngol Head Neck Surg*, **114**, 898–906.

Luna, M.A., Tortoledo, M.E., Ordonez, N.G., Frankenthaler, R.A., and Batsakis, J.G. (1991) Primary sarcomas of the major salivary glands. *Arch Otolaryngol Head Neck Surg*, **117**, 302–6.

Murray, R.D., Brennan, B.M., Rahim, A., and Shalet, S.M. (1999) Survivors of childhood cancer: long-term endocrine and metabolic problems dwarf the growth disturbance. *Acta Paediatr Suppl*, **88**, 5–12.

Schuller, D.E. and McCabe, B.F. (1977) Salivary gland neoplasms in children. *Otolaryngol Clin North Am*, **10**, 399–412.

Shalet, S.M. (1993) Radiation and pituitary dysfunction. *N Engl J Med*, **328**, 131–3.

Shalet, S.M. and Brennan, B.M. (1998) Growth and growth hormone status following treatment for childhood leukaemia. *Horm Res*, **50**, 1–10.

Shikhani, A.H. and Johns, M.E. (1988) Tumors of the major salivary glands in children. *Head Neck Surg*, **10**, 257–63.

Wright, G.L., Smith, R.J., Katz, C.D., and Atkins, J.H., Jr (1985) Benign parotid diseases of childhood. *Laryngoscope*, **95**, 915–20.

Audience discussion

Mr Bradley (Nottingham, UK): What is the life expectancy of children with salivary cancers?

Dr Frankenthaler: The high-risk patients, the very few patients with undifferentiated carcinoma (3–4%), have a very poor outcome. The vast majority of children (90–95%) have a good outcome.

Dr Brennan: A question to Dr Franthenthaler, do you routinely use cross-sectional imaging in children or perhaps, put another way, do you use cross-sectional imaging more frequently in children that adults?

Dr Frankenthaler: If it is a submandibular tumour or a lateral lobe tumour, as in the adult, I have not found that imaging provides additional useful information over and above clinical examination. I agree with Dr Brennan that in tumours that are frankly malignant or where there is something unusual, then such investigations are essential.

Dr Brennan: I would like to reiterate a point. I listened this morning to Professor McGurk listing his selective indications for the use of FNAC. He included children, clarifying that an FNAC indicating a non-neoplastic process, e.g. in a lymph node, would avoid unnecessary surgery. I actually disagree with this approach. I listed three reasons why FNAC is not very useful; the most important is that it is not very practical. I add a further comment. When children present with lumps anywhere in the body, parents immediately think 'cancer'. They equate 'cancer' with 'tumour', as in their mind, all childhood tumours are malignant. Parents are not reassured by the results of an FNAC—they need reassurance with the definitive answer by histological biopsy.

Editorial comment

Childhood tumours place the clinician on the horns of a dilemma. On the one hand there is the rarity of childhood parotid tumours. Most parotid lumps in children are of inflammatory or developmental origin and there is a risk of inadvertently treating an inflammatory lump by parotidectomy. However, neoplasms do occur and, compared with adults, there is an increased risk of encountering a low-grade cancer. Inappropriate treatment carries greater consequences than in an adult. The other horn of the dilemma is that the patient is a child and this gives rise to a well intended but mistaken propensity towards surgical conservatism. This can create a cascade of errors commencing with a report of inadequate excision of (say) low-grade mucoepidermoid carcinoma and the option either to re-excise with its attendant morbidity or radical radiotherapy with complications of defective growth. The careful planning of treatment is therefore essential, and this requires clear evidence of cancer to be obtained at the outset. In this regard, the multidisciplinary team is a prerequisite, and in the difficult case there may be a real role for FNAC.

CHAPTER 12

Morbidity following surgery for benign parotid disease

Christopher O'Brien

Introduction

The aim of parotid surgery is to cure the patient of the pathological process and preserve normal function of the facial nerve. In the management of benign parotid diseases, there is no latitude for facial nerve sacrifice. Benign parotid tumours and inflammatory conditions rarely cause facial nerve dysfunction and, in this setting, nerve preservation is virtually mandatory.

Successful preservation of facial nerve anatomy and function depends on the factors listed in Box 12.1, and are the focus of this chapter.

Facial nerve identification

A number of techniques have been described for identification of the facial nerve at the time of parotid surgery. This author believes that the safest technique involves the use of fixed bony landmarks and the most useful of these is the *tympanomastoid fissure* (O'Brien *et al.* 1993). The tympanomastoid fissure is best identified following initial

Box 12.1 **Successful preservation of the facial nerve**

- ◆ An understanding of the anatomy, permitting safe identification of the facial nerve
- ◆ Meticulous surgical technique facilitating gentle dissection of the facial nerve
- ◆ An awareness that local anatomical and pathological factors may mitigate against normal post-operative facial nerve function
- ◆ Utilization of available techniques and technology to guarantee a good outcome

dissection and identification of the anterior border of the *sternomastoid* muscle and the upper border of the posterior belly of *digastric* muscle. A plane carried vertically through the tympanomastoid fissure will mark the entry of the facial nerve into the parotid gland. This is an exceedingly reliable landmark allowing identification of the trunk of the facial nerve. This author does not use the cartilaginous pointer to assist with nerve localization, and techniques involving retrograde dissection following identification of peripheral facial nerve branches are difficult.

Dissection of the facial nerve

Surgeons will have their own techniques for parotid dissection. The author prefers a technique which makes use of curved mosquito forceps. This allows gentle and accurate dissection on the facial nerve, during which parotid tissue is lifted and separated from the nerve in a single movement. The elevated tissue is then incised with bipolar diathermy scissors. Haemostasis should be achieved by application of small haemostatic clips or bipolar diathermy. Unipolar diathermy should not be used. Magnification is preferred by some surgeons to assist with identification of facial nerve branches. In general, the author only uses magnification in re-do parotid surgery.

Anatomical and pathological considerations

In a previous report, the author published his experience with 259 parotidectomies among 248 patients (Bron and O'Brien 1997). The aim was to correlate the incidence of post-operative facial nerve dysfunction with the clinical and pathological setting. In that study, localized previously untreated tumours lying in the superficial lobe of the parotid gland were treated by 'limited superficial parotidectomy'. This involved removal of the tumour with a surrounding cuff of normal parotid tissue, recognizing that in the majority of cases a 'bare area' of tumour, not covered by parotid tissue, would be present, as this frequently was the narrowest plane of separation from the facial nerve. Patients with sialadenitis were treated either with complete superficial parotidectomy, removing all tissue superficial to the plane of the facial nerve, or 'near total' parotidectomy, removing the entire superficial lobe and as much of the deep lobe as could be extirpated from between the branches of the facial nerve. Patients with deep lobe tumours, that is those lying deep to the plane of the facial nerve, were also treated with near total parotidectomy, removing the superficial lobe initially. The tumour was then dissected carefully and delivered from beneath the branches of the facial nerve. Patients with massive, aggressively invasive, or recurrent malignant tumours were treated with radical total parotidectomy where the entire parotid gland was removed and the facial nerve intentionally sacrificed. Some patients with malignant disease also had a neck dissection with the parotidectomy.

Analysis of the outcome of facial nerve function, judged clinically, is demonstrated for our series and a number of other studies in Table 12.1. In our study, there were 221 patients who had normal facial nerve function pre-operatively, a total of 62 (28%) with initial post-operative weakness, and 11 (5%) with permanent facial nerve injury.

Table 12.1 Incidence of facial nerve injury encountered following parotid surgery for benign disease

	Permanent nerve injury			Transient nerve injury		
	Sydney series (n = 221)	Mehle et al. (n = 256)	Laccourreye et al. (n = 256)	Sydney series (n = 221)	Mehle et al. (n = 256)	Laccourreye et al. (n = 256)
Limited superficial parotidectomy	0/122	–	–	18/122 (15)	–	–
Superficial parotidectomy	0/13	6/173 (3)	–	4/13 (30)	118/256 (46)*	–
Near total parotidectomy	–	4/69 (6)	9/256 (4)	–	–	161/256 (63)
Benign deep lobe tumours	1/31 (4)	–	–	11/31 (34)	–	–
Sialadenitis	0/32	–	–	10/32 (31)	–	–
Parotidectomy with neck dissection	10/23 (43)	–	–	19/23 (83)	–	–

Values in parentheses are percentages.

* No distinction was made between rates for different surgical procedures.

Among those with permanent weakness, the majority (10/11) involved only as far as the lower lip due to injury to the marginal mandibular nerve during a combined parotidectomy and neck dissection for malignant disease. These results compare favourably with other reported series. Mehle *et al.* (1993) reported a 50% incidence of initial postoperative facial weakness in 256 patients treated over a 15-year period for benign parotid conditions at the Cleveland Clinic. Laccourreye *et al.* (1994) described postoperative facial weakness in 66% of (also) 256 patients undergoing total parotidectomy for parotid pleomorphic adenoma over a 25-year period. Permanent facial nerve weakness was approximately 4% in both series.

This author's current experience is that patients with a previously untreated, localized, superficially located tumour have an approximately 10% risk of temporary facial weakness with 100% likelihood of recovery within 3 months of surgery. It is important, however, that patients with chronic sialadenitis, recurrent tumours, tumours involving the deep lobe of the parotid gland, those with invasive malignant tumours, and those patients requiring a neck dissection with their parotidectomy are warned that the risk of initial facial nerve dysfunction is likely to be 30% or more. Permanent dysfunction is uncommon, although parotidectomy combined with neck dissection remains a problem, with weakness of the marginal mndibular branch of the nerve being common and recovery slow.

Reducing operative risk

More recently, the author has made use of continuous intra-operative facial nerve monitoring using a Nerve Integrity Monitor (Xomed™) in order to reduce the likelihood of facial nerve injury in high-risk patients. In a relatively small experience of 20 patients, the Nerve Integrity Monitor has proved useful, but it remains unclear whether this makes parotid surgery safer in the hands of experienced surgeons. It has, however, been shown to be most useful as a training tool for surgical registrars and residents, and may improve the safety of parotid surgery in the hands of qualified but less experienced surgeons. It may also improve the safety of parotid surgery where the facial nerve can be clearly seen but the pathological process dictates the need for dissection and manipulation of individual facial nerve branches.

REFERENCES

Bron, L.P. and O' Brien, C.J. (1997) Facial nerve function after parotidectomy. *Arch Otolaryngol Head Neck Surg*, **123**, 1091–6.

Laccourreye, H., Laccourreye, O., Cauchois, R., Jouffre, V., Menard, M., and Brasnu, D. (1994) Total conservative parotidectomy for primary benign pleomorphic adenoma of the parotid gland: a 25-year experience with 229 patients. *Laryngoscope*, **104**, 1487–94.

Mehle, M.E., Kraus, D.H., Wood, B.G., Benninger, M.S., Eliachar, I., Levine, H.L. *et al.* (1993) Facial nerve morbidity following parotid surgery for benign disease: the Cleveland Clinic Foundation experience. *Laryngoscope*, **103**, 386–8.

O'Brien, C.J., Malka, V.B., and Mijailovic, M. (1993) Evaluation of 242 consecutive parotidectomies performed for benign and malignant disease. *Aust NZ J Surg*, **63**, 870–7.

Audience discussion

Professor Snow (Amsterdam, The Netherlands): You alluded to the high incidence of permanent facial nerve deficit when neck dissection was added to a parotidectomy. An in continuity parotid neck dissection is a wrestling match with respect to the *ramus mandibularis* branch of the facial nerve. Speaking for myself, I am not at all persuaded that continuity is essential oncologically and I am certain that discontinuity dissection makes it easier to preserve the ramus.

Professor O'Brien: Yes, our dissections are done in continuity with the neck but I agree there is no oncological argument against a discontinuous procedure for we do it all the time in the oral cavity. I agree, the nerve can be preserved more predictably with a discontinuous procedure.

Mr Renehan (Manchester, UK): Increasing age has been reported as a negative predictor for facial nerve injury, and it is proposed that this may be due to is ischaemic damage to the nerve (Mra *et al.* 1993). Do you think this is a real issue in the athero-sclerotic patient and, if so, should we refrain from using hypotensive anaesthesia?

Professor O'Brien: I do not know why age is a factor, I think the scientific basis for that observation is pretty thin really.

Professor Snow: Did you say you never use retrograde dissection of the nerve?

Professor O'Brien: The only time I would use it is when I had to re-operate on the gland and I had difficulty identifying the nerve by antegrade dissection. The facial nerve is almost always identifiable using fixed bony landmarks whereas the peripheral branches are one-eighth the size and have no precise landmarks, so it does not make a lot of sense to me.

Professor Snow: In the case of large tumours wedged between the mandible and mastoid, I do not understand how you get them out without a retrograde dissection.

Professor O'Brien: All I can say is that I have not found myself in a position where I wanted to use the retrograde technique.

Question from the floor: In elderly patients who may be on aspirin for cardiovascular prophylaxis, do you take any special precautions?

Professor O'Brien: No. If I get a haematoma I think it is my fault. There are so many people on aspirin it is not practical to delay treatment for 3 months. In my opinion, it is the elderly hypertensive who is at risk of haematoma.

Mr Bradley (Nottingham, UK): What is your policy on informed consent with regards the risk of facial nerve injury and other complications?

Professor O'Brien: I inform each individual that virtually all patients get an area of numbness at the angle of the jaw. I do not routinely preserve the greater auricular nerve. The area of numbness tends to reduce with time and I do not believe it is a serious issue. I do not warn them about Frey's syndrome although its incidence is much higher than 8% or 15%, especially if you search for it prospectively. In relation to facial nerve injury, I provide the figures from my own data rather than use published data.

Mr Webb (Bristol, UK): Do you think the use of a nerve stimulator or suction drainage at the end of the procedure has an effect on facial nerve weakness?

Professor O'Brien: No, I do not think you can blame the drain. I do not use a facial nerve stimulator to find the nerve. We occasionally use it in difficult circumstances but I do not think that contributes to the weakness either really.

Mr Thomas (London, UK): I would like to discuss elective node dissection in the management of melanoma. You had 172 melanoma parotidectomies and 100 of them were elective?

Professor O'Brien: Approximately yes. Initially it was our practice in the Sydney Melanoma Unit to undertake elective parotidectomy if the parotid gland lay in the drainage field of the melanoma. We analysed the data and published the results. Following this paper, we changed our policy and no longer do elective parotidectomy.

Mr Bradley: Could we revisit this issue of selective deep lobe dissection which Professor Snow has described? The inference is that dissection can be accomplished without recourse to any form of superficial parotid dissection. Your approach seems to be a superficial dissection first followed by a deep lobe dissection.

Professor O'Brien: I think there are a couple of issues here. There is an entity which I do not think should be called a deep lobe tumour but probably a retromandibular tumour. You could describe it as a parapharyngeal lump when the tumour grows mainly medially and presents as a parapharyngeal mass. I believe these tumours can be removed via the neck above the posterior belly of the digastric without looking for the nerve. If it presents as a superficial lump but at the time of dissection you find that it is deep to the plane of a nerve, then I find the main trunk of the facial nerve, dissect the superficial lobe as far as I think is appropriate to gain access to the main bulk of the tumour, and deliver it from under the nerve. I am sure that it is not terribly different from what Professor Snow has described; perhaps he undertakes less dissection of the superficial lobe.

Mr Webb: With deep lobe tumours it is not possible to predict the position of the nerve no matter how sophisticated the imaging modality one uses. You have to do identify the nerve surgically before you can tackle the lesion.

Professor Snow: Of course you need to know where the nerve is and you need to lift the superficial lobe but only when the tumour is extending between the two main divisions of the nerve into the superficial lobe. Then the superficial lobe has to be sacrificed as well. But otherwise there is no reason to remove the superficial lobe. You only need to lift it as far as the distal margin of the deep lobe tumour which is then removed and the superficial lobe replaced. I can guarantee they have no Frey's syndrome. The extent to which you lift the superficial lobe depends on the position of the tumour. If the tumour is deep to only the cervical facial division of the nerve, then the superficial lobe has only to be lifted a very short distance. If the lesion is deep to the zygomatic and temporal branches, you have to lift the superficial lobe to a greater extent. But if you replace the superficial lobe you spare the patient Frey's syndrome and produce a better facial contour.

Dr Frankenthaler (Boston, USA): Isn't the defining anatomical landmark the stylo-mandibular ligament? If the tumour is in the parapharyngeal space deep to the stylo-mandibular ligament, that is when you can cut the digastric, the stylohoid muscles and come straight up through the neck, pull the mandible up and take out that tumour. If the tumour is more superficial to the stylomandibular ligament, that is when the superficial lobe of the parotid has to be lifted up or the more traditional method of superficial parotidectomy is used to remove it. Do you have any comments?

Professor Snow: It is hard to make a comment because there are many surgical varia-tions. But I believe you are saying there are situations where you do not need to lift the superficial lobe.

Dr Frankenthaler: That is correct.

Mra, Z., Komisar, A., and Blaugrund, S.M. (1993) Functional facial nerve weakness after surgery for benign parotid tumors: a multivariate statistical analysis. *Head Neck*, **15**, 147–52.

Editorial comment

The facial nerve dominates parotid surgery, and superficial parotidectomy is in fact a dissection of the facial nerve. Several ill-defined factors influence facial nerve damage but the one consistent feature that correlates with nerve injury is the mag-nitude of surgery. The more the nerve is handled, the greater the risk of injury. It follows that any surgical technique that minimizes exposure or handling of the nerve will reduce morbidity.

One of the current proposals to reduce injury is continuous intra-operative facial nerve monitoring. However, Professor O'Brien's contribution has shown that while continual facial nerve monitoring has reduced the transient neuropraxia from 60 to 30%, the data from hospital departments with long experience of parotid surgery is temporary paralysis of 30% without such monitoring. In short, this is another example of one of the leitmotifs of this conference, that skill of the individual surgeon is important to obtain good results. The other factors that influence facial nerve palsy include advanced age; this is not to be taken as an increased risk arising from operative surgery but rather a failure of regeneration following injury due to the ageing process. The size of the tumour affects facial nerve palsy, which is not surprising since the greater the dissection of the nerve the more the risk of nerve damage. A third factor is the duration of symptoms in patients with chronic paroti-tis, as the longer the illness the greater the likelihood of fibrosis within the gland, with all its attendant difficulties in obtaining a dissection plane. The risk in inflammatory disease is more than with benign tumours for this reason. Finally, and self-evidently, a history of previous parotid surgery increases the risk of facial nerve damage.

Malignant Neoplasms

CHAPTER 13

Factors affecting survival in salivary gland cancers

Ronald Spiro

Is clinical staging for salivary cancer too complex?

Regardless of their persuasion, oncologists today will agree that clinical staging plays a critical role in the management of the cancer patient. Stage is essential for proper treatment planning. Moreover, assessments of results are meaningless unless patients with similarly staged tumours are compared. Only 25 years ago, surgeons operating for salivary gland tumours relied almost exclusively on the histological diagnosis when selecting the procedure to be performed. This was obvious in 1975, when Conley published his classic text entitled *Salivary Glands and the Facial Nerve* (Conley 1975). Of the 278 patients with malignant parotid tumours treated by surgeons on the staff of the Pack Medical Foundation, 187 (67%) had an operation which involved resection of the facial nerve. Later in his book, Conley asserted that the 'minimal procedure' in patients with adenoid cystic carcinoma in the parotid gland should be total radical parotidectomy.

Coincidentally, it was also in 1975 that we published a review of 288 patients who received their initial, definitive treatment for parotid gland carcinoma at Sloan-Kettering Memorial Cancer Center (Spiro *et al.* 1975). In this series, the facial nerve was preserved in more than two-thirds of the patients and 58% had less than a total parotidectomy. It was obvious that the extent of the surgery performed had been based, at least partly, on the extent of the tumour.

This observation led us to stage these patients retrospectively. We proposed a simple system which defined 3 and 6 cm as the break points for T stages 1–3 (including facial nerve involvement and extraglandular extension as T3), and suggested N negative versus N positive for classification of the neck. This system had the enormous advantage of simplicity, and our statistical analysis indicated a strong correlation between local recurrence, distant metastasis, and cumulative survival with increasing tumour stage. With modification to bring it in line with T–N–M classification in other sites, this staging system was adopted by the American Joint Committee for Cancer Staging

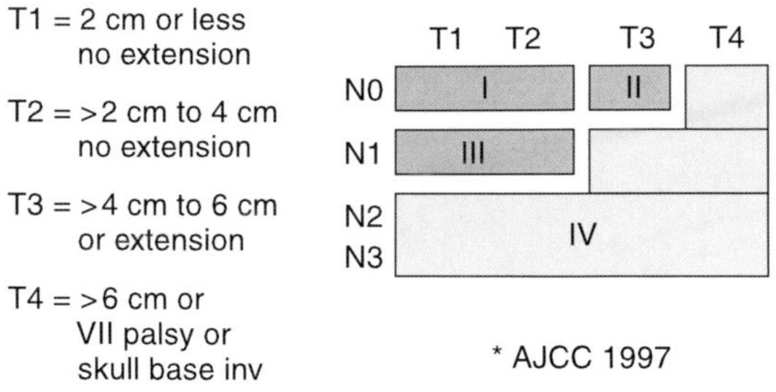

T1 = 2 cm or less
no extension

T2 = >2 cm to 4 cm
no extension

T3 = >4 cm to 6 cm
or extension

T4 = >6 cm or
VII palsy or
skull base inv

	T1	T2	T3	T4
N0	I		II	
N1	III			
N2	IV			
N3				

* AJCC 1997

Fig. 13.1 Clinical staging of major salivary gland carcinoma according to the 1997 version of the American Joint Committee for Cancer (AJCC) staging system.

(AJCC 1978; Levitt *et al.* 1981). Subsequent revisions added to the complexity, but this seems to have been at least partially resolved in the latest version published in 1997 (AJCC, 1997) (Fig. 13.1).

More recently, we reviewed a 45-year experience with 378 previously untreated minor salivary gland cancers in order to verify a long-standing presumption that criteria for staging oral squamous were suitable for minor salivary carcinomas (Spiro *et al.* 1991). Sufficient data were available to stage retrospectively all but 25 of these tumours. Multivariate analysis confirmed that these criteria were just as useful for predicting results in patients who received treatment for minor salivary gland carcinomas in comparable sites. The lower survival rate previously noted in univariate analysis of patients with sinus tumours (Spiro 1986) was not substantiated in this multifactorial assessment, indicating that the difference is primarily related to staging bias.

Tumour grade

The concept of tumour grading can probably be dated back to the 1945 report of Stewart *et al.* (1945) in which the term 'mucoepidermoid' was coined for a neoplasm which previously had been poorly characterized and described under a variety of names. For many years thereafter, pathologists would still argue whether some of these mucoepidermoid tumors were benign, despite the fact that Stewart had divided his patients into 'relatively favourable' and 'highly unfavourable' groups with the caveat that the term 'benign' was '... scarcely ever applicable in the absolute sense'.

Most treatment centres now categorize mucoepidermoid carcinomas as low, intermediate or high grade. Data also exist for a three-tiered grading system for acinic cell carcinoma; we regard the uncommon tumour called papillocystic carcinoma as a high-grade variant of this tumour type (Spiro *et al.* 1978). Based on retrospective re-evaluation, we believe we are able to grade many adenocarcinomas despite a bewildering variety of subtypes such as mucinous, papillary, trabecular, clear cell, apocrine, or sebaceous (Spiro *et al.* 1982). In some instances, the tumour type may define the grade. For example, solid adenocarcinoma (also called duct carcinoma) is considered high grade, whereas terminal duct adenocarcinoma is always a low-grade lesion.

With respect to adenoid cystic carcinomas, there is considerable controversy about the importance of grading. Some of these tumours have a histological pattern that is predominantly *cribriform*, *tubular*, and *solid*, and others have a mixture of cystic and

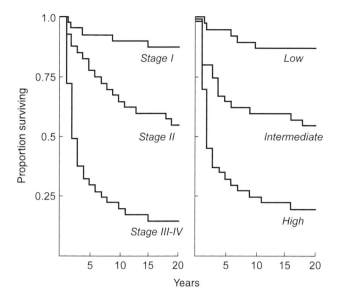

Fig. 13.2 Left: survival differs significantly, regardless of anatomical site or histology, when salivary gland carcinomas are grouped according to clinical stage ($P < 0.0001$). Right: similar survival differences are noted when patients with adenocarcinoma, mucoepidermoid carcinoma, or squamous carcinoma are analysed according to histological grade.

solid features. The cribriform or tubular pattern is designated as grade 1, solid tumours as grade 3, and grade 2 describes tumours containing varying proportions of the two patterns. We are unable to confirm the impression of others that cribriform tumours have a significantly better prognosis. In our experience, the early advantage conferred by a cribriform or tubular appearance tends to disappear when adenoid cystic carcinoma patients are followed for more than 10 years (Spiro and Huvos 1992).

There is no question that stage and grade are both significant predictors of survival (Fig. 13.2) (Spiro 1986), but clinicians who are not prepared to accept clinical stage as the dominant prognostic factor in patients with salivary gland carcinoma should be aware that there are inherent limitations with respect to tumour grading. Not every malignant salivary tumour type is gradeable. Moreover, different pathologists may disagree about the grade of a given tumour even when similar criteria are used. It is important to remember that the classification of salivary gland tumours is an evolving art. We find that diagnoses are not infrequently changed when the histological material is reviewed retrospectively, which only confirms that identification of these tumours can be a formidable challenge.

Relative importance of stage versus grade

Considering the argument further, our retrospective investigation of a sizeable cohort of minor salivary gland carcinomas provided a unique opportunity to assess the relative importance of clinical staging versus tumour grading. In earlier studies which focused on major salivary gland carcinomas, we found that histological diagnosis alone was of limited value. Low-grade and anaplastic/high-grade cancers defined the high and low range of survivorship, but the survival curves for all other carcinomas were quite similar (Spiro 1986).

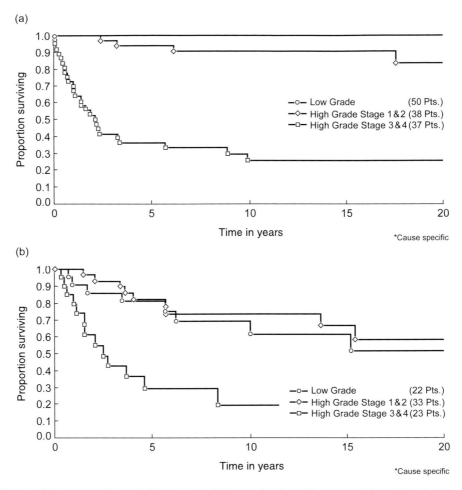

Fig. 13.3 (A) Cause-specific survival for patients with low-grade minor salivary mucoepidermoid carcinoma compared with those with high-grade, but low clinical stage lesions (stage I/II). (B) Cause-specific survival for patients with low-grade minor salivary adenocarcinomas compared with those with high-grade, but low clinical stage lesions (stage I/II).

Based on this information, we divided our 125 patients with mucoepidermoid carcinomas of minor salivary origin into three subgroups: (i) low grade; (ii) intermediate or high grade but low stage; and (iii) intermediate or high grade but high stage. The same subgrouping was done with 78 others who had minor salivary gland adenocarcinomas. The cause-specific survival curves were generated for the mucoepidermoid and adenocarcinoma subpopulations at 5, 10, 15, and 20 years (Fig. 13.3). Although results were clearly better in patients with low-grade lesions, intermediate or high tumour grade had no significant impact on survival unless the tumour was also high stage. To put it differently, low tumour grade was predictive of the best survival, but the impact of higher grade was not significant when the treatment was directed against stage I or II tumours (Armstrong *et al.* 1990).

Table 13.1 Studies using multivariate analyses in assessing prognostic factors in salivary gland cancers

	Institute	n	Sites	Prognostic factors						
				T size	Nodes	Fixity	VII nerve	Grade	Age	Male sex
O'Brien et al. (1986)	Alabama	113	P,SM,M	+++*				++	++	
Theriault and Fitzpatrick (1986)	Toronto	271	P only	+++	+++				+	
Spiro et al. (1989)	SKMCC	463	P, SM	+++*				+++	++	
North et al. (1990)	John Hopkins	87	P, SM			+	++	+		+
Frankenthaler et al. (1991)	MD Anderson	178	P only	++	++		++†	++		
Kane et al. (1991)	Mayo Clinic	194	P only	+*				+	+	+
Leverstein et al. (1998)	Vrije Univ, Amsterdam	65	P only	+	+					
Calaero et al. (1998)	Ferrara	167	P only	++						
Vander Poorten et al. (1999)	NCI, Amsterdam	151	P only	+	++‡	+			+	
Renehan et al. (1999)	Manchester	103	P only	++	++			++		
Kirkbride et al. (in press)	Toronto	184	P only	+++					+++	

P, parotid gland; SM, submandibular gland; M, minor salivary glands. + = P < 0.05; ++ = P < 0.001; +++ = P < 0.0001.

* AJCC (3rd edn) staging.

† Perineural invasion.

‡ Included histologically positive nodes.

SKMCC Sloan-Kettering Memorial Cancer Center.

NCI National Cancer Institute.

Because of the conflict of opinions about grading of adenoid cystic carcinomas, we performed a similar analysis in our patients with this malignancy. This time, the survival in patients with grade 2 and 3 adenoid cystic carcinomas which were small (stage I) was higher than recorded in those with grade 1 tumours without qualification about size (Spiro *et al.* 1991). In a subsequent publication, we confirmed that the prognosis in patients with small adenoid cystic carcinomas is actually better than has been appreciated (Spiro and Huvos 1992).

Other prognostic factors

Several factors have been identified which have an unfavourable impact on survival. These include the histological appearance, the site of origin, tumour size, initial facial nerve palsy, cervical lymph node involvement, male gender, and age more than 50 years. Table 13.1 shows that not all of these are universally independently significant. On multivariate analysis, however, it is the clinical stage of the tumour (based on size, facial nerve involvement, and nodal status) which seems most important, and this is reflected in the current AJCC staging classification.

Staging and treatment

The relative importance of stage versus grade emerges prominently when questions are raised about the need for adjunctive radiotherapy following surgery. In some centres, radiotherapy is given to almost every patient after resection of a malignant salivary gland tumour, particularly if the diagnosis proves to be adenoid cystic carcinoma. The literature contains several studies which claim significant reduction in locoregional recurrence and improved survival with adjunctive radiotherapy. Unfortunately, most of these reports involve relatively small patient populations, do not compare outcome stage by stage, and the follow-up is usually limited.

We addressed these questions by using matched-pair analysis. A cohort with resected salivary gland carcinoma who received post-operative radiation was compared retrospectively with non-irradiated patients from an earlier time frame, carefully matched according to site, age, histological diagnosis, tumour grade, and clinical stage. Survival benefit was apparent only in those who had received post-operative radiotherapy for stage III, IV tumours (Armstrong *et al.* 1990).

Prognosis is generally good in patients with early stage salivary gland cancer, provided a satisfactory resection has been accomplished. Regardless of the histological diagnosis in this favourable cohort, post-operative radiotherapy is probably best reserved for those whose tumour margins are inadequate. In borderline situations, the balance should tip towards adjunctive radiotherapy when there are ominous histological findings characteristic of high tumour grade, such as marked anaplasia or extensive perineural/perivascular infiltration.

148

REFERENCES

American Joint Committee for Cancer Staging and End Results Reporting (1977) *Manual for Staging of Cancer*, 1st edn. American Joint Committee, Chicago.

American Joint Committee for Cancer Staging (1997) *Manual for Staging of Cancer*, 5th edn. American Joint Committee, Chicago.

Armstrong, J.G., Harrison, L.B., Spiro, R.H., Fass, D.E., Strong, E.W., and Fuks, Z.Y. (1990) Malignant tumors of major salivary gland origin. A matched-pair analysis of the role of combined surgery and postoperative radiotherapy. *Arch Otolaryngol Head Neck Surg*, **116**, 290–3.

Calearo, C., Pastore, A., Storchi, O.F., and Polli, G. (1998) Parotid gland carcinoma: analysis of prognostic factors. *Ann Otol Rhinol Laryngol*, **107**, 969–73.

Conley, J.J. (1975) *The Salivary Glands and the Facial Nerve*. Grune and Stratton, New York.

Frankenthaler, R.A., Luna, M.A., Lee, S.S., Ang, K.K., Byers, R.M., Guillamondegui, O.M. *et al.* (1991) Prognostic variables in parotid gland cancer. *Arch Otolaryngol Head Neck Surg*, **117**, 1251–6.

Kane, W.J., McCaffrey, T.V., Olsen, K.D., and Lewis, J.E. (1991) Primary parotid malignancies. A clinical and pathologic review. *Arch Otolaryngol Head Neck Surg*, **117**, 307–15.

Kirkbride, P., Liu, F.-F., O'Sullivan, B., Payne, D., Warde, P., Gullane, P. *et al.* Outcome of curative management of malignant tumours of the parotid gland. *J Radiot Oncol*, in press.

Leverstein, H., van der Wal, J.E., Tiwari, R.M., Tobi, H., van der Waal, I., Mehta, D.M. *et al.* (1998) Malignant epithelial parotid gland tumours: analysis and results in 65 previously untreated patients. *Br J Surg*, **85**, 1267–72.

Levitt, S.H., McHugh, R.B., Gomez Marin, O., Hyams, V.J., Soule, E.H., Strong, E.W. *et al.* (1981) Clinical staging system for cancer of the salivary gland: a retrospective study. *Cancer*, **47**, 2712–24.

North, C.A., Lee, D.J., Piantadosi, S., Zahurak, M., and Johns, M.E. (1990) Carcinoma of the major salivary glands treated by surgery or surgery plus postoperative radiotherapy. *Int J Radiat Oncol Biol Phys*, **18**, 1319–26.

O' Brien, C.J., Soong, S.J., Herrera, G.A., Urist, M.M., and Maddox, W.A. (1986) Malignant salivary tumors—analysis of prognostic factors and survival. *Head Neck Surg*, **9**, 82–92.

Renehan, A.G., Gleave, E.N., Slevin, N.J., and McGurk, M. (1999) Clinico-pathological and treatment-related factors influencing survival in parotid cancer. *Br J Cancer*, **80**, 1296–300.

Spiro, R.H. (1986) Salivary neoplasms: overview of a 35-year experience with 2,807 patients. *Head Neck Surg*, **8**, 177–84.

Spiro, R.H. and Huvos, A.G. (1992) Stage means more than grade in adenoid cystic carcinoma. *Am J Surg*, **164**, 623–8.

Spiro, R.H., Huvos, A.G., and Strong, E.W. (1975) Cancer of the parotid gland. A clinicopathologic study of 288 primary cases. *Am J Surg*, **130**, 452–9.

Spiro, R.H., Huvos, A.G., and Strong, E.W. (1978) Acinic cell carcinoma of salivary origin. A clinicopathologic study of 67 cases. *Cancer*, **41**, 924–35.

Spiro, R.H., Huvos, A.G., and Strong, E.W. (1982) Adenocarcinoma of salivary origin. Clinicopathologic study of 204 patients. *Am J Surg*, **144**, 423–31.

Spiro, R.H., Armstrong, J., Harrison, L., Geller, N.L., Lin, S.Y., and Strong, E.W. (1989) Carcinoma of major salivary glands. Recent trends. *Arch Otolaryngol Head Neck Surg*, **115**, 316–21.

Spiro, R.H., Thaler, H.T., Hicks, W.F., Kher, U.A., Huvos, A.H., and Strong, E.W. (1991) The importance of clinical staging of minor salivary gland carcinoma. *Am J Surg*, **162**, 330–6.

Stewart, F.W., Foote, F.W. Jr, and Becker, W.F. (1945) Muco-epidermoid tumors of salivary glands. *Am Surg*, **122**, 820–84.

Theriault, C. and Fitzpatrick, P.J. (1986) Malignant parotid tumors. Prognostic factors and optimum treatment. *Am J Clin Oncol*, **9**, 510–6.

Vander Poorten, V.L., Balm, A.J., Hilgers, F.J., Tan, I.B., Loftus Coll, B.M., Keus, R.B. *et al.* (1999) The development of a prognostic score for patients with parotid carcinoma. *Cancer*, **85**, 2057–67.

Editorial comment

Professor Spiro's analysis of the data from the Sloan-Kettering Memorial Cancer Center has shown that tumour size is more important that histological type in determining outcome. Thus, adequately treated, small tumours do well irrespective of the histology. Effectively, there has been a revolution in the management of salivary gland cancers over the last 20 years. For reasons elaborated in this chapter, the poor results of surgery in the past were attributed to the unchangeable pathological features of the disease. It followed that treatment was based on the histological type of cancer. This has now changed with the analysis of clinical experience from large treatment centres, as shown in Table 13.1. Now, it is quite clear that treatment should be governed by the clinical features, notably size and tumour extent. This individualizes treatment, and reduces the risk of overtreatment. This will be discussed further in the next chapter.

This chapter highlights that although the general principle of management can be given, the actual application for an individual depends importantly on rather an ill-defined but real factor, *experience*. It is experience that engenders confidence and permits a more conservative approach to selected cases.

CHAPTER 14

Management of salivary gland cancer: clinically or pathologically based?

Carcinomas of the parotid gland and intraoral salivary glands
Isaac van der Waal and Gordon Snow

Pecularities of submandibular carcinomas
Ronald Spiro

Overview
Mark McGurk

Carcinomas of the parotid gland and intraoral salivary glands Issac van der Waal and Gordon Snow

Primary tumours of the parotid

In parotid and submandibular gland neoplasms, the pre-operative diagnosis is usually based on the clinical presentation, although there is an additional diagnostic role for fine needle aspiration cytology (Philips and Jones 1994). Preferably, magnetic resonance imaging (MRI) examination should be performed, particularly in the case of reduced mobility of the tumour since such a phenomenon may indicate location in the deep lobe.

When dealing with a benign tentative diagnosis, based on cytology, and in the absence of clinical signs of malignancy, such as rapid growth, pain, facial nerve disturbance, or lymph node metastasis, a standard surgical excision may be carried out. The patient should be informed that a more accurate histopathological diagnosis can only be made after availability of the surgical specimen.

Fresh frozen sections of a primary salivary gland tumour, even after complete removal, are in general discouraged, since accurate histopathological typing of salivary gland neoplasms sometimes does require more time than is available during a fresh frozen section procedure. On the other hand, per-operative lymph node sampling with immediate frozen section analysis is a common and valuable precautionary measure in cases of suspected malignancy of a parotid or submandibular gland neoplasm.

When dealing with a tentative diagnosis of a malignant epithelial tumour of the parotid gland and a preoperatively intact function of the facial nerve, the surgeon may be confronted with a treatment dilemma. The two objects of parotid surgery, i.e. removal of the tumour and preservation of the facial nerve, are then in conflict. In our series, we encountered this dilemma in 16 patients (Leverstein *et al.* 1998). Our surgical philosophy in such cases is conservative. However, if the facial nerve is surrounded by tumour, and this happened to be the case in six of these patients, and preservation of the nerve would indicate that macroscopic remnants of tumour would be left behind, the nerve ought to be resected with a healthy margin. Usually this requires resection of the main trunk and its primary branches. In such cases, an immediate microsurgical reconstruction of the continuity of the nerve is carried out using a graft, provided that the size of the defect and the age of the patient provide a reasonable chance of success of such a procedure. However, if the tumour extends close to the nerve, the facial nerve is peeled carefully off the tumour although this transgresses the classical oncological principle that malignant tumours ought to be removed with a wide healthy margin. After a full course of post-operative radiotherapy, none of these 10 patients, with a median follow-up of 68 months, developed locoregional recurrence, while in each patient facial nerve function remained completely intact. These results support a conservative approach with regard to the facial nerve in selected cases, and confirm the efficacy of post-operative radiotherapy in eradicating microscopic remnants of tumour after surgery. Others have reported similar findings (Spiro *et al.* 1989; Renehan *et al.* 1999).

When the final histopathological diagnosis of a salivary gland tumour differs from the tentative one, additional local or regional treatment may be required, by surgery and/or irradiation.

Intraoral salivary glands

Location in the soft tissues

Due mainly to its limited size, an incisional biopsy specimen of an (intraoral) salivary gland tumour may be difficult to interpret. Therefore, in well-encapsulated small (up to ~1–2 cm.) swellings, located in the soft tissues such as the lips, the cheek mucosa, the tongue, and the floor of the mouth, the taking of an excisional biopsy should be considered, with or without previous fine needle aspiration cytology for determination of the tissue type. The patient should be informed that additional treatment might be required after the histopathological examination of the surgical specimen, consisting of either local surgery or post-operative radiotherapy. As with salivary cancers at other sites, stage (ostensibly the size of the primary tumour) is a reliable predictor of outcome (Vander Poorten *et al.* 2000).

Location in the hard palate

When dealing with an often well-circumscribed, palatal tumour, it is recommended to obtain a preliminary histopathological diagnosis based on an incisional biopsy

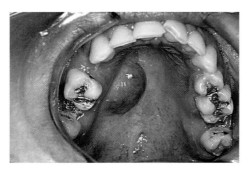

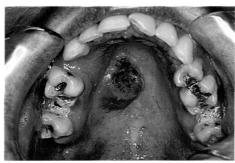

Fig. 14.1 Typical appearance of a pleomorphic adenoma of the palate before and after an incision biopsy. In the palate, where a wide excision is possible, this does not increase the risk of recurrence.

(Fig. 14.1) and also to perform appropriate imaging of the underlying palatal bone, preferably by computerized tomography (CT) scans.

In the absence of underlying bone destruction or nasal or paranasal involvement, a histologically benign palatal salivary gland tumour located at the hard palate may be removed by a rather conservative surgical procedure, leaving the underlying palatal bone intact by performing subperiosteal removal. Such a procedure does not seem to be justified for histologically malignant salivary gland tumours at this site, including the so-called polymorphous low-grade adenocarcinoma. Instead, wider mucosal margins should be observed and the underlying palatal bone, even when uninvolved at the CT scans, should be removed since it is known that salivary gland carcinomas may extend well beyond the clinically and radiographically visible margins (Fig. 14.2). In the case of an adenoid cystic carcinoma in this site, post-operative irradiation is recommended, even when free surgical margins have been obtained (van der Wal *et al.* 1989).

When the removal of palatal bone is foreseen, a prosthetic appliance should be made in advance that can be used per-operatively in order to obtain a provisional closure of the palatal defect. However, others may prefer to perform a primary reconstruction of the defect.

In the event of local recurrence on the hard palate, which is rare in the authors' experience of some 75 cases of primary salivary gland tumours of the palate of all types (median follow-up = 10 years), one should be able to detect such recurrence by clinical inspection at an early stage.

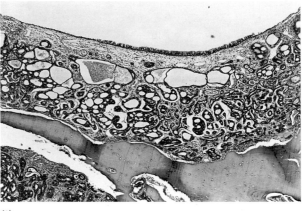

(A)

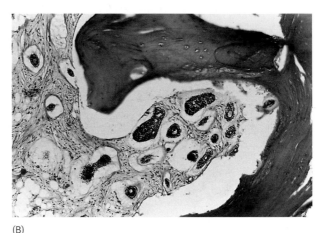

Fig. 14.2 (A) Low power view of a surgical specimen of the maxilla. The CT scans showed no bone involvement; nevertheless, numerous tumour islands of adenoid cystic carcinoma were found on histopathological examination (H&E; original magnification ×10). (B) In another part of the surgical specimen, the tumour had spread into the antral lining (H&E; original magnification ×40).

(B)

Peculiarities of submandibular carcinomas Ronald Spiro

The need for a comprehensive dissection

Sound oncological principles dictate that removal of the submandibular gland is adequate surgical treatment only for those patients who have small cancers that are confined within the capsule of the gland. Unfortunately, this is the exception when dealing with these uncommon neoplasms. More often, the carcinoma is found to be adherent to, or even invading, adjacent muscles and nerves, and occasionally even the floor of the mouth and the mandible.

All too often, surgeons proceed with a radical neck dissection when a malignant diagnosis is obtained, but ignore involvement of the structures adjacent to the gland. Lymphadenectomy is certainly indicated when nodes are involved, and may be appropriate in selected N0 patients who have aggressive tumours. More importantly, the surgeon and the patients must always be prepared for a more extensive procedure which removes that portion of the bed of the gland which is adherent to, or invaded by, the tumour. This may include: the mylohyoid and digastric muscles; the hypoglossal, lingual, or lowest branch of the facial nerve; the floor of the mouth; and a portion of the mandible. Extensive submandibular gland carcinomas will require a composite resection with segmental mandibulectomy quite similar to that performed in patients with locally advanced squamous carcinoma arising in the floor of the mouth.

Overview Mark McGurk

Introduction

Our understanding of salivary gland cancer has trailed behind neoplastic disease from other sites because of the relative rarity of these cancers and the dispersal of experience between hospital departments. In addition, the disease has a long natural history which means that patients have to be followed for 20–30 years before the full course of events is exposed. It is not surprising with this paucity of data that it took most of the 20th century to accumulate sufficient information to enable identification of the main biological factors that ultimately govern the management of this disease. A number of misunderstandings have accumulated along the way, and some myths still persist. In the previous chapter (Chapter 13), Professor Spiro has clearly shown that the clinical features of salivary gland cancer are the most powerful prognostic indicators, and are more relevant than conventional pathological characteristics. Clinical features should therefore dictate treatment options, and this is emphasized in this section.

As a prelude, an understanding of the historical background is helpful.

Historical perspective

During the first half of the 20th century, confusion reigned concerning the exact nature of salivary gland cancers. This was entirely understandable as the histological appearances of salivary tumours are so diverse. Neither clinical nor histological features could reliably distinguish slow growing and relatively indolent cancers from non-cancerous pleomorphic adenoma. A further complication at that time was the view that mixed parotid tumours (pleomorphic adenoma—the most common parotid tumour) were considered hamartomas (Wood 1904; Wilson and Willis 1912). These assumptions, together with the limitations imposed by the fear of damaging the facial nerve, were a natural discouragement to comprehensive parotid surgery (as we know it today). Local excision (Figs 14.3 and 14.4) with high recurrence rates prevailed and subsequently, repeated courses of radiotherapy were required (McFarland 1936). Among this heterogeneity of treatment policies, some tumours appeared to behave as malignant, but it was unclear if this was inherent to the nature of the tumour, or was a consequence of repeated treatment.

By the mid-century, it became clear that the parotid gland could be dissected safely and reliably without danger to the facial nerve, and *superficial parotidectomy* was popularized by Janes of Toronto (Janes 1940), Bailey in London (Bailey 1941), and Redon

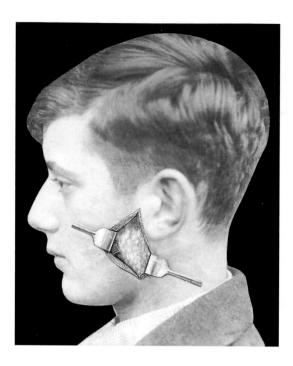

Fig. 14.3 Historical pictures, recorded by Hamilton Bailey, showing two patients with recurrent parotid tumours after local excision. Note incision directly over tumour.

at Paris (Redon 1942). Interest subsequently was generated among pathologists, and the debate on the histogenesis and classification of salivary tumours was taken forward by the accumulating archive of tumour specimens (Foote and Frazell 1953). However, the rate of accumulation of information was unequal, because although pathological specimens were available immediately for histological examination and categorization, the clinical data took years to collect. Treatment thus was naturally discussed in terms of the histological classification of salivary tumours. This situation prevailed until the late 1980s and even early 1990s, until data (much of it from the Sloan-Kettering Memorial Cancer Center, New York) showed that clinical factors were a better discriminator of outcome (Spiro 1986, 1995). This work has been replicated by many more studies and is summarized in Table 13.1.

The problem of a pathological approach to the treatment of salivary gland cancer

Histologically, the first source of confusion is one of multiple histological types and subtypes of salivary cancers (Chapter 3). Clearly there cannot be a separate treatment approach to each. The second problem is a practical one; the lack of a precise histological diagnosis prior to surgical resection. The third point of confusion is the conflicting use of the term 'grade' when applied as a prognostic term in salivary cancer. The word is used in three separate ways. (i) Traditionally, this term is used with reference to histological features that predict outcome but only applies to a limited number of salivary tumour types, for example low- and high-grade mucoepidermoid carci-

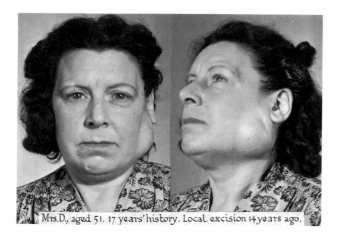

Mrs. D., aged 51. 17 years' history. Local excision 14 years ago.

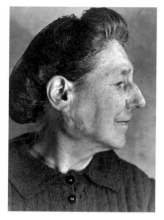

Fig. 14.4 An illustration made by Hamilton Bailey of a common technique used to approach parotid tumours prior to 1940. The limited exposure afforded by this approach predisposed to rupture and spillage of tumour (verbal communication B. Hancock)

noma. (ii) In the remaining tumours, the prognosis is predicted more readily from historical outcome analysis by tumour type or class. Thus, acinic cell cancers tend to be indolent with a low metastasis rate, and so are considered low grade, whereas carcinoma in-pleomorphic adenomas frequent metastasize and are considered high grade. (iii) The third way is in its clinical usage. Here clinical features indicative of bad tumour biology (early fixity, rapid diffuse growth, nerve dysfunction, and cervical metastasis) describe the high-grade lesion. It is the latter which is relied on more and more by surgeons when planning treatment, and its dominance is reflected by its incorporation in the staging system for salivary cancer.

Against this background of problems, we have attempted to simplify this pathological diversity of histological types (Renehan *et al.* 1999). Following retrospective review of 103 previously untreated parotid cancers, we found that the survival curves for many different histological types fell into three broad patterns or biological groups: those with a good prognosis (acinic cell carcinoma, low-grade mucoepidermoid carcinoma, and low-grade adenocarcinoma); those with a poor prognosis (squamous cell carcinoma, anaplastic carcinoma, carcinoma ex-pleomorphic adenoma, high-grade mucoepidermoid carcinoma, and high-grade adenocarcinoma); and adenoid cystic

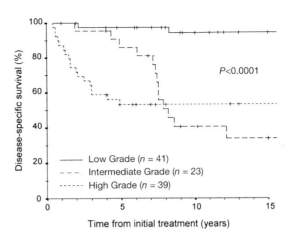

Fig. 14.5 Survival by tumour grade (Christie Hospital 1952–1992). Low-grade: acinic cell carcinoma, low-grade mucoepidermoid carcinoma, and low-grade adenocarcinoma; intermediate grade: adenoid cystic carcinoma and epithelial mypoepithelial carcinoma; high-grade: squamous cell carcinoma, anaplastic carcinoma, carcinoma ex-pleomorphic adenoma, high-grade mucoepidermoid carcinoma, and high-grade adenocarcinoma.

carcinoma (together with the rare epithelial myoepithelial carcinoma) which forms a distinct intermediate group characterized by a protracted course, with late recurrences and metastases (Fig. 14.5).

A clinical approach to the treatment of salivary gland cancers

Over the past two decades, the surgical management of salivary cancer has been shaped by two developments. First, there has been the realization that bigger more extensive surgical resection does not equate with improved local control. Adjuvant radiotherapy now has a major role in controlling minimal residual disease (Chapter 15). The effect of adjuvant radiation on survival is more controversial due to the inherent propensity of salivary gland cancers to metastasize. Secondly, there has been consistent evidence demonstrating that tumour size and extent are the major determinants of survival.

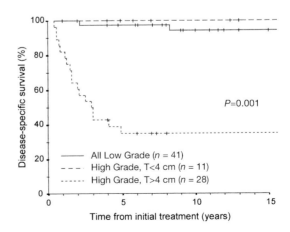

Fig. 14.6 Survival in low grade versus high grade; high grade subdivided by size, Christie Hospital 1952–1992.

Thus, for example, small histologically high-grade cancers have a prognosis greater than 90% (Fig. 14.6). This has led to an individual patient approach to treatment determined mainly by the clinical features in each patient. Thus, a blanket policy based on histological classification is not tenable.

The importance of tumour size: the 4 cm rule

For parotid gland tumours (the most common presentation), the distinction between size less than or greater than 4 cm is an important determinant of outcome. This is echoed throughout Chapters 13–18 in the present volume. Thus, Spiro has shown that 5-year survival for tumours less than 4 cm (1987 AJCC stage I, II) is better than 50%, compared with less than 25% for larger tumours (Chapter 13). Dr Slevin shows evidence that adjuvant radiotherapy improves not only local control but also survival for tumours greater than 4 cm in size (Chapter 15), and Dr Frankenthaler includes data demonstrating that the risk of occult neck disease is 20% for tumours greater than 4 cm, compared with only 4% for smaller tumours (Chapter 16). Finally, Dr Gallo shows that tumour size is a major determinant of distant metastases, and that distant disease is indeed rare for tumours less than 4 cm in size (Chapter 18).

Taken together, the simplest and most important pre-operative evaluation is tumour size. Lumps that are greater than 4 cm in size fall into a class of high-risk or complex tumour. These tumours are candidates for careful and thorough investigation, and both the surgeon and patient should be mentally prepared for the possible use of post-operative radiotherapy.

REFERENCES

Bailey, H. (1941) Treatment of tumours of the parotid gland with special reference to total parotidectomy. *Br J Surg*, **28**, 337–46.

Foote, F.W. and Frazell, E.L. (1953) Tumours of the major salivary glands. *Cancer*, **6**, 1065–133.

Janes, R.M. (1940) The treatment of tumours of the salivary gland by radical excision. *Can Med Assoc J*, **43**, 554–9.

Leverstein, H., van der Wal, J.E., Tiwari, R.M., Tobi, H., van der Waal, I., Mehta, D.M. *et al.* (1998) Malignant epithelial parotid gland tumours: analysis and results in 65 previously untreated patients. *Br J Surg*, **85**, 1267–72.

McFarland, J. (1936) Three hundred mixed tumours of the salivary glands, of which sixty-nine recurred. *Surg Gynecol Obstet*, **63**, 457–68.

Phillips, D.E. and Jones, A.S. (1994) Reliability of clinical examination in the diagnosis of parotid tumours. *J R Coll Surg Edinb*, **39**, 100–2.

Redon, H. (1942) *Mem Acad de Chir*, **68**, 338.

Renehan, A.G., Gleave, E.N., Slevin, N.J., and McGurk, M. (1999) Clinico-pathological and treatment-related factors influencing survival in parotid cancer. *Br J Cancer*, **80**, 1296–300.

Spiro, R.H. (1986) Salivary neoplasms: overview of a 35-year experience with 2,807 patients. *Head Neck Surg*, **8**, 177–84.

Spiro, R.H. (1995) Changing trends in the management of salivary tumors. *Semin Surg Oncol*, **11**, 240–5.

Spiro, R.H., Armstrong, J., Harrison, L., Geller, N.L., Lin, S.Y., and Strong, E.W. (1989) Carcinoma of major salivary glands. Recent trends. *Arch Otolaryngol Head Neck Surg*, **115**, 316–21.

Vander Poorten, V.L.M., Balon, A.J.M., Hilgers, F.J.M., Tau, B., Keus, R.B., and Hart, A.A.M. (2000) Stage as major long term outcome predictor in minor salivary gland carcinoma. *Cancer*, **89**, 1195–204.

van der Wal, J.E., Snow, G.B., Karim, A.B., and van der Waal, I. (1989) Intraoral adenoid cystic carcinoma: the role of postoperative radiotherapy in local control. *Head Neck*, **11**, 497–9.

Wilson, L.B. and Willis, B.C. (1912) The so-called mixed tumors of the salivary glands. *Am J Med Sci*, **143**, 656–70.

Wood, F.C. (1904) The mixed tumors of the salivary glands. *Ann Surg*, **39**, 57–97 and 207–39.

Audience discussion

Mr D. Adlam (Cambridge, UK): I would like to ask Professor van der Waal a question. I like your approach to the hard palate tumour, but the difficulty I have sometimes is very small tumours in the hard palate. I have actually performed an excisional biopsy rather an incisional because it is difficult to get a tiny biopsy. How do you feel about the very small tumours in the palate?

Professor van der Waal: It depends perhaps on the definition of small of course. Say 3–4 mm, well then that is probably okay. Greater than 1 cm, and you should do an incisional biopsy.

Professor Spiro: Just a comment. This is a hobbyhorse of mine, and I am glad the question was asked. All too frequently I see patients who have had a limited excisional biopsy of a small salivary lesion, perhaps up to 1 cm, and what comes out of that when you get a malignant diagnosis is that the patient inevitably ends up with a larger defect than they would have had, had there been a definitive excision in the first place. I do think there are selective situations with small tumours where an experienced clinician can take one look and say: I am not sure whether this is benign or malignant, but I can do an excision and probably a conservative one right down to the periosteum. However, what if this then necessitates a frozen section checking the deep margin—then you would have to have the patient prepared for a palatal defect, as you might then extend the procedure to include bone based only on a frozen section result.

Professor van der Waal: The only comment I have on your comment is that I would be very reluctant to work with fresh frozen sections of salivary gland tumours. They can be so terribly difficult even when you have a long time to make your diagnosis. With a frozen section, you have to make your diagnosis within a few minutes and make a surgical decision based on that.

Professor Spiro: I think your point is well taken but, in this situation, you are not looking for a specific diagnosis, but merely for the presence of tumour at the deep margin.

Mr Fardy (Cardiff, UK): Professor van der Waal, in one of your slides, you mention peri-operative evaluation of lymph nodes by lymph node sampling and frozen section. I am slightly concerned about this. I just wondered what you thought of pre-operative evaluation of the lymph node status by ultrasound and FNAC plus CT scanning. The work by van der Brekel and colleagues (1999) showed that you get very good specificity plus sensitivity. For intraoral cancers, Woolgar *et al.* (1994, 1995) has clearly shown that you get skip lesions in the neck chain, and this is probably the same for salivary gland cancers. How do you know if an upper neck node is negative on frozen section that the next node along is not positive?

Professor Snow: We are very keen on staging the neck, and particularly for squamous cell disease of the head and neck in order to avoid unnecessary neck dissections. I feel that, in the past, we did too many elective neck dissections. During his talk, Professor van der Waal was alluding to peri-operative sampling in a parotid cancer with an N0 neck. In patients with a tentative diagnosis of malignancy, we would always image the neck very carefully first with MRI, not only the parotid but also the whole neck down to the clavicles. If after that the neck is considered negative, we would still sample the upper neck node in a malignant case. In addition, I always feel with my finger above the digastric area and if I feel something that is a little too solid I take it out and send it for frozen section.

Question from the floor: About not using FNAC for the minor salivary glands and in and around the mouth. I just wonder whether it might be worthwhile re-addressing this.

Professor Spiro: I just wanted to offer a suggestion that I find very useful; a 3 mm cutaneous punch is one of the very best ways to sample intraoral minor salivary tumours.

Comment from floor: I get the impression that cytology is not performed routinely amongst our oral pathology colleagues in this country. Professor Spiro's suggestion is a welcome one.

van den Brekel, M.W., Reitsma, L.C., Quak, J.J., Smeele, L.E., van der Linden, J.C., Snow, G.B. *et al.* (1999) Sonographically guided aspiration cytology of neck nodes for selection of treatment and follow-up in patients with N0 head and neck cancer. *AJNR Am J Neuroradiol*, **20**, 1727–31.

Woolgar, J.A., Vaughan, E.D., Scott, J., and Brown, J.S. (1994) Pathological findings in clinically false-negative and false-positive neck dissections for oral carcinoma. *Ann R Coll Surg Engl*, **76**, 237–44.

Woolgar, J.A., Beirne, J.C., Vaughan, E.D., Lewis Jones, H.G., Scott, J., and Brown, J.S. (1995) Correlation of histopathologic findings with clinical and radiologic assessments of cervical lymph-node metastases in oral cancer. *Int J Oral Maxillofac Surg*, **24**, 30–7.

CHAPTER 15

The role of radiotherapy in the management of salivary gland cancer

The evidence

Nicholas Slevin

Patient selection and use of fast neutrons

Robert Frankenthaler

The evidence   Nicholas Slevin

Introduction

The main role of radiotherapy for salivary gland cancer is in the post-operative adjuvant setting. Other applications include definitive irradiation of unresectable disease, initial management for some minor salivary gland carcinomas, and palliative radiotherapy for symptomatic primary or metastatic disease.

Adjuvant radiotherapy improves locoregional control: the evidence

Single centre retrospective series (Fitzpatrick and Thetriault 1986; Piedbois *et al.* 1989; Harrison *et al.* 1990), matched-pair analysis (Armstrong *et al.* 1990), and historical reviews consistently demonstrate an improvement in local control when a combined approach is compared with surgery alone, particularly for advanced stage disease, high-grade tumours, and including adenoid cystic disease.

Similar conclusions were reached following a retrospective analysis of 104 patients treated with radical radiotherapy over a 10-year period between 1977 and 1986 at the Christie Hospital (Sykes *et al.* 1995). Surgery was performed at a large number of District General Hospitals in the North West of England as well as the Christie Hospital. A combination of surgery and post-operative radiotherapy was used in 87 patients, whilst the remaining 17 patients were treated with radiotherapy alone (15 were considered inoperable, one was unfit for surgery, and one refused surgery). Of the 87 patients who had surgery, 25 had lumpectomy only, 50 had a superficial parotidectomy, and 12 had a total parotidectomy. Thirty-five of 104 patients were considered to have gross residual disease, comprising 11 with recurrent disease after earlier surgery, seven with obvious macroscopic residual disease at completion of surgery, and the 17 treated by radiotherapy alone. There were 34 patients with minimal residual disease referred either because of tumour spillage during operation or with histologically positive excision margins. Thirty-five patients were classified as having no residual disease and were usually referred because of large primary size or/and high-grade histology. The majority of patients (84 out of 104) received external beam megavoltage photon therapy using a beam-directed shell, whilst the remaining patients had electron or neutron beam treatment, and a single patient had a radium needle implant. The standard dose was 50 Gy in 15–16 daily fractions over 3 weeks.

The 5- and 10-year survival figures corrected for intercurrent death were 60 and 49%, respectively, with primary control of 68 and 58%. The prognostic factors for survival included T and N stage, whether resection had been attempted previously, extent of residual disease, presence of 7th nerve palsy or pain at presentation, and age. Local control for patients who were considered to have no residual disease before radiotherapy was 80–90% at 10 years compared with 30–40% for patients considered to have gross disease prior to radiotherapy. The survival figures from this series are consistent with other large reported series bearing in mind the different patient selection criteria and different management policies; 5-year determinant survival figures of 60–75% (Spiro *et al.* 1975; Pedersen *et al.* 1992). Outcome from a radiotherapy series will obviously be prejudiced by inclusion of patients who have both inoperable and recurrent disease, as in this review.

A separate review has been made of 103 patients with primary parotid cancer treated surgically at the Christie Hospital (1952–1992), two-thirds of whom received post-operative radiotherapy (Renehan *et al.* 1999). The 5-year disease-specific survival was 78%. It is evident from examination of these two overlapping data sets that most patients with small tumours (completely excised) of low-grade histology were not referred for post-operative radiotherapy. Consequently, any examination of the role of radiotherapy must acknowledge these variable patterns of referral added to the already heterogeneous patient population, variable stage, histological subtypes, and grade and

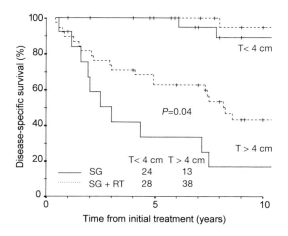

Fig. 15.1 Comparison of survival in patients treated with surgery alone versus combined therapy according to tumour size (T) and tumour grade. Numbers in the lower half of the graphs are the number of patients per group at time zero. SG, surgery alone; SG + RT, surgery with adjuvant radiotherapy.

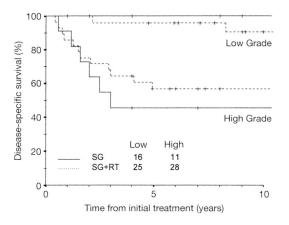

Fig. 15.2 Comparisons of locoregional recurrence rates in patients treated by surgery alone versus combined therapy considered by tumour grade. Numbers below the horizontal line are the number of patients per group. SG, surgery alone; SG + RT, surgery with adjuvant radiotherapy.

adequacy of previous surgical management. From these two studies, however, one can conclude that adjuvant radiotherapy significantly reduced locoregional recurrence (16% versus 62%) and significantly improved 5-year survival (63% versus 33%) in tumours larger than 4 cm compared with treatment by surgery alone (Fig. 15.1). The disease-specific survival for the combined approach in high-grade tumours was superior to that for surgery alone, even accepting the likely negative bias towards adverse prognostic factors in the combined modality group. However, this difference of 56% versus 45% at 5 years did not reach statistical significance (Fig. 15.2).

In the Christie radiotherapy series, the referral base was from both the Christie and a large number of District General Hospitals, so that the adequacy of surgical excision was extremely variable. In this situation, all patients referred were accepted for postoperative radiotherapy. Centralization of management for this uncommon malignancy is warranted.

Adjuvant radiotherapy may improve survival in high-risk groups: the evidence

Accepting the limitations of retrospective analysis and historical comparisons, postoperative radiotherapy seems to confer a survival benefit for patients with higher stage disease (Table 15.1). The lack of survival benefit seen in some reports is likely to be due to a bias of adverse prognostic factors underlying the referral for post-operative radiotherapy, as well as small numbers in many series (e.g. Shingaki *et al.* 1992). The detection of a survival benefit from radiotherapy will be undermined by including patients with early stage disease whose prognosis with adequate surgery alone is excellent anyway, as well as patients with multiple adverse prognostic factors who have a high risk of distant metastases, in most of whom locoregional management will not influence survival. The capacity of radiotherapy for prevention of systemic disease by reducing locoregional relapse (and distant seeding thereof) is also being studied in breast cancer, and it is of interest that two recent randomized studies of post-operative

Table 15.1 Impact of adjuvant radiotherapy on local control and 5-year survival

	Local control		5-year survival	
	SG + RT	SG	SG + RT	SG
Tumour stage (>4 cm)				
Armstrong *et al.* (1990)	51%	17%	51%	10%*
Renehan *et al.* (1999)	84%	37%**	63%	33%*
High grade				
Armstrong *et al.* (1990)	63%	44%	57%	25%*
Frankenthaler *et al.* (1991)†	85%	55%*	65%	45%
Renehan *et al.* (1999)	92%	58%*	56%	45%

SG, surgery alone; RT, radiotherapy.

Log-rank test, *P <0.05; **P <0.001.

† Local recurrence rates and survival rates estimated from Kaplan–Meier curves.

radiotherapy demonstrated a significant survival benefit in high-risk premenopausal women (Overgaard *et al.* 1997; Ragaz *et al.* 1997).

Radiotherapy alone for salivary cancer

There are two situations in which radiotherapy is used for the primary management of salivary gland cancer, i.e. inoperable cases and initial management for some minor salivary gland carcinomas.

Radiotherapy for inoperable disease

With the advent of microscopic reconstructive techniques, cases considered to be inoperable are now uncommon. In the Christie Hospital radiotherapy series where radical radiotherapy was given for gross disease, the local control was about 30–40% at 10 years (Sykes *et al.* 1995). This potential for long-term local control of salivary gland cancer using radiotherapy alone confirms an earlier study from this hospital (Stewart *et al.* 1968), and coincides with the most commonly quoted local control figures of 25–50% (Spiro *et al.* 1989).

Definitive radiotherapy for minor salivary gland carcinomas

The commonest sites of occurrence are the oral cavity and nasal cavity/sinuses, and the histology is adenoid cystic in 50–60% of cases. In view of the uncertain radiosensitivity of minor salivary gland cancer, surgery remains the treatment of choice followed by adjuvant radiotherapy in many cases. A large series of 51 patients treated with radiotherapy alone for minor salivary gland carcinoma confirms that radiotherapy alone can produce long-term local control for patients who are unfit for surgery, have unresectable disease, or prefer radiotherapy for better function (Parsons *et al.* 1996). The potential for long-term local control of adenoid cystic carcinoma with radiotherapy alone was also seen in a historical series of 82 patients treated at the Christie Hospital (Cowie and Pointon 1984).

Palliative radiotherapy

Palliative radiotherapy can be utilized for locally advanced disease in a patient with poor performance status or for symptomatic metastatic disease. Despite improvements in local disease control, distant metastases occur in about 30% of patients with salivary gland carcinomas. The commonest type of metastatic disease in a series of 72 patients from the Christie Hospital was pulmonary (61%), followed by osseous (18%), brain (18%), and hepatic (11%) (Chapter 18).

Palliative radiotherapy for lung and hepatic disease is unlikely to be contributory towards quality of life, whereas bone and brain irradiation may be worthwhile, particularly in the context of a long natural history of disease.

Carcinoma of the submandibular gland

Unfortunately, all too often, our experience with submandibular gland cancer involves patients who are referred after a gland enucleation (the 'wrong operation') elsewhere yields an unsuspected diagnosis of carcinoma. A full course of radiation therapy may be appropriate for some individuals, but it is not the treatment of choice for those who have gross residual tumour. When small tumours are confined within the capsule, gland enucleation followed by a full course of radiation therapy is an attractive option. As yet, there are no data to confirm that this conservative approach will yield results comparable with those achieved with a more radical extirpation.

The most common submandibular gland cancer is adenoid cystic carcinoma and, because of the difficulty of ensuring complete resection, all such patients should be referred for post-operative radiotherapy. In a series of 30 patients from the Christie Hospital treated by radiotherapy, the overall 5-year survival rate was 70% and local control was 85% at 5 years (Sykes *et al.* 1999).

The approach used at the Christie is to subtend the whole submandibular compartment with margins of 2–3 cm on the pre-operative bulk of disease. Another study reported a local recurrence of 35% in surgically treated submandibular gland cancer compared with 15% when post-operative radiotherapy was added (Weber *et al.* 1990). For post-operative radiotherapy in adenoid cystic disease, some authors advocate irradiating the entire path of the facial nerve including the base of skull, but this is not justified in the majority of cases (enlarging target volumes reduces radiation tolerance).

Patient selection and fast neutrons   Robert Frankenthaler

Adjuvant radiotherapy as a supplement to surgery

The treatment of salivary neoplasms is complicated by the unique anatomy of the various sites and the myriad of tumours that can be found at these sites. Each tumour

167

has its own particular pathophysiology and interacts with each site in a characteristic way. Understanding the regional anatomy as well as the clinical behaviour of the various tumour types is an essential part in creating and executing an appropriate operative plan. We must acknowledge and understand the limits of surgery, especially in the setting of poor prognostic factors.

Today there is no effective chemotherapy for the treatment of these tumours, and surgery and radiation remain the only two modalities available to treat salivary neoplasms. The indiscriminate use of radiation not only takes away a future potential treatment but also can lead to unnecessary added side effects. Up until the 1960s, surgery was the only available treatment for salivary gland tumours as it had been felt that these tumours were radioresistant. However, retrospective reviews from excellent clinical centres began to report high rates of local and regional recurrence in high-risk patients (Guillamondegui *et al.* 1975; Spiro *et al.* 1975; Fu *et al.* 1977). The initial report from the M.D. Anderson Hospital in 1975 (Guillamondegui *et al.* 1975; McNaney *et al.* 1983) demonstrated a 50% decrease in local failures when post-operative radiation was utilized for patients with aggressive histologies. Several other institutions then reported similar findings, with local failure rates between 10 and 30%. Garden and colleagues (1994) reported an overall local failure rate of only 12%, with paranasal sinus sites having the highest rate (17%). These values should be taken as today's accepted norms. Similar figures were reported from the Sloan-Kettering Memorial Cancer Center (Armstrong *et al.* 1990).

Patient selection for adjuvant radiotherapy

These data, together with the evidence outlined by Dr Slevin, have firmly established radiation as an effective modality for decreasing local recurrence in high-risk patients. Currently, the indications for post-operative radiation are: high grade, perineural inva-

Box 15.1 **Indications for post-operative radiation**

Absolute indications

◆ Positive or doubtful histological margins

◆ Equal or greater than 4 cm

If either of the above do not apply, the following should also considered*

◆ High-grade histology

◆ Adenoid cystic carcinoma

◆ Perineural invasion

◆ Perilymphatic invasion

◆ Extraparotid extension

*Tumour size ≥4 cm itself will cover the majority of indications.

sion, lymphatic vessel invasion, extraparotid extension, close (<2 mm) or positive margins, recurrent lesions, and deep lobe tumours (Box 15.1). Although the risk of regional disease is low, there are patients at high risk for occult and clinical disease. Currently, the indication for the treatment of the neck are clinical neck disease, high grade, tumours >4 cm, facial paralysis, lymphatic channel invasion, and extraparotid extension (Frankenthaler *et al.* 1993).

Fast neutron therapy

Photons and electrons remain the mainstay of radiation treatment. Occasionally, the treatment of oropharyngeal and tongue tumours requires the use of interstitial implants.

What is the role of neutron therapy, and what advantage does it hold over conventional treatment? Neutrons have a decreased dependency on the oxygen effect, having a low oxygen enhancement ratio. With neutrons, there is a reduction in the variation of radiosensitivity across the cell cycle. Cells have a decreased ability to repair neutron-related sublethal and potentially lethal damage. The radiobiological effectiveness for salivary gland tumours has been found to be higher than for other solid tumours. The indications for neutron therapy are the treatment of unresectable disease and advanced recurrent disease. The limiting factor to its broader utilization is the high frequency of severe late and acute complications. In the RTOG/MRC study (Laramore *et al.* 1993), the efficacy of photons was compared directly with that of neutrons for treating advanced disease; the control rate was so much better with neutrons that the study had to be stopped and photons were no longer used for advanced cases. Other North American experiences have been similar (Koh *et al.* 1989; Buchholz *et al.* 1992). There have even been some data to support improved survival for these patients, and complete responses have been reported to be as high as 85%. However, neutron therapy was associated with unacceptable normal tissue morbidity. In the context of a diminishing number of neutron facilities and the lack of clear evidence for survival benefit, it seems likely that photon therapy will continue to be used in most centres. Moreover, the increasing use of modified fractionated photon regimes seems to be improving the outcome for this group of patients (Wang and Goodman, 1991).

REFERENCES

Armstrong, J.G., Harrison, L.B., Spiro, R.H., Fass, D.E., Strong, E.W., and Fuks, Z.Y. (1990) Malignant tumors of major salivary gland origin. A matched-pair analysis of the role of combined surgery and postoperative radiotherapy. *Arch Otolaryng ol Head Neck Surg*, **116**, 290–3.

Buchholz, T.A., Shimotakahara, S.G., Weymuller, E.A., Jr, Laramore, G.E., and Griffin, T.W. (1993) Neutron radiotherapy for adenoid cystic carcinoma of the head and neck. *Arch Otolaryngol Head Neck Surg*, **119**, 747–52.

Cowie, V.J. and Pointon, R.C. (1984) Adenoid cystic carcinoma of the salivary glands. *Clin Radiol*, **35**, 331–3.

Fitzpatrick, P.J. and Theriault, C. (1986) Malignant salivary gland tumors. *Int J Radiat Oncol Biol Phys*, **12**, 1743–7.

Frankenthaler, R.A., Luna, M.A., Lee, S.S., Ang, K.K., Byers, R.M., Guillamondegui, O.M. *et al.* (1991) Prognostic variables in parotid gland cancer. *Arch Otolaryngol Head Neck Surg*, **117**, 1251–6.

Frankenthaler, R.A., Byers, R.M., Luna, M.A., Callender, D.L., Wolf, P. and Goepfert, H. (1993) Predicting occult lymph node metastasis in parotid cancer. *Arch Otolaryngol Head Neck Surg*, **119**, 517–20.

Fu, K.K., Leibel, S.A., Levine, M.L., Friedlander, L.M., Boles, R., and Phillips, T.L. (1977) Carcinoma of the major and minor salivary glands: analysis of treatment results and sites and causes of failures. *Cancer*, **40**, 2882–90.

Garden, A.S., Weber, R.S., Ang, K.K., Morrison, W.H., Matre, J., and Peters, L.J. (1994) Postoperative radiation therapy for malignant tumors of minor salivary glands. Outcome and patterns of failure. *Cancer*, **73**, 2563–9.

Guillamondegui, O.M., Byers, R.M., Luna, M.A., Chiminazzo, H., Jr, Jesse, R.H., and Fletcher, G.H. (1975) Aggressive surgery in treatment for parotid cancer: the role of adjunctive postoperative radiotherapy. *Am J Roentgenol Radium Ther Nucl Med*, **123**, 49–54.

Harrison, L.B., Armstrong, J.G., Spiro, R.H., Fass, D.E., and Strong, E.W. (1990) Postoperative radiation therapy for major salivary gland malignancies. *J Surg Oncol*, **45**, 52–5.

Koh, W.J., Krall, J.M., Peters, L.J., Maor, M.H., Laramore, G.E., Burnison, C.M. *et al.* (1993) Neutron vs. photon radiation therapy for inoperable regional non-small cell lung cancer: results of a multicenter randomized trial. *Int J Radiat Oncol Biol Phys*, **27**, 499–505.

Laramore, G.E., Krall, J.M., Griffin, T.W., Duncan, W., Richter, M.P., Saroja, K.R. *et al.* (1993) Neutron versus photon irradiation for unresectable salivary gland tumors: final report of an RTOG-MRC randomized clinical trial. Radiation Therapy Oncology Group. Medical Research Council. *Int J Radiat Oncol Biol Phys*, **27**, 235–40.

McNaney, D., McNeese, M.D., Guillamondegui, O.M., Fletcher, G.H., and Oswald, M.J. (1983) Postoperative irradiation in malignant epithelial tumors of the parotid. *Int J Radiat Oncol Biol Phys*, **9**, 1289–95.

Overgaard, M., Hansen, P.S., Overgaard, J., Rose, C., Andersson, M., Bach, F. *et al.* (1997) Postoperative radiotherapy in high-risk premenopausal women with breast cancer who receive adjuvant chemotherapy. Danish Breast Cancer Cooperative Group 82b Trial. *N Engl J Med*, **337**, 949–55.

Parsons, J.T., Mendenhall, W.M., Stringer, S.P., Cassisi, N.J., and Million, R.R. (1996) Management of minor salivary gland carcinomas [see comments]. *Int J Radiat Oncol Biol Phys*, **35**, 443–54.

Pedersen, D., Overgaard, J., Sogaard, H., Elbrond, O., and Overgaard, M. (1992) Malignant parotid tumors in 110 consecutive patients: treatment results and prognosis. *Laryngoscope*, **102**, 1064–9.

Piedbois, P., Bataini, J.P., Colin, P., Durand, J.C., Jaulerry, C., Brunin, F. *et al.* (1989) Conventional megavoltage radiotherapy in the management of malignant epithelial tumours of the parotid gland. *Radiother Oncol*, **16**, 203–9.

Ragaz, J., Jackson, S.M., Le, N., Plenderleith, I.H., Spinelli, J.J., Basco, V.E. *et al.* (1997) Adjuvant radiotherapy and chemotherapy in node-positive premenopausal women with breast cancer. *N Engl J Med*, **337**, 956–62.

Renehan, A.G., Gleave, E.N., Slevin, N.J., and McGurk, M. (1999) Clinico-pathological and treatment-related factors influencing survival in parotid cancer. *Br J Cancer*, **80**, 1296–300.

Shingaki, S., Ohtake, K., Nomura, T., and Nakajima, T. (1992) The role of radiotherapy in the management of salivary gland carcinomas. *J Craniomaxillofac Surg*, **20**, 220–4.

Spiro, R.H., Armstrong, J., Harrison, L., Geller, N.L., Lin, S.Y., and Strong, E.W. (1989) Carcinoma of major salivary glands. Recent trends. *Arch Otolaryngol Head Neck Surg*, **115**, 316–21.

Spiro, R.H., Huvos, A.G., and Strong, E.W. (1975) Cancer of the parotid gland. A clinicopathologic study of 288 primary cases. *Am J Surg*, **130**, 452–9.

Stewart, J.G., Jackson, A.W., and Chew, M.K. (1968) The role of radiotherapy in the management of malignant tumors of the salivary glands. *Am J Roentgenol Radium Ther Nucl Med*, **102**, 100–8.

Sykes, A.J., Logue, J.P., Slevin, N.J., and Gupta, N.K. (1995) An analysis of radiotherapy in the management of 104 patients with parotid carcinoma. *Clin Oncol R Coll Radiol*, **7**, 16–20.

Sykes, A.J., Slevin, N.J., Birzgalis, A.R., and Gupta, N.K. (1999) Submandibular gland carcinoma; an audit of local control and survival following adjuvant radiotherapy. *Oral Oncol*, **35**, 187–90.

Wang, C.C. and Goodman, M. (1991) Photon irradiation of unresectable carcinomas of salivary glands. *Int J Radiat Oncol Biol Phys*, **21**, 569–76.

Weber, R.S., Byers, R.M., Petit, B., Wolf, P., Ang, K., and Luna, M. (1990). Submandibular gland tumors. Adverse histologic factors and therapeutic implications. *Arch Otolaryngol Head Neck Surg*, **116**, 1055–60.

Audience discussion

Question from the floor: Why had fast neutron therapy not become more widely available?

Dr Slevin: I think that the randomized study (Laramore *et al.* 1993) did show significant improvement in locoregional control which did not translate into survival benefits. In part, the reason for this may have been the particular advantage for neutrons over photons in adenoid cystic disease. In radiobiological terms, the ability of neutrons actually to target cells in different parts of the cell cycle, perhaps even the resting phase, is better. We know that adenoid cystic carcinoma is a slow growing tumour but, unfortunately, in the context of treating locally advanced disease, most of those patients will actually have metastatic disease. In fact, the randomized trial showed an increased metastatic death compared with the photon arm of the trial. In the UK, we had a neutron facility in Liverpool; Liverpool advertised the facility for these patients with advanced salivary gland disease but, in the absence of a survival benefit for patients in the clinic, I think people in the UK were reluctant to send a patient a long way for this treatment. This is a shame because it does seem to have a place for adenoid cystic disease.

Dr Henk (London, UK): Yes. We also had a problem with neutrons where they were used at the Hammersmith Hospital, London (Catterall and Errington 1987). In particular, there were cases with disastrous necrosis 4–5 years after therapy. Some of these were fatal, and I imagine there are many surgeons in the audience who have had to deal with these patients. The problem is that the neutrons do indeed affect the resting cell, and this applies to normal cells as well as bone, cartilage, and connective tissues.

Professor Spiro (New York, USA): I just want to emphasize the point that Nick Slevin made very appropriately in his first reference to the match-paired analysis. The most important result of that study was that post-operative radiation therapy did not offer anything in terms of survival in patients with low-stage disease. That would also pertain to adenoid cystic carcinoma. Again, I make the point not to make treatment decisions based on histology alone. A 0.5 cm adenoid cystic carcinoma adequately removed does not necessarily need adjunctive radiation therapy.

Question from the floor: I would just like to ask the clinical oncologists, in the presence of perineural invasion, how far do you extend your fields?

Dr Henk: Well, for adenoidcystic carcinoma which is notorious for neural spread, I will take my fields up to the origin where the major nerve exits the skull base. I know the M.D. Anderson have talked about extending the field to the skull base if a major named nerve is involved (Garden *et al.* 1994). I never quite understood that philosophy; I do not know whether anybody here who could explain it.

Dr Frankenthaler: I guess I can respond on behalf of the M.D. Anderson. The reason for the radiation to the skull base is that when the lingual nerve branch was invaded there was evidence of invasion towards the skull base. We had a number of patients where tumour spread into the trigeminal ganglion, and disease came back. This caused pain and numbness of the forehead and of the cheek. I think it behoves the salivary gland surgeon to consider nerve invasions other than the facial nerve, and biopsy if necessary—such as the mylohyoid nerve in submandibular cancer surgery, and the auriculotemporal nerve in parotid cancer surgery.

Catterall, M. and Errington, R.D. (1987) The implications of improved treatment of malignant salivary gland tumors by fast neutron radiotherapy. *Int J Radiat Oncol Biol Phys*, **13**, 1313–8.

Editorial comment

The role of radiotherapy in the management of salivary cancer is no longer a controversial subject. There is indisputable evidence that residual microscopic disease at the site of the primary salivary tumour is best controlled by full doses of postoperative radiotherapy. What does remain a question is whether or not despite improvements in local control there are any differences in survival. Overall, radiotherapy seems to have no impact on survival. A possible exception to this rule is the large histologically aggressive salivary cancer—there is evidence emerging that adjuvant radiotherapy may provide both improved local control and improved survival in this group.

CHAPTER 16

Factors that predict for neck metastases and their treatment

Robert Frankenthaler

Introduction

In considering the subject of neck metastases from salivary gland cancers, two separate issues must be discussed. First, the incidence of neck metastases at the time of initial presentation, either clinically detectable or occult. Central to this, as with other head and neck cancers, is the prediction of occult disease and when to treat electively, and much of this chapter is dedicated to this debate. The oncological importance of the presence of neck metastases has been highlighted in many studies as a major negative predictor of survival (Chapter 13). More recent studies have been able to show that the presence of microscopic disease in lymph nodes is also very important and highly predictive for distant metastases (Chapter 18). Second is the development of neck metastases subsequent to initial definitive treatment, and this will be discussed in the latter part of the chapter.

Incidences of clinical detectable and occult neck metastases

As a group, regional lymphatic involvement from salivary gland malignancies is relatively uncommon. Overall, the reported incidence of clinically positive lymph nodes

Table 16.1 Incidence of neck metastases by anatomic site from various series

	Parotid	Submandibular	Minor
Spiro (1986)	125/623 (20)	43/129 (33)	68/526 (13)
McGuirt (1989)	20/71 (28)	3/13 (23)	1/5 (20)
Rodriguez Cuevas et al. (1995)	21/103 (20)	4/26 (15)	4/18 (22)
Renehan et al. (1996)	18/141 (13)	4/11 (36)	0/23 (0)

Values in parentheses are percentages.

ranges from 13 to 28% in studies which include all comers (Table 16.1). Rates of nodal involvement may vary between anatomic sites, but it is unclear whether this represents true differences in lymphatic drainage or is determined by the cancer types associated with specific glands. Thus, it is thought that neck node involvement from minor glands is less than that from the major glands, and that this in turn reflects the high prevalence of adenoid cystic carcinoma, a distinctive cancer known to have a low risk of neck metastases. In contrast, a predominance of mucoepidermoid carcinoma, salivary duct carcinoma, squamous cell carcinoma, and anaplastic carcinoma, known to have a potency for lymphatic spread, may increase the likelihood of regional disease from parotid tumours. In some series, rates of cervical nodal involvement appear higher for submandibular gland and sublingual gland cancers, as earlier extraglandular extension places these sites at a greater risk. However, among carcinomas in these glands, adenoid cystic carcinoma is also prevalent, which negates against a high rate of nodal spread; so clearly the factors related to lymphatic spread are complex and multifactorial.

Other factors have also been noted to predict for clinically positive nodes, notably the presence of facial nerve involvement in parotid cancers. Older series reported 60–70% associations (Eneroth 1972; Conley and Hamaker 1975).

A true assessment of risk of occult nodal metastases has only been possible over the past two decades as the use of elective neck dissections has become more widespread, not only for salivary malignancies, but for head and neck cancer in general. As parotid carcinoma is the most common salivary cancer, the most robust data relate to this gland. The incidence of occult disease thus ranges from 5 to 14% (Table 16.2). As imaging modalities for examining the neck improve in accuracy, there may be an upward shift in rates from clinically detectable pre-operative nodes with a consequent decrease in occult disease. This may explain the lower rates in the recently reported Italian series (Chapter 18). Spiro (Kelley and Spiro 1996) has pointed out that the rates of occult disease should be expressed as a percentage of patients with N0 (rather than all patients) and, accordingly, occult disease rates range from 7 to 15%.

Table 16.2 Percentage of clinically detectable and occult nodal metastases in patients with surgically treated parotid carcinomas

	n	Clinically detectable nodes	Occult nodes*
Kane et al. (1991)	194	9 (5)	28 (14){15}
Frankenthaler et al. (1991)	178	25 (14)	–
Kelley and Spiro (1996)	121	16 (13)	10 (8){10}
Leverstein et al. (1998)	65	10 (15)	6 (9){11}
Gallo et al. see Chapter 18	148	22 (15)	8 (5){7}

Values in parentheses are percentages.

* Percentages of occult nodal metastases are expressed in terms of all patients treated ( ) and number of patients with a clinically negative neck { }.

Predictive factors for occult neck metastasis

While a number of studies have examined prognostic factors that may be predictive for the presence of occult disease, there have been two notable studies, from the M.D. Anderson Hospital (Frankenthaler *et al.* 1991, 1993) and the Sloan-Kettering Memorial Cancer Center (SKMCC) (Armstrong *et al.* 1992), which have been particularly detailed and comprehensive, and are described in some detail here (Table 16.3).

Table 16.3 Predictors of occult lymph node metastases

	M.D. Anderson* ($n = 97$)	SKMCC† ($n = 407$)
Tumour size		
T1	8/117 (8)	
T2	7/79 (9)	11/252 (7)
T3	7/44 (16)	
T4	5/20 (25)	21/88 (24)
	$P = 0.11$	$P = 0.0004$
Facial nerve paralysis		
Absent	7/84 (8)	
Present	5/15 (33)	
	$P = 0.02$	
Histological type		
Mucoepidermoid carcinoma		26/179 (14)
Low grade	0/20	
Intermediate/high grade	4/22 (18)	
Acinic cell carcinoma	0/12 (0)	2/53 (4)
Adenocarcinoma	2/8 (25)	7/38 (18)
Adenoid cystic carcinoma	0/13 (0)	2/54 (4)
Carcinoma ex-pleomorphic adenoma	0/6 (0)	0/58 (0)
Epidermoid carcinoma	1/2 (50)	9/22 (41)
Salivary duct carcinoma	4/5 (80)	
Undifferentiated carcinoma	–	1/1 (100)
Tumour grade		
Low	1/37 (3)	2/125 (2)
Intermediate	–	13/96 (14)
High	11/62 (18)	29/59 (49)
	$P = 0.06$	$P < 0.0001$
Perilymphatic invasion		
Absent	4/74 (5)	
Present	8/25 (32)	
	$P = 0.001$	

* Parotid gland only (Frankenthaler *et al.* 1993).

† Major salivary glands (Armstrong *et al.* 1992).

Figures in brackets represent percentages.

SKMCC Sloan-Kettering Memorial Cancer Center.

The SKMCC series reported on 407 patients with clinically negative necks, and found tumour size and grade to be the key predictive factors. A quarter of patients with T4N0 had occult disease in the neck; almost half of patients with high-grade tumours had a risk of occult metastases. Specifically, when considered in terms of tumour size, tumours larger than 4 cm had a 20% risk of occult disease compared with only 4% for the smaller tumours ($P < 0.0001$).

In our study from the M.D. Anderson Hospital (Frankenthaler *et al.* 1993), we tried to take a step by step approach. We asked what would be most predictive pre-operatively, during the procedure, and then post-operatively. We assessed the following factors as potential predictors of occult neck metastases: age at presentation, clinical stage, tumour size, gender, facial nerve paralysis, grade, site, extraparotid extension, positive margins, and perineural and intralymphatic invasion. The analysis focused on 99 patients with previously untreated parotid cancer who underwent elective neck dissection as part of their initial definitive treatment. By univariate analysis, we found clinical nerve involvement, extraparotid extension, and perilymphatic invasion to be most predictive. When we looked at the factors available prior to surgery, facial paralysis and tumour grade were the most predictive. After surgery, when the results of the pathology and clinical factors can be coalesced, age greater than 54 years, extraparotid extension, and intralymphatic invasion were the most predictive. In common with the SKMCC data, we found that regional spread was associated more often with adenocarcinoma classified as Not Otherwise Stated (NOS), salivary duct carcinoma, squamous cell carcinoma, undifferentiated carcinoma, and high-grade mucoepidermoid carcinoma, whereas nodal involvement is uncommon for adenoid cystic carcinoma, acinic cell carcinoma, carcinoma in-pleomorphic adenoma, and epithelial myoepithelial carcinoma.

Other studies have demonstrated the presence of p53 mutation (Brennan *et al.* 1995) and a high proliferating cell nuclear antigen (PCNA) level (Frankenthaler *et al.* 1994) are associated with a higher incidence of occult nodes.

Clinical decisions: elective treatment of N0 necks

There is no controversy over the need to perform a neck dissection for the N+ patient. I believe that once there is a measurable node, the rationale for selective node dissection is lost. Lymph flow patterns change and skip areas are more frequent. It is for this reason that I prefer a complete lymphadenectomy. By this, I do not recommend a radical neck dissection for all of these patients. The neck dissection should preserve the *sternocleidomastoid muscle*, the *jugular vein*, and the *spinal accessory nerve*, if it is technically and oncologically feasible to leave these structures intact. I also recommend post-operative radiation to the neck in the presence of multiple lymph nodes, multiple lymph node level involvement, extracapsular invasion, and for any neck with a node greater than 2 cm in size.

The difficulty comes in deciding who should be treated electively and, if they are to be treated, by what modality and to which regions? The study by Armstrong *et al.* (1992) greatly assists us in defining the levels more at risk for parotid and submandibular occult disease (Fig. 16.1). Post-operative radiation or an extended supra-

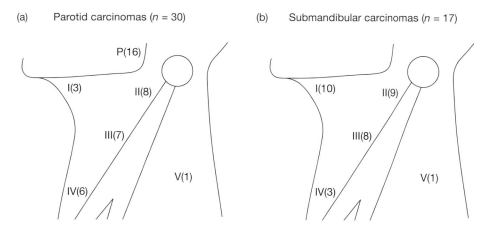

(a) Parotid carcinomas (*n* = 30)

(b) Submandibular carcinomas (*n* = 17)

Fig. 16.1 Distribution of nodal metastases for (A) parotid cancers and (B) submandibular cancers. Data taken from Armstrong *et al.* (1992).

omohyoid dissection is equally effective in treating occult disease at these sites. Levels I, II, III, and the upper portion of V are removed routinely during a supra-omohyoid dissection. I would then extend the dissection by cutting the omohyoid muscle and including level IV in the dissection.

Elective regional treatment must be considered for all salivary cancers which are large (>4 cm) and high grade. Extracapsular extension, intralymphatic invasion, and pre-operative facial paralysis are other indications, but often co-exist with either large size and/or high grade. An elective neck dissection should be chosen when it facilitates the approach to the primary tumour, and for patients who cannot receive a therapeutic dose of post-operative radiation due to previous treatment. It is imperative that either computerized tomography or a magnetic resonance scan is obtained prior to surgery for all high-risk patients. This is especially important in the neck that is difficult to examine, one with a large sternocleidomastoid muscle, abundant fat, or short length. Any findings on the imaging studies that suggest pathological lymphadenopathy, such as extracapsular invasion, central necrosis, or size greater than 1.5 cm, must be addressed surgically.

Peri- and intra-operative assessment

Prior to preparing and towelling, and when the patient has been anaesthetized, the patient's neck should be examined to take advantage of the completely relaxed musculature. For all high-risk patients, the incision should allow for possible extension of the procedure to include a neck dissection. The lymph nodes in the upper neck should be assessed and, if they appear abnormal, they should be biopsied. This is my practice and is advocated by many others in the literature (Ball *et al.* 1992; Leverstein *et al.* 1998). A positive lymph node on frozen section will necessitate a neck dissection. Generally, most of the large, high-risk primary tumours will require some neck exposure and removal of lymph nodes in level II and the upper portion of level V. It is for this reason that all N0 patients at high risk for lymph nodes should be prepared and consented for a possible neck dissection.

The use of fine needle aspiration cytology (FNAC) has been discussed in detail (Chapter 4). As a supplementary pre-operative test, I find it helpful to define high-risk patients. If there is a well-trained, experience cytopathologist who is knowledgeable about head and neck pathology, I obtain the pathology for all high-risk patients. I do not do this routinely for the more common well-circumscribed masses of the superficial lobe of the parotid.

Elective treatment of the neck with post-operative radiation

Although the discussion of management of the N0 neck in this chapter has concentrated on the role of surgery (elective neck dissection), one may argue equally for a role for post-operative radiotherapy in the same setting. When we analysed the M.D. Anderson Hospital series (Frankenthaler *et al.* 1993), the factors which predicted for the presence of occult neck disease were almost identical to those associated with increased local recurrence, and thus dictated the need for post-operative radiotherapy. While this approach is widely practised, to my knowledge, there are limited data describing the effectiveness of this approach. As the rate of neck failure is relatively low (<10%, see below), it is likely to require large patient numbers to show differences (either positive or negative) between this approach and elective neck dissection. As staging the neck status in the treatment of salivary gland cancers is not required, post-operative radiotherapy offers an alternative to surgery for the treatment of the N0 neck.

Neck failures: incidences and treatment

In contrast to what has been discussed so far in this chapter, there is a paucity of data focusing specifically on neck failure rates following the treatment of salivary cancers (it

Table 16.4 Disease recurrence in the neck with and without primary failure

	Overall			Without primary site failure
	Parotid	Submandibular	Minors	Parotid
North *et al.* (1990)	3/87 (3)	–	–	–
Shah and Ihde (1990)	31/623 (5)	5/129 (4)	47/526 (9)	–
Frankenthaler *et al.* (1991)	11/178 (6)	–	–	5/178 (3)
Pedersen *et al.* (1992)	22/110 (20)	–	–	–
Spiro *et al.* (1993)	2/65 (3)	–	–	–
Rodriguez Cuevas *et al.* (1995)	9/153 (6)			
Renehan *et al.* (1999)	9/103 (9)	–	–	8/103 (8)

Values in parentheses are percentages.

is usually indeterminable from quoted 'locoregional failure rates'). Table 16.4 shows that for most studies, neck failure rates are less than 10% and, in many instances, these occur without failure at the primary site. There are equally few data on subsequent salvage rates and the effect on prognosis although, anecdotally, the price of failure is high. In most cases, the preferred treatment option is a radical neck dissection if the patient is fit for general anaesthetic.

REFERENCES

Armstrong, J.G., Harrison, L.B., Thaler, H.T., Friedlander Klar, H., Fass, D.E., Zelefsky, M.J. et al. (1992) The indications for elective treatment of the neck in cancer of the major salivary glands. *Cancer*, **69**, 615–9.

Brennan, J.A., Mao, L., Hruban, R.H., Boyle, J.O., Eby, Y.J., Koch, W.M. et al. (1995) Molecular assessment of histopathological staging in squamous-cell carcinoma of the head and neck. *N Engl J Med*, **332**, 429–35.

Conley, J. and Hamaker, R.C. (1975) Prognosis of malignant tumors of the parotid gland with facial paralysis. *Arch Otolaryngol*, **101**, 39–41.

Eneroth, C.M. (1972) Facial nerve paralysis. A criterion of malignancy in parotid tumors. *Arch Otolaryngol*, **95**, 300–4.

Frankenthaler, R.A., Luna, M.A., Lee, S.S., Ang, K.K., Byers, R.M., Guillamondegui, O.M. et al. (1991) Prognostic variables in parotid gland cancer. *Arch Otolaryngol Head Neck Surg*, **117**, 1251–6.

Frankenthaler, R.A., Byers, R.M., Luna, M.A., Callender, D.L., Wolf, P., and Goepfert, H. (1993) Predicting occult lymph node metastasis in parotid cancer. *Arch Otolaryngol Head Neck Surg*, **119**, 517–20.

Frankenthaler, R.A., el Naggar, A.K., Ordonez, N.G., Miller, T.S., and Batsakis, J.G. (1994) High correlation with survival of proliferating cell nuclear antigen expression in mucoepidermoid carcinoma of the parotid gland. *Otolaryngol Head Neck Surg*, **111**, 460–6.

Kane, W.J., McCaffrey, T.V., Olsen, K.D., and Lewis, J.E. (1991) Primary parotid malignancies. A clinical and pathologic review. *Arch Otolaryngol Head Neck Surg*, **117**, 307–15.

Kelley, D.J. and Spiro, R.H. (1996) Management of the neck in parotid carcinoma. *Am J Surg*, **172**, 695–7.

Leverstein, H., van der Wal, J.E., Tiwari, R.M., Tobi, H., van der Waal, I., Mehta, D.M. et al. (1998) Malignant epithelial parotid gland tumours: analysis and results in 65 previously untreated patients. *Br J Surg*, **85**, 1267–72.

McGuirt, W.F. (1989) Management of occult metastatic disease from salivary gland neoplasms. *Arch Otolaryngol Head Neck Surg*, **115**, 322–5.

North, C.A., Lee, D.J., Piantadosi, S., Zahurak, M., and Johns, M.E. (1990) Carcinoma of the major salivary glands treated by surgery or surgery plus postoperative radiotherapy. *Int J Radiat Oncol Biol Phys*, **18**, 1319–26.

Pedersen, D., Overgaard, J., Sogaard, H., Elbrond, O., and Overgaard, M. (1992) Malignant parotid tumors in 110 consecutive patients: treatment results and prognosis. *Laryngoscope*, **102**, 1064–9.

Renehan, A.G., Gleave, E.N., Slevin, N.J., and McGurk, M. (1999) Clinico-pathological and treatment-related factors influencing survival in parotid cancer. *Br J Cancer*, **80**, 1296–300.

Rodriguez Cuevas, S., Labastida, S., Baena, L., and Gallegos, F. (1995) Risk of nodal metastases from malignant salivary gland tumors related to tumor size and grade of malignancy. *Eur Arch Otorhinolaryngol*, **252**, 139–42.

Shah, J.P. and Ihde, J.K. (1990) Salivary gland tumors. *Curr Probl Surg*, **27**, 775–883.

Spiro, I.J., Wang, C.C., and Montgomery, W.W. (1993) Carcinoma of the parotid gland. Analysis of treatment results and patterns of failure after combined surgery and radiation therapy. *Cancer*, **71**, 2699–705.

Spiro, R.H. (1986) Salivary neoplasms: overview of a 35-year experience with 2,807 patients. *Head Neck Surg*, **8**, 177–84.

Audience discussion

Professor O'Brien (Sydney, Australia): Can I just ask you about terminology. I know that Bob Byers (1985) first used the term *extended supra-omohyoid neck dissection*, but I suggest that this term is dispensed of and replaced with selective dissection of levels I to IV.

Mr Carter (London, UK): I noted on your parotid surgery, you suggested using a level I–IV neck dissection, yet for submandibular cancers, you only did levels I–III and biopsied underneath the omohyoid. It is my personal belief that supra-omohyoid neck dissections are actually oncologically unsafe. I cannot quite understand why you do not in fact just take level IV. There is no increased morbidity, and if you are doing it for the parotid why not do it for the submandibular?

Dr Frankenthaler: I have no argument with that. I think you could approach it either way. I agree with you that there is no increased morbidity taking the lower nodes and so I have no argument with your comment.

Question from the floor: What level of risk do you think necessitates an indication for doing elective neck dissection?

Dr Frankenthaler: I think, in general, it is considered about 20%; how we reach that figure is another issue.

Question from the floor: Do you think there is an indication for elective radiotherapy? I mean do most of the tumours for which you would do an elective neck dissection also need post-operative radiotherapy?

Dr Frankenthaler: Yes. I think in the situation where the primary does not necessitate a neck dissection, but where there is no indication either intra-operatively or pre-operatively that the neck is involved and yet the primary (histology) demonstrates characteristics that show the neck is at risk, then I think it should be electively radiated.

Question from the floor: You were speaking about sampling the lymph node that is underneath the omohyoid. Do you not sample the subdigastric node, which probably is the first drainage site?

Dr Frankenthaler: The sampling at the time of the surgery! I alluded to our experience at Anderson. When we routinely did a parotid, we sampled the upper neck node, and this is what I do today. I think it is useful if the frozen section is positive, then proceed to a neck dissection. The disadvantage is that if it is negative, and you have a large high-risk tumour, there may be more distally involved nodes, and one has to be careful in the interpretation.

Question from the floor: May I ask a question of the chairman, as he is a head and neck clinical oncologist. What risk percentage for occult nodal metastasis is a reason for you to treat the neck with radiotherapy electively?

Dr Henk (London, UK): My cut-off is 20%. I do not know why this is my figure but I use it for oral squamous cell carcinomas, etc. Probably elective radiotherapy has a lower morbidity than elective neck dissection, so maybe my cut-off should be lower than yours (surgical)—this is a philosophical point really.

Question from the floor: May I go a little bit further on this. What fields do you include in the neck; I am talking about a primary in the parotid gland—surgery has been done just for the primary tumour—and you feel there is an indication for post-op radiotherapy for the primary, and also the risk for occult nodal metastasis is estimated to be 20% or higher. Would you do only level I, II, III, or IV, and do you rule out level V?

Dr Henk: Not with the technique I use. I treat the neck with anterior and posterior fields and include level V. If you use a lateral field, then obviously the field is going to be larger and encompass level V, with increased risk of morbidity, particularly to the spinal cord.

Mr Renehan (Manchester, UK): Finally, may I present a snippet of unpublished data, and it relates to the use of elective radiotherapy post-operatively in high-risk patients. In the Christie series where prophylactic neck dissection was not practised, but an extended radiation field encompassing the upper cervical lymph nodes was widely used, I reviewed the data on 38 patients with T3/T4 tumours; the neck failure rate was only 5%. Similarly, in 28 patients with high-grade tumours treated with post-operative radiotherapy, there were no neck failures.

Byers, R.M. (1985) Modified neck dissection. A study of 967 cases from 1970 to 1980. *Am J Surg*, **150**, 414–21.

Editorial comment

Dr Frankenthaler has shown that cervical lymph node metastasis for salivary cancer is uncommon, and that control of neck disease does not present a significant clinical problem. In Chapter 14, Professor Spiro emphasized that some form of neck dissection is necessary for optimal results with submandibular gland cancer. Thus, the dilemma of whether or not to operate electively on the neck arises mainly with parotid tumours.

Statistical analysis has shown that factors which predict for cervical lymph node metastasis are predominantly tumour size (>4 cm), high grade, extraparotid extension, and perilymphatic invasion. It is a mistake to attempt to predict the presence of occult neck disease on histological type alone. Frankly malignant disease encompasses risk factors which require a neck dissection anyway. In the absence of these signs and where cancer is suspected, Dr Frankenthaler has advocated the use of sampling paraparotid and jugulo-digastric lymph nodes. A positive frozen section report will lead to neck dissection. Finally, in those cases which appear clinically 'benign' and histological examination (unexpectedly) reveals malignancy with risk factors for neck disease, the use of post-operative radiotherapy is still an oncologically effective option to maximize local and regional control.

CHAPTER 17

Can recurrent salivary cancers be salvaged?

The New York experience
Ronald Spiro

The Manchester experience
Andrew Renehan

The New York experience   Ronald Spiro

Local recurrence is a significant problem in the management of salivary gland carcinoma. The incidence varies widely in studies from different centres. Some years ago, we reported that treatment failure occurred overall in about 40% of 1278 patients treated in our hospital for malignant salivary gland tumours (Spiro 1986). Locoregional recurrence rates differed depending on the gland of origin. For the parotid gland, the rate was 39%, with treatment failure almost always involving the primary site and seldom the neck alone. The incidence was much higher in patients with submandibular and minor salivary gland tumours (60 and 65%, respectively), and the disease-free interval tended to be longer, reflecting the higher incidence of adenoid cystic carcinoma in these sites. Remarkably little has been written about the treatment of recurrent salivary gland carcinoma, probably because it is such a challenging and discouraging problem. Older papers contain small numbers of patients and include non-salivary cancers (Hanna *et al.* 1976; Kagan *et al.* 1976).

   Information derived from the Head and Neck Service database at Sloan-Kettering Memorial Cancer Center (SKMCC) indicates that between 1984 and 1995, 191 patients had a parotid or submandibular gland resection for salivary gland carcinoma. In 64 patients (23%), the procedure involved removal of tumour that was recurrent after initial treatment at another hospital. We find that information about prior treatment elsewhere is seldom adequate and often unreliable. This explains why reports from our institution have consistently ignored the patients treated for recurrence and focused instead on those with previously untreated tumours. A notable exception to this policy was a paper which appeared in the *Journal of Surgical Oncology* in 1990, co-authored with our colleagues in radiation oncology (Armstrong *et al.* 1990). This retrospective study dates back to 1966–1982, a time when beam radiation therapy for salivary gland carcinoma was first coming into vogue (Spiro 1995). The information it contains is useful, but limited by its specific focus on the role of radiation therapy in the treatment of salivary recurrence.

Patients and previous treatments

Of the 78 patients included in this study, only 45% gave a history of prior parotidectomy. Presumably, most had only a limited resection of their tumour, a well-recognized predisposing factor for local recurrence. Of interest is the fact that a neck dissection had been performed in one-third of those with recurrent submandibular gland carcinoma. When tumours arising in this gland infiltrate beyond its capsule, many surgeons extend the operation to include a neck dissection, but seem unaware that a lymphadenectomy does not deal with the tumour 'bed'. Sound oncological principles dictate that adjacent muscles and nerves that are adherent to or involved by the tumour should be excised *en bloc* with the specimen.

Re-staging recurrent salivary cancers

Most of the patients treated for recurrent parotid carcinoma required a radical procedure involving total or radical gland resection, occasionally with partial temporal bone resection. Composite resection was common in those with recurrence in the submandibular gland. In this study, it proved useful to divide the cohort into two groups. Group 1 patients had low-grade tumours with negative lymph nodes. Provided clear margins of resection were obtained, no adjunctive treatment was given. Group 2 patients had high-grade tumours, involved lymph nodes, or positive surgical margins. Half of these patients received post-operative radiation therapy. This option was not available in the remainder, who had received prior irradiation.

The role of post-operative radiotherapy

Survival was significantly lower in patients with lesions larger than 3 cm. Based on this experience, post-operative radiation therapy was advised for these patients, and any others with involved nodes, high-grade tumours, or involved resection margins. With increasing use of radiation therapy as an adjunct to the initial resection in recent years, this option is likely to be available in fewer patients. When beam radiation therapy is not feasible, but margins are close or microscopically involved, brachytherapy should be considered.

There are actually two ways to assess treatment failure in patients treated for salivary gland carcinoma. The foregoing deals with patients whose tumours recurred *after* receiving their initial surgery elsewhere. Using our database, we identified 22 patients with locoregional treatment failure (15 with only local recurrence) who received their *first* treatment between 1966 and 1982 in our hospital. It was disappointing to note that only two of these patients were salvaged by subsequent treatment. This reinforces a point which is well recognized in the management of recurrent, benign pleomorphic adenomas: the more adequate and aggressive the initial surgery, the less likely it is that additional treatment will control the tumour.

A word of caution seems appropriate for those who would recommend a major ablative procedure (such as an extended radical parotidectomy with temporal bone resection) for the unfortunate patient who has a sizeable recurrence of a high-grade parotid gland carcinoma. This is a setting in which considerable morbidity can be anticipated, especially if the patient received a full course of radiation therapy after the initial surgery, and very few will be salvaged.

The interval to recurrence (disease-free interval or DFI) is another important consideration when contemplating salvage surgery. When the DFI is measured in months, it is safe to assume that the patient has an aggressive, high-grade tumour with a low probability of salvage. Conversely, the fact that there has been more than one re-treatment does not preclude another effort, particularly when the tumour is low grade and years have elapsed between recurrences.

Fast neutron therapy

More than 6 years ago, a cooperative prospective study established that neutrons are more effective than photons in the treatment of recurrent or inoperable salivary gland carcinoma (Stelzer *et al.* 1994). Subsequent reports from Laramore's group in Seattle, Washington, suggest that locoregional control can be achieved in a significant proportion of these patients (Douglas *et al.* 1999, 2000). These data are based on a relatively small and heterogeneous group of patients with less than adequate follow-up (Chapter 15). The enthusiasm for neutron therapy has to be balanced against the fact that the morbidity of such treatment can be formidable.

Basically, there are several options to consider for patients with recurrent salivary gland carcinoma: best supportive care, chemotherapy, neutron irradiation, or surgery. For the patient who has a small local recurrence after resection of a low-grade carcinoma, re-operation is preferred. This is particularly true when prior treatment has involved a limited resection and no radiation therapy has been given. Facial nerve preservation may even be possible in some of these patients. For all others, the decision will necessarily involve weighing the likelihood of significant morbidity against a very limited prospect of 'cure'. At the very least, patients need to be aware that neutron therapy is an option when a major, deforming surgical intervention is proposed in unfavourable circumstances.

The Manchester experience   Andrew Renehan

Like Professor Spiro, we too realized that the literature on the management of salivary gland cancers was indeed limited. For the purpose of this chapter, within our database of 244 patients with salivary carcinoma treated at the Christie Hospital (Renehan *et al.* 1996), we focused specifically on recurrent parotid gland cancers. Inclusion criteria were *first time* recurrences within the parotid gland and/or regional lymphatic field after a minimum disease-free period of 6 months following initial treatment. Patients with concomitant distant metastases and those referred with microscopic residual disease for immediate post-operative radiation were excluded. Of 103 patients with primary parotid cancer, there were 26 locoregional recurrences (Renehan *et al.* 1999). A further 29 patients with first time recurrences were referred from elsewhere, giving a total sample of 55 patients [males 23, females 32, median age: 62.5 years (range 10–88 years)].

In an attempt to compare the biological nature of recurrent tumours, we included 77 patients with primary parotid cancer without locoregional recurrence, used as a referent. Survival data and disease status were evaluated to 1998 with a median follow-up of 10 years (range 4–28 years).

Patients and previous treatments

Details of initial treatments were available in all but one patient; the majority had been treated by local excision (60%), the remainder by formal parotidectomy (26%) or radical parotidectomy (six patients). Twenty-one patients (39%) initially received radiotherapy and this limited its use in the treatment of recurrent disease.

Of the 55 patients with locoregional recurrence, 44 underwent salvage surgery (with or without radiotherapy) and 11 were treated by radiotherapy alone. Thirty-seven patients had recurrence in the parotid bed, for whom salvage surgery was local dissection, nine; superficial and total parotidectomy, eight; parotidectomy with nerve sacrifice, six; and extended radical parotidectomy, thirteen. Nine patients with nodal disease had a neck dissection, two of which were in combination with parotidectomies. Fourteen (38%) of the fourty four patients also received post-operative radiotherapy. The technique of radiotherapy has been described previously (Sykes *et al.* 1995).

Re-staging of recurrent salivary cancers

We too found that re-staging of recurrences was useful both for predicting prognosis and for determining management. Recurrent tumours were classified into two groups based on fixity, nodal status, and grade, similar to the system described by Armstrong *et al.* (1990): group I consisted of mobile low-grade tumours without lymphadenopathy; and group II comprised recurrences with either (i) tumour fixity, (ii) lymphadenopathy, (iii) adenoid cystic carcinoma, or (iv) high-grade histology. The clinical and pathological characteristics of the patients with recurrences are shown in Table 17.1.

Comparisons with primary cancers

For all 55 patients with recurrent tumours, local recurrence or local disease progression occurred in 17 patients (31%), and distant metastases in 15 patients (27%). The latter compared with 20 patients (26%) out of the 77 primary cases who developed distant metastases without locoregional recurrence. The combined effect of re-emergence of locoregional disease resulted in reduced survival, but the effect was modest and did not differ significantly (Fig. 17.1). An inference is that many of the recurrences seen in our series probably reflected inadequate local treatment rather than truly aggressive biology *de novo*.

Table 17.1 Basic characteristics according to recurrent tumour group I and II, Christie Hospital 1952–1992

	Group I (mobile, LG,N0)	Group II (fixed, IG,HG,N+)
n	19	36
Male:female	6:13	17:19
Median age (years)	59.5 (21–77)	66 (10–88)
Median time, first recurrence (months)	16.5 (6–264)	15 (6–480)
Size of recurrent tumour		
<3 cm	13	11
>3 cm	6	14
Cervical nodes		
Absent	19	23
Present	–	13
Tumour grade		
Low*	19	5
Intermediate†	–	16
High‡	–	15

* LG: low grade; acinic cell, five; LG adenocarcinoma, 10, LG mucoepidermoid, nine.

† IG: intermediate grade; adenoid cystic carcinoma, 16.

‡ HG: high grade; HG adenocarcinoma, three; HG mucoepidermoid, two, carcinoma ex-pleomorphic adenoma, six; undifferentiated, three; epithelial myoepithelial, one.

N+ Cervical lymphadenopathy.

NO No cervical lymphadenopathy.

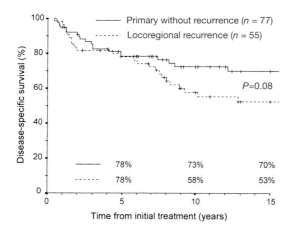

Fig. 17.1 Disease-specific survival for primary parotid cancers without locoregional recurrences versus locoregional recurrences.

In addition, we noted that the development of cervical lymphadenopathy after initial therapy (N^s), although an adverse factor, did not carry the grim prognosis associated with its presence at initial diagnosis (N^i): 5-year survival was 61% for N^s patients compared with 12% for N^i patients (Fig. 17.2).

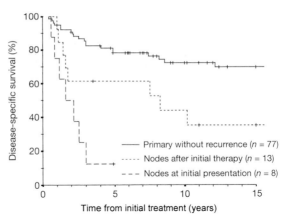

Fig. 17.2 Survival in patients with nodes at initial presentation versus those who subsequently developed nodes. Survival in patients with primary parotid cancers without recurrence is included for comparison. Note: survival estimates are calculated from the date of initial treatment.

Predictors of outcome

We assessed potential factors which may influence outcome (from the date of first recurrence) among all 55 patients with locoregional recurrence (Table 17.2). Important predictors of post-recurrence survival were: initial stage and tumour grade, size of recurrence, presence of nodal recurrence, age at recurrence, and use of radiotherapy. Classification into groups I and II (composites of recurrent tumour size, grade, and nodal status) was highly predictive for subsequent survival; the 5- and 10-year post-recurrence survival rates for group I were 84 and 84%, compared with 52 and 35% for group II ($P = 0.003$) (Fig. 17.3). A subgroup of patients with a particularly poor prognosis were those who had cancers with obvious clinical evidence of malignancy at initial presentation and, despite initial aggressive treatment, their recurrences frequently were diffuse, fixed, and difficult to salvage. The 5-year survival was 28% in this group.

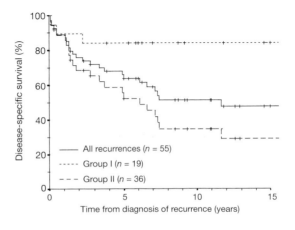

Fig. 17.3 Survival in patients with locoregional recurrence according to group I and II. Note: survival estimates are calculated from the date of diagnosis of first recurrence.

Table 17.2 Clinicopathological factors influencing survival after recurrence

		Survival (%)*		
	n	5-year	10-year	*P*
Initial presentation/treatment				
Clinical stage				
Stage I†	9	100	88	
Stage II	15	72	36	
Stage III/ IV	7	0	<0.001	
Tumour grade				
Low	24	79	79	
Intermediate	16	56	28	
High	15	50	39	0.01
Previous surgery				
No surgery	2			
Nerve-preserving parotidectomy	46	70	58	
Radical parotidectomy	6	28	0	0.006
Recurrent tumour				
Age at first recurrence (years)				
<50	13	92	80	
50–70	22	55	43	
>70	19	53	33	0.02
Tumour size				
<3 cm‡	24	83	71	
>3 cm	20	40	34	0.003
Nodes after initial therapy				
No nodes	42	68	58	
Nodes	13	54	32	0.07
Treatment modality				
Salvage surgery ± RT	44	71	62	
RT alone	11	33	11	0.003

RT: radiotherapy. Only variables which were significant are shown; other factors tested included gender, interval to recurrence, previous RT, and source of referral.

* Calculated from time of diagnosis to recurrence. The *P*-value was determined by log-rank test.

† Calculated on 31 patients with adequate information on initial staging.

‡ Calculated on 44 patients with recurrence confined to primary site.

Outcome following salvage surgery

Focusing solely on the 44 patients with locoregional recurrence treated with salvage intent, the 5-, 10-, and 15-year post-recurrence survival rates were 72, 62, and 58%, respectively. Further local recurrence or progression of local disease occurred in 10 patients (23%), being particularly prevalent in group II (33% versus 11%, $P = 0.12$).

Table 17.3 Further disease following salvage surgery ($n = 44$)

	Second local recurrence		Distant metastasis
	SG	SG + RT	
Group I	1/13	1/6	1/19
Group II	6/17 (35)	2/8 (25)	10/25 (40)†

SG: surgery alone. SG + RT: surgery plus radiotherapy. Values in parentheses are percentages.

† $P = 0.008$, Fisher exact test, two-sided.

Treatment by surgery alone in this high-risk group resulted in poor local control (Table 17.3). Neck disease did not represent a major clinical problem as it was controlled in 89% of cases. Despite salvage therapy, distant metastases occurred in 12 patients (25%); lung was the commonest site (eight patients). Distant failures were more frequent in group II patients (40% versus 5%, $P = 0.008$).

Lessons learned

The analysis from the Manchester series has focused exclusively on patients with first time local and regional recurrences from parotid cancers which afforded an opportunity to compare outcome in patients with and without recurrences, and also evaluate factors which influence prognosis after the development of recurrences. Two main conclusions emerge. First, for recurrent salivary gland cancers in our hands, survival after salvage treatment was modest (>60% at 5 years), which compares favourably with recurrent carcinomas at other head and neck sites, and, indeed, other anatomic sites. While this may, in part, have been attributable to selection bias in this series, in answer to the question set by the chapter title 'Can recurrent salivary cancers be salvaged?'— the answer is, yes. Secondly, in patients with recurrence, prognosis was determined both by factors related to the initial tumour (namely tumour stage and grade) and by factors related to the recurrent tumour (namely group I and II status), and these parameters are not mutually exclusive.

REFERENCES

Armstrong, J.G., Harrison, L.B., Spiro, R.H., Fass, D.E., Strong, E.W., and Fuks, Z.Y. (1990) Observations on the natural history and treatment of recurrent major salivary gland cancer. *J Surg Oncol*, **44**, 138–41.

Douglas, J.G., Lee, S., Laramore, G.E., Austin Seymour, M., Koh, W., and Griffin, T.W. (1999) Neutron radiotherapy for the treatment of locally advanced major salivary gland tumors. *Head Neck*, **21**, 255–63.

Douglas, J.G., Laramore, G.E., Austin Seymour, M., Koh, W., Stelzer, K., and Griffin, T.W. (2000) Treatment of locally advanced adenoid cystic carcinoma of the head and neck with neutron radiotherapy. *Int J Radiat Oncol Biol Phys*, **46**, 551–7.

Hanna, D.C., Dickason, W.L., Richardson, G.S., and Gaisford, J.C. (1976) Management of recurrent salivary gland tumors. *Am J Surg*, **132**, 453–8.

Kagan, A.R., Nussbaum, H., Handler, S., Shapiro, R., Gilbert, H.A., Jacobs, M. *et al.* (1976) Recurrences from malignant parotid salivary gland tumors. *Cancer*, **37**, 2600–4.

Renehan, A., Gleave, E.N., Hancock, B.D., Smith, P., and McGurk, M. (1996) Long-term follow-up of over 1000 patients with salivary gland tumours treated in a single centre. *Br J Surg*, **83**, 1750–4.

Renehan, A.G., Gleave, E.N., Slevin, N.J., and McGurk, M. (1999) Clinico-pathological and treatment-related factors influencing survival in parotid cancer. *Br J Cancer*, **80**, 1296–300.

Spiro, R.H. (1986) Salivary neoplasms: overview of a 35-year experience with 2,807 patients. *Head Neck Surg*, **8**, 177–84.

Spiro, R.H. (1995) Changing trends in the management of salivary tumors. *Semin Surg Oncol*, **11**, 240–5.

Stelzer, K.J., Laramore, G.E., Griffin, T.W., Koh, W.J., Austin Seymour, M., Russell, K.J. *et al.* (1994) Fast neutron radiotherapy. The University of Washington experience. *Acta Oncol*, **33**, 275–80.

Sykes, A.J., Logue, J.P., Slevin, N.J., and Gupta, N.K. (1995). An analysis of radiotherapy in the management of 104 patients with parotid carcinoma. *Clin Oncol*, **7**, 16–20.

Audience discussion

Professor Snow (Amsterdam, The Netherlands): Having heard these talks of Professor Spiro and Mr Renehan, there seems to be some discrepancy. Mr Renehan, it appears that your patients did moderately well following salvage surgery. Is it that many of these represented inadequate first surgery? Surely our concern most be those who have had adequate initial treatment but now have a recurrence.

Mr Renehan: Yes. I agree totally. There was considerable heterogeneity among this cohort, and I suspect a number of them did have inadequate surgical resection to start off with. However, overall, I must emphasize that the salvage rates reported by the Sloan-Kettering data and ours were similar and, even accepting selection bias, etc., salvage rates in recurrent salivary cancers are considerably better than other head and neck cancers. In answer to the title of the lecture 'Can recurrent salivary cancers be salvaged?', I feel the answer is yes in a substantial number.

I will comment finally and concur with Professor Spiro that at one end (the bad end) of the spectrum of recurrences are patients with aggressive and sizeable recurrent disease. The morbidity associated with major ablative surgery is considerable and the salvage rate very low.

Editorial comment

Taken together, the Sloan-Kettering Memorial and Christie Hospital series present the most detailed data to date on the management of recurrent salivary cancers in the literature. There is considerable heterogeneity among recurrent tumours, but two groups are recognizable; truly aggressive cancers that have recurred despite adequate treatment and small low-grade lesions that have failed due to inadequate initial treatment. The catergorization (re-staging) of recurrent tumours into groups I and II (defined in terms of recurrent tumour mobility, nodal status, and grade) is highly predictive of outcome, but overall the salvage rate is modest compared with other head and neck cancers.

The use of re-staging is also relevant in a broader context. At initial presentation, up to half of parotid cancers are clinically 'benign'. In turn, 70% of these have a low-grade histology. The prognosis in this group is good and, if they recur, they invariably fall into group I. Surgical salvage of this group is highly effective, distant metastasis is rare (only one patient in this series), and survival rates high. In comparison, a majority of high-grade tumours are advanced at initial presentation, with frank evidence of malignant disease. Recurrence rates in this group are high, often extensive, and constitute half of group II. In these cases, recurrent disease is not easy to salvage and the morbidity of treatment is high.

CHAPTER 18

Factors predicting distant metastasis and subsequent management

Predictive factors

Oreste Gallo

Outcome following the development of distant metastasis

Andrew Renehan

Predictive factors   Oreste Gallo

Introduction

Distant metastases from carcinoma arising in the head and neck are generally considered to be infrequent (Spiro *et al.* 1989). However, in patients with cancer of the major salivary gland, the incidence of failures at distant sites is higher, with a rate as high as 20–50% (Johns 1980; Spiro 1986). Distant disease may also appear after a considerable time from the initial diagnosis and treatment, particularly in some of the rather slow-growing indolent tumours.

Over the last 20 years, advances in surgical techniques and the combination with post-operative radiation therapy have resulted in greater locoregional control in patients with malignant tumours of the parotid gland (Tu *et al.* 1982; Spiro *et al.* 1989). Concomitantly, it appears that the overall rate of distant metastases from salivary gland cancers has remained the same but the proportion of those arising in the presence of local cure has probably increased (Witten *et al.* 1990; Frankenthaler *et al.* 1991). Against this background, there are limited data about the risk factors associated with the development of distant disease in these patients. Here, we report the relative frequency of distant metastases (DM) in relation to several histopathological and clinical parameters in a series of consecutive parotid cancer patients treated in a single institution. This updates an earlier report (Gallo *et al.* 1997).

The Florence study

From a database of 921 patients with previously untreated parotid neoplasms treated surgically at the Institute of Otolaryngology Head and Neck Surgery, University of

Table 18.1 Clinicopathological characteristics of 148 patients treated at the University of Florence (1970–1994)

	Low-grade	High-grade	Total
Age			
Mean (years)	49.1	58.6	55.2
Range (years)	13–78	11–87	11–87
Gender			
Male	25	57	82 (55)
Female	27	39	66 (45)
Histology			
Mucoepidermoid carcinoma	22	12	34 (23)
Acinic cell carcinoma	23	–	23 (16)
Adenocarcinoma	7	12	19 (13)
Adenoid cystic carcinoma	–	29	29 (20)
Malignant mixed tumour	–	7	7 (5)
Squamous cell carcinoma	–	24	24 (16)
Undifferentiated carcinoma	–	12	12 (8)
Stage (UICC 1978)			
I	25	23	48 (32)
II	17	17	34 (23)
III	8	40	48 (33)
IV	2	16	18 (12)

Values in parentheses are percentages.

Table 18.2 T and N status (TNM staging, UICC1978)

	T1	T2	T3	T4	Total
N0	30	54	27	8	119 (80)
N1	2	9	9	2	22 (15)
N2	1	2	1	3	7 (5)
Total	33 (22)	65 (44)	37 (25)	13 (9)	148

Values in parentheses are percentages.

Florence (1970–1994), this analysis focuses on 148 patients (16%) with a histological diagnosis of carcinoma. The clinical and pathological characteristics are shown in Table 18.1. Patients were divided by tumour grade into low- and high-grade cancers (intermediate grade was not used); almost two-thirds were high grade and included high-grade mucoepidermoid, adenoid cystic carcinoma, undifferentiated carcinoma, high-grade adenocarcinoma, and malignant mixed tumour. The T and N stages are shown in Table 18.2.

All patients were surgically treated: nine had superficial parotidectomy (in three cases associated with facial nerve sacrifice); 139 received a total parotidectomy, with facial nerve preservation in 98 cases, partial nerve sacrifice in seven cases, and complete resection of facial nerve branches in 34 cases. A radical neck dissection was performed in a total of 29 previously untreated patients (all N1–N2). During follow-up, additional cases developed recurrences in the neck. A functional neck dissection was performed in 25 out of 119 cases with clinically negative necks.

Histological examination confirmed the presence of neck metastases in 15 out of 22 (68%) N1 and in seven out of seven (100%) N2 patients. Moreover, occult neck disease was demonstrated in eight out of 25 dissected N0 patients (i.e. occult rate 7 or 8/119). Thus, of the 148 patients, 30 (20%) had pN$^+$ disease. One, two, three, and more than three positive nodes were found in the dissected neck specimens of nine, eight, two, and seven patients, respectively.

Local extension, defined as clinical or macroscopic evidence of an invasion of the skin, soft tissue, and bone, was documented in 33 patients (22%), and seven cases were associated with facial nerve impairment. Moreover, partial or complete facial nerve paralysis alone was documented in 15 (10%) cases at presentation. Most of the patients with pathologically involved neck nodes and most of those with signs of local tumour extension received post-operative radiation therapy. Overall, a total of 46 patients (31%) received post-operative radiation therapy to the primary and to the neck. A dose of 54 Gy or more was delivered to the primary in all these patients.

Follow-up was for a minimum of 5 years or to death in all patients (range: 60–224 months, mean: 88.6 months). For each patient, routine radiographs of the chest were made yearly, supplemented when necessary by a computed tomographic scan of the thorax. Special investigations, such as bronchoscopy with sputum cytology, bone scanning, serum liver function tests, abdominal ultrasound scanning, and brain scans, were performed when indicated.

Rates of distant metastasis

Distant metastases were demonstrated clinically in 35 (24%) of the 148 parotid cancer patients. Twenty-one patients with DM were male, 14 were female [median age = 55 (range 11–76) years]. Of the 35 patients with DM, 15 (43%) were lung metastases (Fig. 18.1), four were brain, and three each for liver, skin, and bone. Five patients had multiple-site DM.

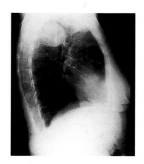

Fig. 18.1 Large cannon ball metastasis in the apex of the lung.

The distribution of DM according to the histology of the primary tumour is shown in Table 18.3. In our series, patients with undifferentiated parotid cancer showed the highest incidence of DM (67%), while acinic cell carcinoma had the lowest risk (13%). Overall, patients with high-grade cancers had a higher occurrence of DM than those with low-grade cancers (32% versus 16%). The lungs were the preferential site of DM in squamous cell carcinoma (four out of five cases) and adenoid cystic carcinomas (four out of six cases).

Table 18.3 Risk of distant metastasis (DM) by histological type

Histological type	n	DM
Mucoepidermoid carcinoma	34	5 (15)
Acinic cell carcinoma	23	3 (13)
Adenocarcinoma	19	6 (32)
Adenoid cystic carcinoma	29	7 (24)
Malignant mixed tumour	7	2 (29)
Squamous cell carcinoma	24	4 (17)
Undifferentiated carcinoma	12	8 (67)
Total	148	35 (24)

Values in parentheses are percentages.

In considering the diagnosis of DM in this cohort, with particular reference to differentiation from subsequent primary cancers, the particular criteria we considered for distinguishing lung metastases from primary parotid cancer and a second primary lung cancer were: (i) a period greater than 5 years for the development of a lung lesion, in the presence of a squamous cell carcinoma; and (ii) different clinical and histopathological features.

Stage is a more important predictor of distant metastasis than histological grade

Using Kaplan–Meier life tables and log-rank tests, we assessed various factors as potential predictors of DM. The four main determinants were clinical stage, nodal status, tumour extension, and tumour grade (Fig. 18.2).

Interestingly, post-operative radiation therapy ($P = 0.29$), local ($P = 0.21$) or regional ($P = 0.37$) tumour control, did not affect the risk of DM, despite their significant prognostic impact on overall survival in our series (log-rank test; $P = 0.06$, $P < 0.0001$, and $P < 0.0001$, respectively). In fact, among 35 patients with DM, only 13 also had locoregional failure.

Multivariate Cox proportional hazards analysis, considering all the above-mentioned prognostic variables, showed that clinical stage and histologically positive neck nodes were the most important factor in predicting the risk of DM (Model 1 in Table 18.4). Since clinical staging incorporates the principal characteristics of the primary tumour, such as tumour size, local extension, and regional lymph node involvement, these factors relate to the risk of DM on univariate analysis. When we broke down this variable in a second Cox model (Model 2 in Table 18.4), it became clear that tumour size, local extension, and the presence of pathologically involved nodes had an independent prognostic significance in determining the likelihood of occurrence of DM.

To our knowledge, this is one of the largest and most comprehensive series addressing factors which influence the development of DM from parotid gland cancers. It is of relevance that the patients were treated within a modern era dictated by comprehensive primary surgery supplemented with the widespread and protocol-directed use of post-operative radiation therapy. We found that a number of factors predict the development of DM by univariate analysis, but that only clinical stage and the histological evidence

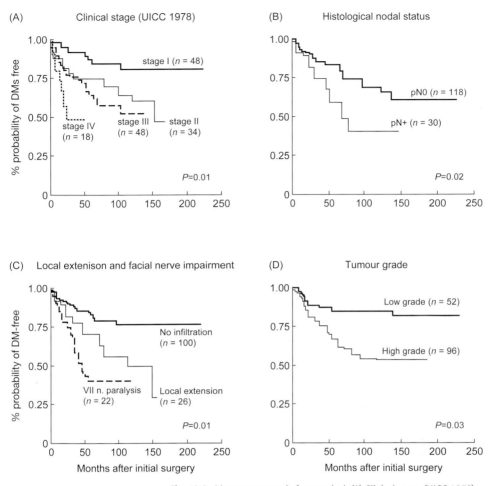

Fig. 18.2 Distant metastasis-free survival. (A) Clinical stage (UICC 1978), (B) histological nodal status, (C) tumour local extension and facial nerve paralysis, and (D) tumour grade.

of neck disease were independently significant on multivariate analysis. By implication, we believe that differential rates of DM expressed according to histological type in previous studies (Batsakis 1982; Batsakis and Bautine 1990) may be misleading, and probably reflect tumour stage.

Towards adjuvant systemic therapies

This report updates a previous report from our institute in which we failed to find a correlation between locoregional failure and the occurrence of DM in a series of 124 subjects (Gallo *et al.* 1997). Here, we confirm this original observation in a larger number of subjects and with a longer follow-up; only 13 (37%) out of 35 patients who developed DM had disease locally (primary site, nine; regional nodes, four) which

Table 18.4 Cox model for distant metastases for the Florence series

Variable	Hazard ratio	95% CI	*P*-value
Model 1			
Stage (I, II versus III, IV)	1.94	1.23, 305	0.04
pN+ (yes versus no)	2.40	1.00, 5.73	0.05
Model 2			
T size (T1, 2 versus T3, 4)	1.60	1.07, 2.39	0.02
Local extension (yes versus no)	1.50	1.02, 2.20	0.04
pN+ (yes versus no)	3.12	1.37, 7.10	0.007

Forward stepwise method used in Cox multivariate analysis.

preceded or was associated with evidence of distant disease. Taken together, these suggest a different biological behaviour for salivary gland carcinoma compared with other cancers of the head and neck area.

Our results are at variance with those reported by others (Spiro *et al.* 1989; Spiro 1997) but, if our data are replicated, the implication of this concept would be that the probabilities of locoregional control and DM are frequently independent in parotid gland cancer. Consequently, the proportion of patients who achieve local control but develop DM is constant, as local failures decrease with the use of more effective local treatment (e.g. higher radiation doses). The clinical importance is this—only the use of *adjuvant therapeutic strategies* (chemotherapy, immunotherapy, or radio-immunoconjugates) after initial surgery and radiation therapy potentially can improve survival in parotid gland cancer patients with subclinical distant disease. Our data suggest that the patients at greatest risk and thus the most suitable candidates for concomitant systemic therapy are those with advanced clinical stage and histologically positive neck nodes. To date, however, there has been some reluctance to using this pathway of management as the clinical results of several phase II studies using different chemotherapeutic agents in patients with advanced salivary cancers have been universally disappointing (Vermorken *et al.* 1993; Verweij *et al.* 1996; Hill *et al.* 1997).

Outcome following the development of distant metastasis   Andrew Renehan

Like the team from the University of Florence, we were also interested in factors which influence the development of distant metastases from salivary cancers, and these will be summarized with reference to patients with previously untreated parotid cancer attending the Christie Hospital, Manchester. Moreover, we were interested in factors which affect subsequent outcome, and these will be dealt with on a broader basis including distant metastases from all salivary cancers and those referred from other institutes.

Predictors of distant metastasis

In our reported series of 103 patients with previously untreated parotid cancers (1952–1992) (Renehan *et al.* 1999), 25 (24%) patients had clinically recognizable DM. On univariate analysis, tumour size (T1, 0%; T2, 5%; T3, 38%; T4, 73%; *P* <0.0001) and tumour grade (low, 2%; intermediate, 44%; high, 36%; *P* <0.001) were significant predictors for the development of DM. Multivariate analysis revealed that the occurrence of DM was best predicted by tumour size, nodal status, and local extension (Table 18.5). Despite apparent local cure in 77 patients, 20 (26%) patients still developed DM, suggesting that in many patients microscopic dissemination had already occurred at presentation.

The notable aspect of these data is the similarity to those reported in the first half of this chapter by Gallo. We agree that while at the extremes, certain histological types may have increased rates of DM (e.g. rare with acinic cell carcinoma), overall this is not an independent influence. Tumour size and extent appear to be the most important predictors of DM.

Classification of distant metastases

From a broader set of 244 patients (primary, secondary; curative, and palliative) with salivary gland carcinoma attending the Christie Hospital (1952–1992), 72 patients (29%) had clinically recognizable DM, defined as disease occurring outside the primary site and the cervical lymph nodes. These patients comprise the focus of the second analysis in this report (Table 18.6). The median follow-up was 10 years in survivors.

For the purpose of analysis, DM were classified at four levels using a classification for nasopharyngeal cancers adopted from Teo *et al.* (1996): (i) either present at or

Table 18.5 Cox model for distant metastases for the Christie Hospital series (n = 103)

Variable	Hazard ratio	95% CI	*P*-value
T size (≥4 cm versus <4cm)	8.49	1.9, 37	0.005
Cervical nodes (yes versus no)	4.49	1.3, 15	0.01
Local extension (yes versus no)	3.87	1.1, 7.2	0.02
Grade*			
(ADCC versus low)	7.98	1.0, 36	0.05
(high versus low)	7.64	1.0, 30	0.05
Perineural invasion (yes versus no)+	–	–	NS
Post-operative RT	–	–	NS

Data adapted from Renehan *et al.* (1999).

ADCC, adenoid cystic carcinoma; RT, radiotherapy; NS, not significant.

* Non-binary variables were treated as categorical to avoid contamination of the *P*-value caused by searching for the most informative cut-point.

† Based on a model of 91 patients due to incomplete data.

CI = Confidence Interval

Table 18.6 Clinicopathological characteristics of 72 patients with distant metastases

	Total cohort	Distant metastases
No. of patients	244	72
M:F		40:32
Median age at diagnosis of first distant metastasis (years)		71 (range 33–87)
Metastasis type		
M1 (at initial presentation)		11
M0 (after initial treatment)		61
Preceding/accompanying disease		
Locoregional disease-free		26 (43)
Locoregional recurrence		35 (57)
Salivary gland origin		
Parotid gland	190	59 (31)
Submandibular gland	20	5 (25)
Minor salivary glands	34	8 (24)
Histological type		
Adenoid cystic carcinoma	75	31 (41)
Undifferentiated carcinoma	38	15 (39)
Carcinoma ex-pleomorphic adenoma	24	8 (33)
Squamous cell carcinoma	14	4 (27)
Acinic cell carcinoma	22	5 (23)
Aadenocarcinoma	30	4 (13)
Mucoepidermoid carcinoma	38	3 (8)
Epithelial–myoepithelial carcinoma	2	1
Salivary duct carcinoma	1	1

Values in parentheses are percentages.

within 2 months of initial presentation (M1) or developed subsequently (M0); (ii) histological type, namely adenoid cystic carcinoma versus other types; (iii) the site of DM in accordance with the AJCC definitions (AJCC 1997); and (iv) where M0 metastases occurred in the absence of locoregional recurrence or where metastases were preceded by and/or accompanied with locoregional recurrence.

Post-metastasis survival

Distant metastasis at presentation has a grave prognosis

Of the 72 patients with DM, 11 had DM at presentation (M1). The outcome in these patients was poor; median post-metastasis survival was 5 months [95% confidence interval (CI): 4, 9] compared with 16 months (95% CI: 5, 32) in the remaining 61 patients with M0.

Adenoid cystic carcinoma has a unique post-metastasis course

The largest histological group with DM was adenoid cystic carcinoma (31 out of the 72 patients). This tumour behaved as a comparatively slow growing cancer with a long natural progression (intermediate grade) and, in the context of distant metastatic disease, had a better prognosis compared with other carcinomas. The 1-, 3-, and 5-year post-metastasis survival rates were 69, 35, and 14%, respectively ($P < 0.0001$) (Fig. 18.3). However, prolonged post-metastasis survival to 10 years as reported by Spiro (1997) was not seen.

Pattern of metastasis

The commonest site of metastasis was pulmonary (61%) followed by osseous (18%), brain (18%), and hepatic (11%). Other sites accounted for 15%, and included five cases with lymph node involvement outside the head and neck, five cases with intra-abdominal disease, and three cases with skin metastases. Metastasis to the lungs frequently (74%) occurred without dissemination of disease to other sites, but isolated pulmonary lesions were uncommon (only two patients). In contrast, hepatic metastases were invariably associated with disseminated disease (Fig. 18.4).

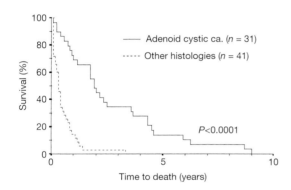

Fig. 18.3 Post-metastasis survival in adenoid cystic carcinoma versus other histologies.

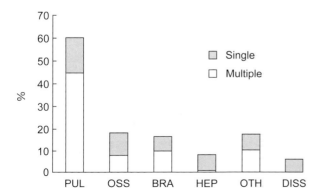

Fig. 18.4 Distribution of metastasis sites. Pulmonary (PUL) included lung fields, pleura, and mediastinal nodes; osseous (OSS) included bone marrow as well as skeletal bone; brain (BRA) is defined as clinical and/or radiological evidence of intracranial pathology attributable to the presence of tumour whether associated or not with direct extension from a deep-seated base of skull disease; hepatic (HEP) and miscellaneous (OTH) included lymph nodes other than head and neck and mediastinal group, and disseminated disease (DISS).

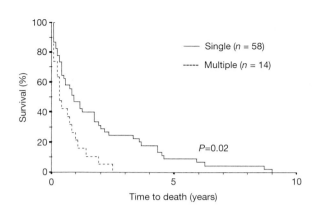

Fig. 18.5 Post-metastasis survival by single versus multiple organ metastases. Single site (as opposed to solitary) was defined as involvement of only one organ (e.g. lung, bone, etc.) within the 2-month period after the first date of diagnosis of distant metastasis; multiple sites involved more than one organ. In the latter categorization, metastases diagnosed subsequent to this temporal window did not affect the definition of the number of sites of distant metastases and were ignored.

Post-metastasis survival was significantly better for single organ involvement compared with multiple organ metastases (log-rank test, $P = 0.02$); 25% of the former patients survived 3 years whereas all patients with multiple organ involvement died within this time period (Fig. 18.5). If a single organ was involved, there was no statistical difference in survival between the three main sites of metastases (pulmonary, osseous, and brain) though occasional long-term survival was observed in patients with lung disease.

The presence of locoregional disease did not influence outcome

Twenty-six patients (43%) developed DM without preceding or accompanying locoregional recurrence. The median time to the diagnosis of DM in these patients was 17 months (range 6–67 months). Compared with those patients in which distant disease was preceded or accompanied by locoregional recurrence [median = 42 months (range 6–247) months], this was significantly shorter ($P = 0.01$). However, this did not translate into a poorer outcome in the former group, and indeed there was no correlation between time delay to the appearance of distant disease and the subsequent interval to death ($r = 0.34$).

A variety of other clinicopathological factors were evaluated for their influence on post-metastasis survival and found to be not significant. These included gender, age at diagnosis of metastasis, referral pattern, and salivary gland site.

Clinical implications

Accepting that this study is retrospective, spanning four decades, during which time modalities for detecting metastatic disease have improved, there are still four important and relevant messages.

1. The presence of distant disease *ab initio* carries a grave prognosis.
2. The clinical course from metastases to death in adenoid cystic carcinoma was longer than for other salivary carcinomas although the attainment of prolonged survival may be overstated in the literature.

3. The separation of metastases into single versus multiple organ disease is highly predictive of post-metastasis survival.

4. Almost half of distant metastases from salivary cancers occur in the presence of apparent local cure, arguing for the need to explore systemic treatment approaches. This has clinical implications for directing investigations and in counselling on prognosis. It also acts as a baseline to judge responses between different chemotherapy regimes for advanced salivary cancer.

The final comment relates to pulmonary metastatectomy, in particular for patients with metastases from adenoid cystic carcinoma. This operation was not used in our series and, therefore, its effect cannot be addressed directly here. However, there are trends towards performing pulmonary metastatectomy for certain malignancies, such as extremity soft tissue sarcomas (Lewis *et al.* 2000), and even metastases from head and neck origin (Mazer *et al.* 1988). We feel that surgeons should be cautious in advocating this approach in asymptomatic patients with adenoid cystic carcinoma for two reasons: first, lung metastases are seldom solitary; and secondly, it is unlikely that pulmonary resection would substantially alter the natural history of this disease.

REFERENCES

American Joint Committee for Cancer Staging (1997) *Manual for Staging of Cancer*, 5th edn. American Joint Committee, Chicago.

Batsakis, J.G. (1982) Pathology consultation. Metastatic patterns of salivary gland neoplasms. *Ann Otol Rhinol Laryngol*, **91**, 465–6.

Batsakis, J.G. and Bautina, E. (1990) Metastases to major salivary glands. *Ann Otol Rhinol Laryngol*, **99**, 501–3.

Frankenthaler, R.A., Luna, M.A., Lee, S.S., Ang, K.K., Byers, R.M., Guillamondegui, O.M. *et al.* (1991) Prognostic variables in parotid gland cancer. *Arch Otolaryngol Head Neck Surg*, **117**, 1251–6.

Gallo, O., Franchi, A., Bottai, G.V., Fini Storchi, I., Tesi, G., and Boddi, V. (1997) Risk factors for distant metastases from carcinoma of the parotid gland. *Cancer*, **80**, 844–51.

Hill, M.E., Constenla, D.O., A' Hern, RP, Henk, J.M., Rhys Evans, P., Breach, N. *et al.* (1997) Cisplatin and 5-fluorouracil for symptom control in advanced salivary adenoid cystic carcinoma. *Oral Oncol*, **33**, 275–8.

Johns, M.E. (1980) Parotid cancer: a rational basis for treatment. *Head Neck Surg*, **3**, 132–41.

Lewis, J.J., Leung, D., Espat, J., Woodruff, J.M., and Brennan, M.F. (2000) Effect of reresection in extremity soft tissue sarcoma. *Ann Surg*, **231**, 655–63.

Mazer, T.M., Robbins, K.T., McMurtrey, M.J., and Byers, R.M. (1988) Resection of pulmonary metastases from squamous carcinoma of the head and neck. *Am J Surg*, **156**, 238–42.

Renehan, A.G., Gleave, E.N., Slevin, N.J., and McGurk, M. (1999) Clinico-pathological and treatment-related factors influencing survival in parotid cancer. *Br J Cancer*, **80**, 1296–300.

Spiro, R.H. (1986) Salivary neoplasms: overview of a 35-year experience with 2,807 patients. *Head Neck Surg*, **8**, 177–84.

Spiro, R.H. (1997) Distant metastasis in adenoid cystic carcinoma of salivary origin. *Am J Surg*, **174**, 495–8.

Spiro, R.H., Armstrong, J., Harrison, L., Geller, N.L., Lin, S.Y., and Strong, E.W. (1989) Carcinoma of major salivary glands. Recent trends. *Arch Otolaryngol Head Neck Surg*, **115**, 316–21.

Teo, P.M., Kwan, W.H., Lee, W.Y., Leung, S.F., and Johnson, P.J. (1996) Prognosticators determining survival subsequent to distant metastasis from nasopharyngeal carcinoma. *Cancer*, **77**, 2423–31.

Tu, G., Hu, Y., Jiang, P., and Qin, D. (1982) The superiority of combined therapy (surgery and postoperative irradiation) in parotid cancer. *Arch Otolaryngol*, **108**, 710–3.

Vermorken, J.B., Verweij, J., de Mulder, P.H., Cognetti, F., Clavel, M., Rodenhuis, S., Kirkpatrick, A. and Snow, G.B. (1993) Epirubicin in patients with advanced or recurrent adenoid cystic carcinoma of the head and neck: a phase II study of the EORTC Head and Neck Cancer Cooperative Group. *Ann Oncol*, **4**, 785–8.

Verweij, J., de Mulder, P.H., de Graeff, A., Vermorken, J.B., Wildiers, J., Kerger, J. *et al.* (1996) Phase II study on mitoxantrone in adenoid cystic carcinomas of the head and neck. EORTC Head and Neck Cancer Cooperative Group. *Ann Oncol*, **7**, 867–9.

Witten, J., Hybert, F., and Hansen, H.S. (1990) Treatment of malignant tumors in the parotid glands. *Cancer*, **65**, 2515–20.

Audience discussion

Professor Spiro (New York, USA): Perhaps I did not hear it, but I think it might be good for this audience to ask the question 'What do you do with the patient with adenoid cystic carcinoma and, on follow-up, one finds nodules on a chest X-ray? The patient is asymptomatic.' I just insert here that our practice is very conservative. Reports are few and the data often lumped together with all head and neck sites. Resection of metastatic lung nodules is particularly difficult to justify in patients with adenoid cystic carcinoma, either as a curative or palliative effort. Pulmonary metastases in these patients are almost never solitary, and untreated patients may survive for many years without symptoms. Our practice is not to treat unless they are symptomatic because it is only palliative in the first place. Is this the perception of others?

Mr Renehan: I concur totally. Perhaps I did not illustrate clearly in my talk: there is evidence of benefit from metastatectomy, for instance, for lung metastases from sarcomas, or hepatic metastases from colorectal cancer, but salivary cancers are different, in particular adenoid cystic carcinoma.

Professor Snow (Amsterdam, The Netherlands): During follow-up of patients who have been treated for salivary gland cancer who had no symptoms of distant metastasis, do you regularly ask for a chest X-ray. If you find metastatic disease, do you inform the patient accordingly when the pathology is an adenoid cystic carcinoma?

Dr Gallo: We follow-up the patient regularly and we do perform chest X-rays. I must add that we do have experience of two patients with adenoid cystic carcinoma in whom we performed lung resections. In both cases, unfortunately, we were unsuccessful because we found involved nodes in the lung, and subsequently adminstered chemotherapy but had no response. Now we do not treat these cases.

Professor Snow: And what is the Mediterranean philosophy if you find a metastasis on the X-ray, do you discuss this with the patient? I am talking here only of adenoid cystic carcinoma.

Dr Gallo: Yes. I recently spoke with Professor Spiro about a young woman with adenoid cystic carcinoma with lung metastasis discovered 5 years after initial treatment. She had local cure and was asymptomatic. She had chemotherapy but her nodules continue to increase in size. We were unable to offer her further therapy.

Professor Spiro: I am fascinated that you persist with your question, Gordon. In North America today, the standard of care mandates that the patient has to be informed. If not, you would be subject to a successfully prosecuted suit if you withheld it.

Professor Snow: Well I just want to make sure. However, I still have no satisfactory answer to the situation in which you find a lung metastasis, inform the patient of its presence, but also proceed to inform him/her that there is no effective therapy. What do you say when the patient then asks 'Well, why did you do the test then in the first place?' How is it in Britain?

Mr Renehan: There is truth in many of these arguments. In addition, there is considerable evidence, including from randomized trials, which shows that chest radiology is an ineffective surveillance tool in common cancers such as breast and colorectal cancer. Ineffective, in that it fails to influence survival. And I am sure this is also the case for salivary cancers. We, however, still do perform annual chest radiography, recognizing that one of the main reasons is to document the natural history of salivary cancers as I feel it is now time to start addressing the systemic treatment of these carcinomas. I would like to try and use this forum to discuss whether people felt this was an area of further research. To date, clinical trials of chemotherapy for advanced cases has been generally disappointing. However, I agree with the comments of Dr Gallo and feel that adjuvant systemic chemotherapy may be different. I feel we need more laboratory work on this.

Dr Henk (London, UK): Yes, I think it is fair to say that chemotherapy for salivary cancer had been stuck for 30 years, and is not going anywhere. Is there anyone here who has any experience of response to chemotherapy for metastatic salivary gland cancer? My experience is that they do not respond to any of the normal regimes such as platinum. Our current focus is a study of amphicylone with platinum by continuous ambulatory infusion—so far this appears no better.

Mr Renehan: I would like to finish by trying to look into the crystal ball. I have been very impressed with Dr Gallo's data on the development of distant metastases. In particular, histologically positive cervical nodes is highly predictive. Although occult neck disease is relatively uncommon, I predict that in the future, we may be undertaking elective neck dissections for salivary cancers, say in large tumours, to stage the patient and base treatment decisions about systemic therapy on the findings. This would be analogous to current practice in breast cancer.

Editorial comment

Until recently, the subject of distant metastasis from salivary gland cancers has been broadly ignored. The data from Dr Gallo clearly show that clinical stage and histologcal nodal status are the key predictors for the development of distant disease. The Christie data are in agreement with this. In addition, both series have shown that as locoregional recurrence has improved over the last few decades, the proportion of 'distant metastasis only' has increased. The issue of systemic chemotherapy has been raised, but there appears to be a degree of pessimism as experience to date is that salivary cancers are resistant to most of the common regimes. Adenoid cystic carcinoma stands out as a class on its own, with a relatively high incidence of late distant metastasis. These tumours can be indolent, and the length of survival after metastasis is usually longer than for other salivary tumours. However, even with adenoid cystic carcinoma, fewer than 20% of patients survive 5 years. Finally, pulmonary metastatectomy for adenoid cystic carcinoma has been discussed by many people in the audience. There appears to be a general consensus that this surgical intervention is ineffective, and in general should be discouraged.

CHAPTER 19

The controversial adenoid cystic carcinoma

Is this cancer curable and where does it fail?
Ronald Spiro

The implications of histological grade and perineural invasion
Andrew Barrett and Paul Speight

The role of conservative versus radical surgery
Gordon Snow and Isaac van der Waal

Is this cancer curable and where does it fail?   Ronald Spiro

The nature of adenoid cystic carcinoma

In 1859, Bilroth coined the term 'cylindroma' to describe an unusual sinus tumour, the histological appearance and behaviour of which had been described 3 years previously by Robin and Laboulbene. Not until 1942 was the malignant nature of this neoplasm fully appreciated by Dockerty and Mayo (1942). In Foote and Frazell's classic 1953 paper, this tumour was unequivocally classified as an adenocarcinoma. They expressed a preference for the term 'adenoid cystic carcinoma', which had been used at Sloan-Kettering Memorial Cancer Center by James Ewing for many years (Foote and Frazell 1953).

Adenoid cystic carcinoma (ACC) is the histological diagnosis in less than 10% of patients with salivary gland tumours. It should be remembered that tumours having the identical microscopic appearance occur in a variety of sites, including the lacrimal gland, the skin, the oesophagus, the breast, the tracheobronchial tree, the uterine cervix, Bartholin's gland, and the prostate. In our experience, the incidence of these tumours varies widely according to the salivary gland of origin: minor glands 31%; submandibular gland 14%; and parotid 2%. More than 70% of our ACC patients have tumours which originate in minor salivary glands, with the palate—by far the most common site—accounting for more than 20% of the entire cohort.

ACC has three distinctive growth patterns: cribriform, tubular, and solid. Grading is complicated by the fact that all of these morphological features can be present in the same tumour. The criteria used in our hospital are as follows: grade 1, cribriform or tubular pattern predominates—only occasional solid features; grade 2, approximately equal distribution of cribriform or tubular components and solid features; and grade 3, solid pattern dominates with minimal evidence of glandular features. Much emphasis has been placed on grading of ACC in other centres, but we have found its prognostic value to be limited. As is true for other salivary carcinomas, clinical staging is the most important predictor of outcome (Chapter13). There is as yet no specific staging system for minor salivary gland carcinomas, but the latter can be readily staged using criteria identical to those used for squamous carcinoma in similar sites (Spiro *et al.* 1991; Spiro and Huvos 1992). Imaging is particularly important for staging ACCs of minor gland origin, especially those arising in and around the sinuses. An important caveat with respect to the staging of ACC is that these tumours are *always* more extensive than can be appreciated either clinically or by radiographs. The propensity of these tumours to extend insidiously via perineural and perivascular pathways well beyond visible or palpable tumour explains why many of these patients are understaged even by experienced clinicians.

Where does ACC fail?

In our patient cohort with ACC, local recurrence was by far the most common indication of treatment failure, occurring in about two-thirds of our patients. The time to recurrence or metastasis (disease-free interval or DFI) ranged from 1 month to more than 19 years (median 36 months). Recurrence at the primary site was noted much less often in those with stage I tumours when compared with all other stages. Post-operative radiotherapy significantly reduced the local failure rate, but patient age, gender, extent of surgery, and tumour grade had no appreciable impact (Spiro *et al.* 1991). Neck failure is not a prominent problem in patients with ACC, presumably because cervical lymph node involvement is uncommon on initial presentation (<10%) and occurs overall in about 15%. Distant metastasis occurred in almost 40% of our patients, most often in association with local or neck recurrence. In most of these patients, the lung was the only site of distant spread. When ACC patients with pulmonary metastases are followed until they die, it is impressive that many of these patients remain totally asymptomatic and functional until late in the course of their disease. Once they develop symptoms, or the tumour spreads to viscera, brain, or bone, however, survival seldom exceeds 1 or 2 years. Our experience indicates that large tumour size and locoregional treatment failure are the two factors most predictive of distant metastasis.

Treatment

Surgery

Surgery remains the mainstay in the treatment of ACC, and the extent of the resection depends on the stage and site of the primary tumour. In our experience, fewer than half of patients with stage I, II tumours require a radical resection, compared with more than 80% of those with stage III or IV disease. As for site differences, radical resection is necessary in all but a few who have sinus or laryngeal primaries, whereas this is true in our experience only in about one-half and one-third of those with mouth and major gland tumours, respectively. It is common for early sinus and non-glottic larynx cancers to be asymptomatic, which explains why lesions arising in these relatively inaccessible sites tend to be high stage by the time the histological diagnosis is established.

Only 20% of our patients have required a lymphadenectomy. Elective node dissection is hard to justify unless it facilitates a more adequate resection of the primary tumour (e.g. high stage submandibular gland cancers).

Radiotherapy

Radiation therapy has become increasingly important as an adjunct to the surgical treatment of ACC. As with salivary tumours of other histological type, the evidence suggests that post-operative radiotherapy reduces local recurrence, but does not significantly prolong survival. For radiotherapy to be effective, portals must be generous and the dosage must be adequate. Given the potential for perineural spread along major nerves, treatment directed to the primary must often include the skull base. Unless lymph nodes are involved, a lesser dose is delivered to the neck. The usual indications in patients with salivary gland carcinomas are high tumour stage, which carries an increased risk of locoregional treatment failure, or concern about tumour clearance at the resection margins. More often than not, the patient with ACC receives radiotherapy because of margin concerns, regardless of the clinical stage. Our experience suggests that surgery alone may be sufficient in selected patients with small lesions provided the surgeon is satisfied with the resection and the pathologist confirms that the margins are clear.

Reports in the literature confirm that neutrons are more effective than photons in the treatment of salivary gland carcinomas. Data have been presented which indicate that neutron radiation is a viable option in patients with unresectable or recurrent salivary gland carcinomas, including ACC. The radiation experience, whether with neutrons or photons, needs to be interpreted with caution. Almost all of the studies are retrospective and include relatively few patients with limited follow-up. In reality, 5-year follow-up is almost meaningless in patients with ACC because this tumour can grow very slowly, and it is not unusual for recurrence and distant metastasis to occur after disease-free intervals exceeding 10 years. There is also concern about increased morbidity associated with neutron therapy, which should be weighed in treatment selection.

Is ACC curable?

In our experience, disease-specific survival rates at 5, 10, 15, 20, and 25 years were 79, 54, 46, 38, and 27%, respectively. With this neoplasm, survival curves never level off and tumour-related deaths occur for as long as the patients are followed (Fig 19.1). The

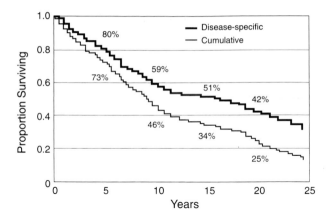

Fig. 19.1 Cumulative versus disease-specific survival in a cohort with salivary gland adenoid cystic carcinoma followed for up to 25 years. The curves continue to decline for as long as the patients are followed.

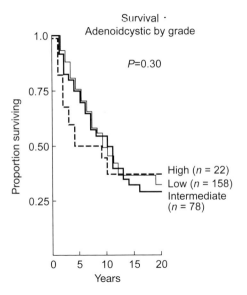

Fig. 19.2 Cumulative survival according to tumour grade. The trend towards lower survival with high-grade tumours disappears after patients have been followed more than 10 years.

clinical stage of the tumour has a highly significant impact on treatment results. Ten, 15-, and 20-year disease-specific survival in patients with stage I tumours was 94, 81, and 73%, respectively, compared with 50, 40, and 33% for stage II, and 18, 10, and 0 for stages III and IV, combined.

We found no significant difference in results when patients with ACC arising in major salivary glands were compared with those having minor gland tumours, except for a significantly lower survival rate in patients with nasal cavity or sinus primaries. These tend to be higher stage tumors which more often require complex, technically challenging resections. With respect to tumour grade, the trend towards better survival noted in those whose tumours showed a predominantly cribriform pattern (grade 1) was less apparent as these patients were followed beyond 10 years (Fig 19.2).

Treatment of distant metastases

On rare occasions, definitive treatment of a primary ACC may be indicated despite the presence of pulmonary metastases initially. Patients with minimal lung involvement may live for years (>10 years in 10%) with minimal symptoms, and control of the potentially symptomatic primary tumour by resection may enhance the quality of survival.

When ACC metastasizes to the lungs, patients are often referred to the medical oncologist and occasionally to the thoracic surgeon. Presently, there are no single agents or drug combinations that have a significant and predictable impact on this tumour. For this reason, it is hard to justify potentially morbid chemotherapy unless there are symptoms to palliate.

In some centres, metastasectomy has been performed in selected ACC patients who develop pulmonary metastases. Those who advocate a thoracotomy in this setting need to appreciate the unique biological behaviour of this unusual tumour (i.e. prolonged survival with or without treatment), as well as the fact that lung metastases in patients with ACC are almost always multiple (Fig. 19.3). At the time of writing, there are no solid data to confirm that resection of metastatic lung lesions from ACC yields a significant survival benefit.

The implications of histological grade and perineural invasion   Andrew Barrett and Paul Speight

ACC is defined by the World Health Organization as 'an infiltrative malignant tumour having various histological features with three growth patterns: glandular (cribriform), tubular or solid. The tumour cells are of two types: duct-lining cells and cells of myoepithelial type. Perineural or perivascular spread without stromal reaction is very characteristic. All structural types of adenoid cystic carcinoma can be associated in the same tumour' (Seifert 1991).

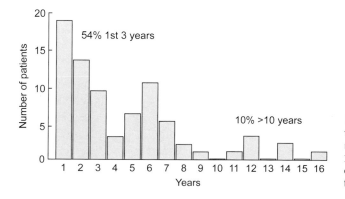

Fig. 19.3 Survival in years after the detection of distant metastasis. Death occurred within 3 years in 54%, but survivals in excess of 10 years were recorded for 10% of the patients.

211

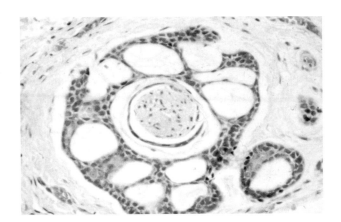

Fig. 19.4 An adenoid cystic carcinoma showing the typical cribriform pattern and perineural infiltration.

There is general agreement that some histological factors are related to the prognosis of this tumour. Most authorities, for example, accept that of the various morphological patterns, the tubular or cribriform subtypes are the best differentiated and offer the best prognosis, while the solid type is the least differentiated and the most aggressive clinically (Perzin *et al.* 1978). The significance of perineural invasion (PNI), however, remains uncertain and disputed (Fig. 19.4). Spiro and co-workers have documented a cohort of ACC amounting to more than 400 cases and have suggested that histological features, including PNI, are not reliable as predictors of ACC behaviour. They conclude that clinical stage is more predictive of distant metastasis and ultimate prognosis (Spiro and Huvos 1992; Spiro 1997).

With respect to PNI, the WHO concur with Spiro's group, but others do not, and neurotropism and spread by PNI would seem a reasonable explanation for the propensity of ACC to recur locally and show occult extension beyond the apparent resection margins. The purpose of this review is to establish if evidence of PNI affects the patient's prognosis.

The incidence of clinically apparent perineural invasion

Other than palsy or numbness, symptoms of PNI are often non-specific, but strong evidence for PNI is a burning pain, such as glossopyrosis (Hemprich and Schmidseder 1988), or stinging sensation, especially in the distribution of the trigeminal (usually) or other cranial nerve (Laine *et al.* 1990). An atypical *tic douloureux* has also been reported as a clinical manifestation of PNI in ACC (Laine *et al.* 1990).

In 18 published studies, the mean percentage of patients with evidence of neurological deficit (other than pain) was 23% (median 18%, range 2–86%) (Table 19.1). That less than a quarter of patients with ACC suffer paralysis or paraesthesia may be attributable to the fact that a major nerve may not be in the vicinity of the tumour (Huang *et al.* 1997), nerves undergo pressure degeneration only in the later stages of disease or in confined spaces (Chomette *et al.* 1982), and finally nerves may be involved without accompanying nerve dysfunction (Ballantyne *et al.* 1963; Witt 1991).

Table 19.1 Frequency of paralysis and/or paraesthesia in adenoid cystic carcinoma of the salivary glands: all affected nerves are cranial nerves (Roman numerals)

Authors	Site	n	% with symptoms	Affected nerve
Smout and French (1961)	Nasopharynx and paranasal sinuses	19	37	I–VII
Smout and French (1961)	Parotid	14	21	VII
Blanck et al. (1967)	Parotid	35	29	VII
Eneroth (1972)	Parotid	49	26	VII
Spiro et al (1974)	All	68	13	VII*
	Parotid	35	20	Not specified
Conley and	Submandibular	18	13	Not specified
Dingman (1974)	Sublingual	3	33	Not specified
	Minor	78	18	Not specified
Cummings (1977)	Parotid	14	57	VII
Perzin et al. (1978)	All	62	5	V, VII, X
Seaver and Kuehn (1979)	All	93	11	VII, X
Marsh and Allen (1979)	All	38	16	III, IV, V, VI, VII, VIII
Nascimento et al. (1986)	All	61	2	VII
Hemprich and Schmidseder (1988)	All	21	10	V
Koka et al. (1989)	All	51	8	Not stated
Weinstein and Conley (1989)	Parotid	43	18	VII
Weber et al. (1990)	Submandibular	86**	12	V, VII, XII
Callender et al. (1992)	Parotid and submandibular	3	33	VII
Huang et al. (1997)	Parotid	14	9	VII
Ginsberg and DeMonte (1998)	Palate	7	86	II, III, IV, V,V I, VII†

* Six patients had parotid ACC, three had submandibular gland ACC.

† Via the greater petrosal nerve.

** All malignant submandibular gland tumours, not just ACC.

Histopathological evidence of perineural invasion and its effect on outcome

If histological evidence of PNI is sought (Table 19.2), the mean frequency is 51% with a median of 46% and range of 8–96%. The effect of this feature on outcome was only recorded in 25 studies; 14 reported an adverse effect and 11 no effect. However, only 15 studies applied statistical tests; of these, nine reported an adverse affect on prognosis and six no effect. In the adverse group, four publications added the qualification that the involved nerves either had to be major, 'named' nerves, or nerves of a minimum diameter (0.25–3 mm; Luna et al. 1990). The relationship is unclear; in some reports, PNI corre-

Table 19.2 Frequency of histological PNI in adenoid cystic carcinoma of the salivary glands, with association with prognosis

Authors	Site	n	% with PNI	Prognostic significance
Moran *et al.* (1961)	All	127	85	Not stated
Smout and French (1961)	All	65	43	Not stated
Bardwil *et al.* (1966)	Minor	48	46	Not stated
Stuteville and Corley (1967)	Intraoral	36	33	Worse*
Blanck *et al.* (1967)	Parotid	35	46	Worse*
Luna *et al.* (1968)	Intraoral	33	51	Not stated
Leafstedt *et al.* (1971)	All	81	46	None*
Byers *et al.* (1973)	Submandibular	21	71	Worse*
Tarpley and Giansanti (1976)	Minor	50	29	Worse*
Osborn (1977)	All	43	14	None*
Perzin *ct al* (1978)	All	62	60	None*
Seaver and Kuehn (1979)	All	93	20	Worse*
Szanto *et al.* (1984)	All	79	76	None
Morinaga *et al.* (1986)	All	61	51	None
Nascimento *et al.* (1986)	All	61	33	None
Shingaki *et al.* (1986)	All	13	8	Not stated
Matsuba *et al.* (1986)	All	71	86	None*
Santucci and Bondi (1986)	All	34	38	Worse
van der Wal *et al.* (1986)	Intraoral	22	72	None
Vrielinck *et al.* (1988)	All	37	51	Worse
Hemprich and Schmidseder (1988)	All	21	33	Not stated
Koka *et al.* (1989)	All	51	31	None
Weber *et al.* (1989)	Lip/buccal	42	38	Worse
Weber *et al.* (1990)	Submandibular	37	84	None
Luna *et al.* (1990)	Submandibular	26	96	Worse[†]
Eibling *et al.* (1991)	All	28	96	Worse[†]
Witt (1991)	Minor	14	29	None*
Kuhel *et al.* (1992)	Palate	41	42	Not stated
Sigal *et al.* (1992)	All	26	23	Not stated
Beckhardt *et al.* (1995)	Palate	43	35[‡]	Worse
Garden *et al.* (1995)	All	198	69	Worse[†]
Toth *et al.* (1996)	All	33	61	Not stated
Gandour-Edwards *et al.* (1997)	All	18	83	Not stated
Huang *et al.* (1997)	All	91	63	Worse
Fordice *et al.* (1999)	All	160	49	Worse[†]

* No statistical tests carried out, or *P*-value for results not given.

[†] If a major nerve (i.e. cranial or branch), or nerve above a certain diameter is involved, not if there is merely focal PNI or involvement of very small nerves.

[‡] This study comprised 116 malignant salivary gland tumours, of which ACC comprised 43; 35% of the entire sample showed PNI. The specific percentage of ACC showing PNI was not stated.

lated to recurrence but not survival (Eibing *et al.* 1991), and in others it was significant at the univariate, but not the multivariate level (Beckhardt *et al.* 1995). A confounding factor is that the sample size is only about 50 cases in most studies. The two largest studies ($n = 198$ and $n = 160$) reported an adverse outcome with PNI provided large nerves were involved (Garden *et al.* 1995; Fordice *et al.* 1999). However, PNI correlates with other factors (Box 19.1) including tumour size and morphology, which are also associated with outcome.

Which nerves are critical?

All prospect of cure is lost once ACC breaches the base of the skull, a situation primarily related to minor gland tumours (Conley and Dingman 1974). The routes via which invasion of the cranial base is most likely to occur are the maxillary (V_2) and the mandibular (V_3) divisions of the trigeminal nerve, and the facial nerve. In reviewing 11 ACC amongst a collection of 80 head and neck tumours which showed PNI, the major nerves involved were named in each case (Ballantyne *et al.* 1963). These were branches of V_3 in seven cases, the facial nerve in one, both the trigeminal and the facial nerves in one, the palatine nerves in one, and in one ACC of the maxillary sinus, the optic nerve. ACC of the submandibular gland can also involve the hypoglossal nerve (Weber *et al.* 1989; Huang *et al.* 1997).

The maxillary (V_2) and mandibular (V_3) divisions of the trigeminal nerve

Intraorbital and, subsequently, intracranial extension of ACC of the palatal and maxillary antral glands may occur via contiguous spread through the pterygopalatine fossa (Bardwil *et al.* 1966; Lee *et al.* 1997), and ocular symptoms have been reported after a palatal tumour permeated the inferior orbital fissure (Ginsberg *et al.* 1998). The infraorbital nerve is at risk from ACC of the maxillary sinus (Vrielinck *et al.* 1988), and may

---

Box 19.1 Clinicopathological correlations with perineural invasion (PNI)

PNI in ACC correlates with:

◆ Tumour size

◆ Duration of disease

◆ Positive margin

◆ In certain sites (e.g. paranasal sinuses), denotes a grave prognosis

But PNI does not correlate with:

◆ Lymphatic metastasis

present with paraesthesia of the maxillary teeth (Beckhardt *et al.* 1995). The vulnerable branches of V_3 are the lingual, inferior alveolar, and mylohyoid nerves when tumour is present in the submandibular gland (Conley and Dingman 1974; Lee *et al.* 1985; Weber *et al.* 1990), tongue, or floor of the mouth (Bardwil *et al.* 1966). The mental nerve is at risk with labial gland ACC (Bardwil *et al.* 1966), and the auriculotemporal nerve from parotid tumours (Ballantyne *et al.* 1963).

Once at the foramen rotundum (in the case of V_2) or the foramen ovale (V_3), neoplastic cells can enter the middle cranial fossa and cavernous sinus to reach other branches of the trigeminal nerve.

The facial nerve

ACC of the parotid have been reported to pass through the stylomastoid foramen, along the facial canal and internal acoustic meatus to gain access into the posterior cranial fossa (Kumar *et al.* 1993). Symptoms of such extensive spread along the facial nerve are uncommon, but facial paralysis is a negative prognostic indicator because it denotes either advanced disease or the presence of a tumour with an aggressive nature. Eneroth (1972) documented 378 patients with malignant parotid tumours, 46 (12%) of whom had facial nerve palsy and the vast majority of whom (98%) died from their disease. In 6/46, this was the only symptom of the tumour. in comparison, only 33% of the 332 patients without facial palsy died. The risk for metastasis was also much higher (77% as opposed to 27%) if facial nerve paralysis had developed, and only 11% of patients with facial nerve paralysis survived 5 years. The rate of facial palsy in ACC was more than twice that of the study cohort as a whole (26%), but paradoxically the mean survival time after onset of paralysis was actually longer in cases of ACC (3.9 years, range 6 months–8.5 years) than the mean for all malignancies (just over 2 years).

Histological grading

Several investigators have looked at possible correlations between morphology and PNI. One group reported that 39% of tumours with a cribriform or solid morphology showed PNI, compared with 23% of tubular lesions, and thus suggested that there is a link between PNI and the histological growth pattern. Statistical analysis showed that the mortality rate was significantly higher in patients whose tumours showed PNI (Santucci and Bondi 1986). These authors also discussed the tumour's growth in terms of 'pushing' or 'infiltrative' fronts, with the former never showing PNI. A combination of infiltrative front and PNI was fatal in 92% of the cases where it occurred. The fact that most ACC were of solid morphology coincided with the highest rates of PNI in the submandibular and sublingual glands, according to another group (Huang *et al.* 1997).

These observations are supported by some (Byers *et al.* 1973), but contradicted by others (Shinganki *et al.* 1986). Whilst PNI occurred in 20/61 ACC, of which nine were solid, 11 cribriform, and three tubular, a trend similar to that noted above (Santucci and Bondi 1986), there was no correlation with outcome (Santucci and Bondi 1986).

216

Does PNI affect prognosis?

Histological evidence of PNI does not appear to be an independent factor but is associated with larger and more aggressive tumours. Clinical evidence on PNI (e.g. facial nerve palsy) is an important prognostic factor and is one of the features taken into account in staging.

The role of conservative versus radical surgery
Gordon Snow and Isaac van der Waal

In the past, the great majority of ACC have been treated by surgery alone. Invariably, high local recurrence rates, varying from 42 up to 67%, have been reported after surgery (Conley and Dingman 1974; Spiro *et al.* 1974; Jones *et al.* 1997). This is attributed to insidious infiltration into soft tissue and bone, and to perineural invasion and extension, making delineation of the surgical margins difficult. Super-radical surgery has been advocated to overcome this problem (Conley and Dingman 1974). Conventionally, these tumours have been considered to have poor radiosensitivity, and radiotherapy has not been used much in the management of this disease in the past. However, in the last three decades, radiotherapy has been applied as a post-operative adjunct to surgery in many centres. From the reported results, it is quite clear that the combination of surgery and post-operative radiotherapy has reduced local recurrence rates dramatically. Based on these experiences, surgery with post-operative radiotherapy has been implemented in many institutions as standard therapy for all but the smallest ACCs with clear margins and without perineural invasion. As a consequence of this important development, the question has come up: Is it really necessary and in the interest of the patient with ACC that the surgeon always aims to obtain tumour-free margins at all costs, or is there a place for conservative, less than radical surgery when this is combined with post-operative radiotherapy? In an attempt to provide an answer to this question, the experiences gained with the combination of surgery and post-operative radiotherapy in the treatment of ACC will be reviewed in more detail, focusing first on the factors which determine the efficacy of radiotherapy in this setting. Subsequently, the role of surgery integrated into combined treatment with radiotherapy will be discussed, in particular for the sites most often involved.

The efficacy of post-operative radiotherapy

The local recurrence rates reported after treatment with surgery and post-operative radiotherapy for ACC vary between 15 and just over 20% (Cowie and Pointon 1984; Simpson *et al.* 1984; Miglianico *et al.* 1987; Kim *et al.* 1994; Fordice *et al.* 1999). Garden *et al.* (1995) analysed in detail the influence of positive margins and nerve invasion in ACC treated with surgery and radiation in a large series of almost 200 patients. Forty-two percent of their patients had microscopic positive margins, and an additional 28% had close (5 mm) or uncertain margins. Eighteen percent of patients with positive margins developed local recurrences, compared with 9% with close or uncertain margins and 5% with negative margins. In the whole series, there was a trend towards better local control with increasing doses. This was significant in patients with positive margins, in whom local control rates were 40 and 88% for doses <56 Gy and ≥56Gy, respectively. Similarly, Simpson *et al.* (1984) found that patients who received a dose ≥60 Gy in addition to surgery had significantly higher local control rates than those who received <60 Gy. Miglianico *et al.* (1987) attempted to define a threshold dose that would allow adequate local control. It appeared that a dose of 65 Gy is required in cases of irradiation after incomplete resection. Garden *et al.* (1995) recommend a dose of 60 Gy to the tumour bed, supplemented to 66 Gy for patients with positive margins. Garden *et al.* (1995) furthermore found that perineural invasion was an adverse factor only when a major (named) nerve was involved. In that situation, they advise treating the base of skull electively.

It is important to note that decrease of local failure by combined therapy does not appear to have had a major impact on survival. The main reason for this is that distant metastases continue to develop in 38–50% of patients (Simpson *et al.* 1984; Spiro 1997). Spiro (1997) has demonstrated that primary tumour size in excess of 3 cm is highly predictive of distant metastases.

The role of surgery integrated into combined treatment with radiotherapy

The aim of cancer surgery is to obtain free margins. Patients in whom the surgeon has succeeded in obtaining clear margins in general do better than those with positive margins. ACC is no exception in this regard. However, in many cases of ACC, it is much more difficult, if not impossible, to obtain free margins than it is for example in squamous cell carcinoma (SCC) of the head and neck. Actually, when margins are taken that are generally considered to be adequate in SCC—depending on the site within the head and neck, 1–2 cm of healthy looking tissue all around the tumour—the margins have been proven to be positive in the majority of patients with ACC. With post-operative radiotherapy, local recurrence rates can be reduced to around 15%. Furthermore, the difference in survival between patients with free margins and those with positive margins appears to be much less in ACC than in SCC because distant failures are much more frequent in ACC. Another unique feature of ACC is that it usually has a prolonged clinical course, spanning a decade or more, despite progressive disease. Quality of life, always important, is a vital issue for the typical patient with ACC, who will live many years after initial therapy. It is against this background that many head and neck surgeons today would agree with the statement expressed by Garden *et al.* (1995) that: 'Surgical management is to be balanced between being aggressive enough to ideally obtain clear margins, but not be overly morbid when all gross disease has been removed.' To illustrate this philosophy of conservative surgery in combination with post-operative radiotherapy, our management policy in ACC at the two most often involved sites, the oral cavity—particularly the palate—and the parotid gland, will be discussed in more detail.

ACC in the oral cavity

The potential local and regional spread of ACC in the oral cavity has been well described and depicted by Conley and Dingman (1974). Bearing in mind the potential spread, these authors state that 'the biggest operation that can be rationally developed is the best. The inability to evaluate the perimeters of this tumour clinically dictates that the boldest attack on the tumour and its environs should be the primary objective; this is the prime opportunity for cure'. From the 1970s, we have implemented a different approach of conservative surgery followed by radiotherapy. Between 1970 and 1988, 20 patients with intraoral ACC were treated initially by surgery (van der Wal *et al.* 1989). A margin of clinically (and radiographically) normal tissue was included in the excision. The width of the margin varied depending on the site of the tumour. For instance, in tumours of the palate, a margin of approximately 1 cm was included, while in other sites (e.g. the upper lip) a more conservative excision was performed.

In four cases, there were negative surgical margins; in 16 cases there were positive margins at histopathological examination. Fourteen of these 16 patients received post-operative radiotherapy. Relatively wide fields along with shrinking fields techniques were used. Dosages, with conventional tumour dose fractions of 2 Gy, five fractions a week, ranged from 66 to 70 Gy. Long-term local control was achieved in all 14 patients with positive surgical margins who underwent post-operative irradiation. These results are consistent with those reported by others (Regine *et al.* 1993). Post-operative radio-therapy seems an adequate treatment to deal with the problem of positive surgical margins at the microscopical level in intraoral ACC, avoiding excessively mutilating surgery. It is of interest to note that nine of these 14 patients died of distant metastases at varying intervals (2–19 years) after primary treatment of their ACCs.

ACC of the parotid gland

One of the most difficult problems which can occur during parotid surgery is that in which the tumour lies very close to the facial nerve, whose function was intact before operation. The two objects of parotid surgery, i.e. removal of the tumour and preserva-tion of the facial nerve, are then in conflict. We encountered this treatment dilemma in six patients with ACC (Leverstein *et al.* 1998). Our surgical philosophy in such cases is conservative. The facial nerve is carefully peeled off the tumour, although this trans-gresses the classical oncological principle that malignant tumours ought to be removed with a wide healthy margin. After a full course of post-operative radiotherapy, only one of the six patients with a median follow-up of more than 5 years developed a local recurrence, while in each patient facial nerve function remained completely intact. Similar favourable experiences with this policy have been reported by others (McNaney *et al.* 1983). However, if the facial nerve is surrounded by tumour and preservation of the nerve would indicate that macroscopic remnants of tumour would be left behind, the nerve ought to be resected.

Finally, it is important to emphasize that combined modality treatment is associated with increased morbidity when compared with single modality treatment. The morbid-ity is site-dependent, patients with primary tumours in the nose and paranasal sinuses suffering more severe morbidity than patients with primary tumours at other sites (Fordice *et al.* 1999). However, it is to be remembered that there is general agreement that in the overwhelming majority of ACC, a combination of surgery and postoperative radiotherapy is absolutely required.

REFERENCES

Ballantyne, A.J., McCarten, A.B., and Ibanez, M.L. (1963) The extension of cancer of the head and neck through peripheral nerves. *Am J Surg*, **106**, 651–67.

Bardwil, J.M., Reynolds, C.T., Ibanez, M.L., and Luna, M.A. (1966) Report of one hundred tumors of the minor salivary glands. *Am J Surg*, **112**, 493–7.

Beckhardt, R.N., Weber, R.S., Zane, R., Garden, A.S., Wolf, P., Carrillo, R. *et al.* (1995) Minor salivary gland tumors of the palate: clinical and pathologic correlates of outcome. *Laryngoscope*, **105**, 1155–60.

Bilroth, T. (1859) Beobachtugen uber Geschwulste der Speicheldrusen. *Virchows Arch Pathol Anat*, **17**, 357–75.

Blanck, C., Eneroth, C.-M., Jacobsson, F., and Jakobsson, P.A. (1967) Adenoid cystic carcinoma of the parotid gland. *Acta Radiol Ther Phys Biol*, **6**, 177–96.

Byers, R.M., Jesse, R.H., Guillamondegui, O.M., and Luna, M.A. (1973) Malignant tumors of the submaxillary gland. *Am J Surg*, **126**, 458–63.

Callender, D.L., Frankenthaler, R.A., Luna, M.A., Lee, S.S., and Goepfert, H. (1992) Salivary gland neoplasms in children. *Arch Otolaryngol Head Neck Surg*, **118**, 472–6.

Chomette, G., Auriol, M., Tranbaloc, P., and Vaillant, J.M. (1982) Adenoid cystic carcinoma of minor salivary glands. Analysis of 86 cases. Clinico-pathological, histoenzymological and ultrastructural studies. *Virchows Archs (Pathol Anat)*, **395**, 289–301.

Conley, J. and Dingman, D.L. (1974) Adenoid cystic carcinoma in the head and neck (cylindroma). *Arch Otolaryngol*, **100**, 81–90.

Cowie, V.J. and Pointon, R.C.S. (1984) Adenoid cystic carcinoma of the salivary glands. *Clin Radiol*, **35**, 331–3.

Cummings, C.W. (1977) Adenoidcystic (sic) carcinoma (cylindroma) of the parotid gland. *Ann Otol Rhinol Laryngol*, **86**, 280–92.

Dockerty, M.B. and Mayo, C.W. (1942) Primary tumours of the submaxillary gland with special reference to mixed tumours. *Surg, Gynecol Obstet*, **74**, 1033–45.

Eibling, D.E., Johnson, J.T., McCoy, J.P., Jr, Barnes, E.L., Syms, C.A., Wagner, R.L. *et al.* (1991) Flow cytometric evaluation of adenoid cystic carcinoma: comparison with histologic subtype and survival. *Am J Surg*, **162**, 367–72.

Eneroth, C.-M. (1972) Facial nerve paralysis—a criterion of malignancy in parotid tumours. *Arch Otolaryngol*, **95**, 300–4.

Foote, F.W. and Frazell, E.L. (1953) Tumours of the major salivary glands. *Cancer*, **6**, 1065–133.

Fordice, J., Kershaw, C., El-Naggar, A., and Goepfert, H. (1999) Adenoid cystic carcinoma of the head and neck: predictors of morbidity and mortality. *Arch Otolaryngol Head Neck Surg*, **125**, 149–52.

Gandour-Edwards, R., Kapadia, S.B., Barnes, L., Donald, P.J., and Janecka, I.P. (1997) Neural cell adhesion molecule in adenoid cystic carcinoma invading the skull base. *Otolaryngol Head Neck Surg*, **117**, 453–8.

Garden, A.S., Weber, R.S., Morrison, W.H., Ang, K.K., and Peters, L.J. (1995) The influence of positive margins and nerve invasion in adenoid cystic carcinoma of the head and neck treated with surgery and radiation. *Int J Radiat Oncol Biol Phys*, **32**, 619–26.

Ginsberg, L.E. and DeMonte, F. (1998) Imaging of perineural tumor spread from palatal carcinoma. *AJNR Am J Neuroradiol*, **19**, 1417–22.

Hemprich, A. and Schmidseder, R. (1998) The adenoid cystic carcinoma. Special aspects of its growth and therapy. *J Craniomaxfac Surg*, **16**, 136–9.

Huang, M., Ma, D.Q., Sun, K., Guangyan, Y., Guo, C., and Gao, F. (1997) Factors influencing survival rate in adenoid cystic carcinoma of the salivary glands. *Int J Oral Maxillofac Surg*, **26**, 435–9.

Jones, A.S., Hamilton, J.W., Rowley, H., Husband, D., and Helliwell, T.R. (1997) Adenoid cystic carcinoma of the head and neck. *Clin Otolaryngol*, **22**, 434–43.

Kim, K.H., Sung, M.W., Chung, P.S., Rhee, C.S., Park, C.I., and Kim, W.H. (1994) Adenoid cystic carcinoma of the head and neck. *Arch Otolaryngol Head Neck Surg*, **120**, 721–6.

Koka, V.N., Tiwari, R.M., van der Waal, I., Snow, G.B., Nauta, J., Karim, A.B.M.F. *et al.* (1989) Adenoid cystic carcinoma of the salivary glands: clinicopathological survey of 51 patients. *J Laryngol Otol*, **103**, 675–9.

Kuhel, W., Goepfert, H., Luna, M., Wendt, C., and Wolf, P. (1992) Adenoid cystic carcinoma of the palate. *Arch Otolaryngol Head Neck Surg*, **118**, 243–7.

Kumar, P.P., Patil, A.A., Ogren, F.P., Johansson, S.L., and Reeves, M.A. (1993) Intracranial skip metastasis from parotid and facial skin tumors: mechanism, diagnosis, and treatment. *J Nat Med Assoc*, **85**, 369–74.

Laine, F.J., Sen, M.E., Braun, I.F., Nadel, L., and Som, P.M. (1990) Perineural tumor extension through the foramen ovale: evaluation with MR imaging. *Radiology*, **174**, 65–71.

Leafstedt, S.W., Gaeta, J.F., Sako, K., Marchetta, F.C., and Shedd, D.P. (1971) Adenoid cystic carcinoma of major and minor salivary glands. *Am J Surg*, **122**, 756–62.

Lee, A.G., Phillips, P.H., Newman, N.J., Hayman, L.A., Schiffman, J.S., Segal, S.E. *et al.* (1997) Neuro-ophthalmologic manifestations of adenoid cystic carcinoma. *J Neuro-Ophthalmol*, **17**, 183–8.

Lee, Y.Y., Castillo, M., and Nauert, C. (1985) Intracranial perineural metastasis of adenoid cystic carcinoma of head and neck. *J Comput Tomogr*, **9**, 219–23.

Leverstein, H., Van der Wal, J.E., Tiwari, R.M., Tobi, H., Van der Waal, I., Mehta, D.M. *et al.* (1998) Malignant epithelial parotid gland tumours: analysis and results in 65 previously untreated patients. *Br J Surg*, **85**, 1267–72.

Luna, M.A., Stimson, P.G., and Bardwil, J.M. (1968) Minor salivary gland tumours of the oral cavity. A review of 68 cases. *Oral Surg*, **25**, 71–86.

Luna, M.A., El-Naggar, A., Batsakis, J.G., Weber, R.S., Garnsey, L.A., and Goepfert, H. (1990) Flow cytometric DNA content of adenoid cystic carcinoma of submandibular gland. *Arch Otolaryngol Head Neck Surg*, **116**, 1291–6.

Marsh, W.L. and Allen, M.S. (1979) Adenoid cystic carcinoma. Biologic behaviour in 38 patients. *Cancer*, **43**, 1463–73.

Matsuba, H.M., Spector, G.J., Thawley, S.E., Simpson, J.R., Mauney, M., and Pikul, F.J. (1986) Adenoid cystic salivary gland carcinoma. A histopathological review of treatment failure patterns. *Cancer*, **57**, 519–24.

McNaney, D., McNeese, M.D., Guillamondegui, O.M., Fletcher, G.H., and Oswald, M.J. (1983) Postoperative irradiation in malignant epithelial tumors of the parotid. *Int J Radiat Oncol Biol Phys*, **9**, 1289–95.

Moran, J.J., Becker, S.M., Brady, L.W., and Rambo, V.B. (1961) Adenoid cystic carcinoma. A clinicopathological study. *Cancer*, **14**, 1235–50.

Miglianico, L., Eschwege, F., Marandas, P., and Wibault, P. (1987) Cervico-facial adenoid cystic carcinoma: study of 102 cases. *Int J Radiat Oncol Biol Phys*, **13**, 673–8.

221

Morinaga, S., Nakajima, T., Shimosato, Y., Saitoh, H., Ebihara, S., and Ono, I. (1986) Histologic factors influencing prognosis of adenoid cystic carcinoma of the head and neck. *Jpn J Clin Oncol*, **16**, 29–40.

Nascimento, A.G., Amaral, A.L.P., Prado, L.A.F., Kligerman, J., and Silveira, T.R.P. (1986) Adenoid cystic carcinoma of salivary glands. A study of 61 cases with clinicopathologic correlation. *Cancer*, **57**, 312–9.

Osborn, D.A. (1977) Morphology and the natural history of cribriform adenocarcinoma (adenoid cystic carcinoma). *J Clin Pathol*, **30**, 195–205.

Perzin, K.H., Gullane, P., and Clairmont, A.C. (1978) Adenoid cystic carcinomas arising in salivary glands. *Cancer*, **42**, 265–82.

Regine, W.F., Mendenhall, W.M., Parsons, J.T., Stringer, S.P., Cassisi, N.J., and Million, R.R. (1993) Radiotherapy for adenoid cystic carcinoma of the palate. *Head Neck*, **15**, 241–4.

Santucci, M. and Bondi, R. (1986) Histologic–prognostic correlations in adenoid cystic carcinoma of major and minor salivary glands of the oral cavity. *Tumori*, **72**, 293–300.

Seaver, P.R., Jr and Kuehn, P.G. (1979) Adenoid cystic carcinoma of the salivary glands. A study of 93 cases. *Am J Surg*, **137**, 449–55.

Seifert, G. (1991) *Histological Typing of Salivary Gland Tumours*, 2nd edn. Springer-Verlag, Berlin.

Shingaki, S., Saito, R., Kawasaki, T., and Nakajima, T. (1986) Adenoid cystic carcinoma of the major and minor salivary glands. A clinicopathological study of 17 cases. *J Maxfac Surg*, **14**, 53–6.

Sigal, R., Monnet, O., de Baere, T., Micheau, C., Shapeero, L.G., Julieron, M. *et al.* (1992) Adenoid cystic carcinoma of the head and neck: evaluation with MR imaging and clinical–pathologic correlation in 27 patients. *Radiology*, **184**, 95–101.

Simpson, J.R., Thawley, S.E., and Matsuba, H.M. (1984) Adnoid cystic salivary gland carcinoma: treatment with irradiation and surgery. *Radiology*, **151**, 509–12.

Smout, M.S. and French, A.J. (1961) Prognosis of pseudoadenomatous basal-cell carcinoma. *Arch Pathol*, **72**, 107–12.

Spiro, R. (1997) Distant metastasis in adenoid cystic carcinoma of salivary origin. *Am J Surg*, **174**, 495–8.

Spiro, R.H. and Huvos, A.G. (1992) Stage means more than grade in adenoid cystic carcinoma. *Am J Surg*, **164**, 623–8.

Spiro, R.H., Huvos, A.G., and Strong, E.W. (1974) Adenoid cystic carcinoma of salivary origin. A clinicopathologic study of 242 cases. *Am J Surg*, **128**, 512–20.

Spiro, R.H., Thaler, H.T., Hicks, W.F., Kher, U.A., Huvos, A.H., and Strong, E.W. (1991) The importance of clinical staging of minor salivary gland carcinoma. *Am J Surg*, **162**, 330–6.

Stuteville, O.H. and Corley, R.D. (1967) Surgical management of tumors of intraoral salivary glands. *Cancer*, **20**, 1578–86.

Szanto, P.A., Luna, M.A., Tortoledo, M.E., and White, R.A. (1984) Histologic grading of adenoid cystic carcinoma of the salivary glands. *Cancer*, **54**, 1062–9.

Tarpley, T.T. and Giansanti, J.S. (1976) Adenoid cystic carcinoma. Analysis of 50 cases. *Oral Surg*, **41**, 484–97.

Toth, A.A., Daley, T.D., Lampe, H.B., Stitt, L., and Veinot, L. (1996) Schwann cell differentiation of modified myoepithelial cells within adenoid cystic carcinomas and polymorphous low-grade adenocarcinomas: clinicopathologic assessment of immunohistochemical staining. *J Otolaryngol*, **25**, 94–102.

van der Wal, J.E., Snow, G.B., and van der Waal, I. (1986) Intraoral adenoid cystic carcinoma. The presence of perineural spread in relation to site, size, local extension, and metastatic spread in 22 cases. *Cancer*, **66**, 2031–3.

van der Wal, J.E., Snow, G.B., Karim, A.B.M.F., and Van der Waal, I. (1989) Intraoral adenoid cystic carcinoma: the role of postoperative radiotherapy in local control. *Head Neck*, **11**, 497–9.

Vrielinck, L.J.G., Ostyn, F., Van Damme, B., Van den Bogaert, W., and Fossian, E. (1988) The significance of perineural spread in adenoid cystic carcinoma of the major and minor salivary glands. *Int J Oral Maxillofac Surg*, **17**, 190–3.

Weber, R.S., Palmer, J.M., el-Naggar, A., McNeese, M.D, Guillamondegui, M., and Byers, R.M. (1989) Minor salivary gland tumors of the lip and buccal mucosa. *Laryngoscope*, **99**, 6–9.

Weber, R.S., Byers, R.M., Petit, B., Wolf, P., Ang, K., and Luna, M. (1990) Submandibular gland tumors. Adverse histologic factors and therapeutic implications. *Arch Otolaryngol Head Neck Surg*, **116**, 1055–60.

Weinstein, G.S. and Conley, J.J. (1989) Adenoid cystic carcinoma of the parotid gland: a review of surgical management with reference to the facial nerve. *Ann Otol Rhinol Laryngol*, **98**, 845–7.

Witt, R.L. (1991) Adenoid cystic carcinoma of the minor salivary glands. *Ear, Nose Throat J*, **70**, 218–22.

Audience discussion

Professor Spiro: Professor Snow, I think your talk was provocative. What troubles me is the word 'conservative' in the treatment of adenoid cystic carcinoma. The surgical approach to ACC is clearly not 'conservative' although the anatomic location may limit the extent of surgery and compromise the margins. Is this what you mean by 'conservative'?

Professor Snow: The word 'conservative' was proposed by Professor McGurk. It may not be perfect but it does confer a theme which I perhaps need to explain further. It does not seem sensible to try at all costs to achieve free margins, as proposed in the past by Conley and Dingman. I really think that with post-operative radiotherapy the argument for super-radical surgery is no longer true. I would take this further and say that if the facial nerve is working pre-operatively (in the case of parotid adenoid cystic carcinoma), it should work post-operatively. By analogy, I have the same philosophy with the eye (in the case of anterior ethmoidal lesions); if there is unimpaired vision and no diplopia, one should aim to leave it (the eye).

Professor O'Brien (Sydney, Australia): May I just ask Professor Snow and Professor Spiro to pursue this facial nerve issue. How do you manage the facial nerve in a parotidectomy for either a known or suspected diagnosis of adenoid cystic, when at the time of operation the nerve is macroscopically abnormal although it was functioning normally pre-operatively? If you divide the nerve, do you use frozen section evaluation? Do you chase the nerve into the mastoids? When and how do you reconstruct?

Professor Spiro: This is a pretty broad question as you frame it. I have been in the position, not for adenoid cystic, where I had an erroneous false-negative frozen section diagnosis of a benign tumour when there was clinical evidence tumour of tumour infiltration of the nerve trunk. Guided by the histology, I opted not to sacrifice the nerve, and the carcinoma recurred. I have discussed this lesson at meetings—there is a body of opinion out there that was horrified that I would contemplate nerve sacrifice without a histological diagnosis. I disagree very strongly with this. I really spend time preparing my patients for the possibility of nerve loss even under the least threatening circumstances. I would much rather be overprepared that underprepared. I think you have to rely on clinical judgement at the end of surgery.

Professor Snow: I have peeled tumour off the facial nerve. To complicate matters, many of these nerves do not look normal—they are thickened and seem to be infiltrated with tumour. Still if I can peel a functioning nerve off the tumour, I do so. However, if a functioning facial nerve is surrounded by tumour, it ought to be resected. In this last situation, I like to have a frozen section just to be sure that it is cancer. We do take a frozen section of the transected nerve but we do not trace the nerve into the mastoid. When the transected nerve is positive, we do not undertake a reconstruction.

Professor Spiro: I would take frozen sections of the transected nerve and take the nerve back as far as the stylomastoid foramen if necessary. Personally, I would not get into an intricate nerve dissection at that point because I think that the deck (playing cards) is stacked against you.

Professor Spiro: I would like to emphasize the point Professor Snow made. I perceive a definite reluctance and a timidity in the surgical community to sacrifice nerves when they need to be sacrificed. What happens is the surgeon just dances and waltzes around the quality issues and the next thing you know he has got tumour contamination of his field. We need to have the resolve to take the nerve when it looks like it has to be taken. If it can possibly be spared, we all subscribe to the idea of conservatism. But you must, on the other hand, not be reticent when the clinical indications are readily apparent.

Professor McGurk (London, UK): Professor Speight, I would like to address the question of the wide local dissemination of ACC and the acknowledged difficulty in obtaining clear surgical margins ostensibly due to the tumour's capacity for perineural infiltration. Is there selective tumour migration down nerves or is neural infiltration just a feature of the individual tumour's propensity to diffuse local dissemination?

Secondly, do you think clinical evidence of nerve infiltration is itself important or is rather a indication of a biologically aggressive tumour?

Professor Speight: As a pathologist, apart from the very small localized ACC you occasionally see in the lip and sometimes in the parotid, I do not think I have ever seen an ACC with clear surgical margins. They are terribly infiltrative tumours. The perineural infiltration is, I think, a manifestation of this infiltrative nature. I do not think selective migration is a particular feature of this tumour. Nerve infiltration is not unique to ACC; other tumours also infiltrate nerves. The evidence we have obtained from the literature indicates that nerve infiltration correlates with large rapidly growing tumours. Obviously these factors are inter-related. So I think perineural infiltration is a manifestation of bad tumour biology.

Professor Spiro: I feel I should inject some optimism into this discussion. I am sure many of you in this audience have had an unpleasant surprise when you removed an apparently benign 1–1.5 cm parotid lump to be informed that it is an adenoid cystic carcinoma. These clinically benign cases can have clear margins. In my book, a standard subtotal parotidectomy, preserving the nerve, is an acceptable conservative procedure, as Professor Snow suggested, and in our experience the patient is likely to do well with a course of adjuvant radiation therapy.

Professor O'Brien: Professor Speight, in your talk you seemed to infer that histological factors predicted outcome. It is contrary to the Memorial Hospital experience.

Professor Speight: No, I showed a series of histological features which are associated with prognosis. I also said that none of these are independent variables. They were included and had to be taken into consideration when designating stage and grade.

Professor O'Brien: Can you tell me how you grade the tumours then?

Professor Speight: I do not, in my report, grade a tumour as low, intermediate or high. But I regard the solid adenoid cystic carcinomas as having a worse prognosis although the situation is confused by the fact that a lot of cribriform-type adenoid cystic carcinomas have solid areas and cannot be graded. So, in practice, the overall grading is really clinicopathologically based. You find out how the tumour has behaved, the speed of growth, clinical evidence of perineural infiltration, and check the radiographs for bone erosion. I do not think the histology features alone are sufficient.

Professor O'Brien: A question to the surgeons. This is a disease with protracted lethality. Would you ever consider carrying out a radical operation, in a very symptomatic patient with local or regional recurrence, in the presence of distant metastatic disease if the natural history of the metastatic disease was very slow?

Professor Spiro: It is a situation we have encounted. We have a small cohort (I cannot give you numbers of patients) who presented with otherwise localized resectable tumours and a few lung nodules. We resected the local disease on the presumption that the surgery was going to give the patient a better quality of life even if they are going to die of the disease eventually.

Professor Snow: I would like to come back to the word conservative for it may have been misinterpreted. I was speaking about the main sites for ACC, i.e. the oral cavity, the palate, and the parotid. The nose and sinuses are completely different, these cases do badly. I note that in Professor Spiro's presentation of intraoral lesions, more than half were major excisions. What margin would you take with a histologically proven adenoid cystic of the palate?

Professor Spiro: I arbitrarily define a radical operation as a maxillectomy; a more conservative operation will be wide local excision. When dealing with a small favourable adenoid cystic carcinoma, I advocate a somewhat aggressive approach in order to get a generous margin. It is not necessarily increasing the morbidity. In the palate, I aim for at least a 10 mm margin. The issue of whether to undertake an *en bloc* resection depends on the individual case. For a small (5 mm) adenoid cystic carcinoma, I could excise it without putting a hole in the palate. But more often than not, as they get larger the only way you can ensure a reasonable deep margin is to fenestrate the palate while you are at it.

Professor Spiro: Dr Slevin, adenoid cystic carcinoma is responsive to radiotherapy. Can these tumours be cured by this modality of treatment?

Dr Slevin (Manchester, UK): We seem to have quite a large series where the patients were treated with definitive radiotherapy out of preference to reduce the morbidity from surgery. My own experience is that with macroscopic disease the response is inconsistent. I would always advocate surgery with adjuvant radiotherapy. I have no experience with targeted radiotherapy in terms of boosting procedures. But in general terms the boosted area is quite large, so I do not think there is a place for such an approach.

Professor Spiro: I saw beam therapy used decades ago. You could certainly get a response but in a matter of months or few years the tumour grew back around the radiation field.

Editorial comment

Adenoid cystic carcinoma is the *bête noir* of salivary gland cancers, with a reputation for perineural spread, a high incidence of local recurrence, and a perception that it is incurable. This has produced a surgical mindset towards radical surgery, especially for the small resectable lesion. These issues have been addressed in this chapter.

What has emerged, and is the theme of this book, is that clinical features are all-important to optimal management of this salivary tumour. As with all tumour families, there is a spectrum of activity. The small, discrete adenoid cystic carcinoma that presents as an apparently benign lump can be cured. Professor Spiro reports disease-specific survival for stage I lesions of 73% at 20 years! Professor Snow's approach is not for radical surgery in this part of the disease spectrum. However, treatment has to be tailored to the clinical findings in each individual patient. In the palate, where tumour clearance is a reality without the threat of added morbidity, Professor Spiro advocates a determined approach to obtain clear margins.

There is general agreement that with large or high stage ACC it is difficult to obtain clear margins. Super-radical surgery is no more effective than adjuvant radiotherapy in reducing the risk of local recurrence, but carries significant morbidity.

Professor Speight has looked at the significance of perineural spread in the context of adenoid cystic carcinoma. On histological examination, about half of the patients will show evidence of perineural infiltration but only 50% of these patients will have clinical evidence of nerve dysfunction. The latter tends to accompany large or clinically high-grade cancers. Histological evidence of extensive nerve involvement appears simply to reflect the invasive or inherent adverse biological nature of the particular cancer and not a propensity to selective migration along nerves. There are, of course, vivid examples of ACC extending along nerves or nerve routes into the cranial cavity; but in the presence of gross local disease. Remarkable for its absence is evidence of late cranial extension in otherwise cured patients (Spiro 1997). Circumstantial evidence (Spiro 1997) would suggest that perineural extension is not a prominent feature of ACC. Perineural infiltration is not synonymous with perineural extension! The link is inferential.

CHAPTER 20

The management of skin metastases to the parotid lymph nodes

The Australian experience
Christopher O'Brien

Towards preserving the facial nerve
Meirion Thomas

The Australian experience   Christopher O'Brien

The patterns of parotid malignancy vary around the world. In North America and Europe, primary parotid malignancies occur more frequently than metastatic disease, and the commonest primary parotid malignancy is mucoepidermoid carcinoma. In Australia, because of the high incidence of cutaneous malignancy, especially involving the skin of the head and neck in areas draining readily to the parotid gland, the commonest form of parotid malignancies is metastatic carcinoma. This is exemplified by the parotid surgery experience of the author at the Department of Head and Neck Surgery, Royal Prince Alfred Hospital, Sydney (January 1987 to June 1999) summarized in Table 20.1. The common malignancies which metastasize to the parotid gland are cutaneous *squamous cell carcinoma*, *malignant melanoma*, and *Merkel cell carcinoma*.

Squamous cell carcinoma

Australia has the highest reported incidence of cutaneous squamous cell carcinoma in the world, estimated to be approximately 250 cases per 100 000 population annually (Marks *et al.* 1993). This incidence rate reflects a high level of recreational and occupational sun exposure in a population largely descended from Anglo-Saxons and Celts. Squamous cell carcinoma (SCC) accounts for approximately 20% of cutaneous malignancies in Australia, the commonest being *basal cell carcinoma*. There is evidence that approximately 5% of cutaneous SCCs metastasize to regional nodes (Rowe *et al.* 1992), but metastatic disease may be more common from primary tumours involving the scalp and external ear (Fig. 20.1), and also in immuno-compromised patients (Glover *et al.* 1994).

In an earlier series of 75 patients from the Royal Prince Alfred Hospital, histological extracapsular spread was found in 71% (O'Brien *et al.* 1991; Khurana *et al.* 1995).

Table 20.1 Histological diagnoses in 676 parotidectomies from the Royal Prince Alfred Hospital, Sydney (January 1987 to June 1999)

Tumour type	*n*
Primary benign	
Pleomorphic adenoma	174 (26)
Warthin's tumour	36 (5)
Monomorphic adenoma	10
Oncocytoma	4
Sialadenitis	73 (11)
Others	26
Primary malignant	All = 55 (8)
Mucoepidermoid carcinoma	12
Acinic cell carcinoma	9
Adenocarcinoma	7
Carcinoma ex-pleomorphic adenoma	6
Adenoid cystic carcinoma	6
Lymphoma	9
Others	6
Metastatic lesions (from skin)	
Malignant melanoma	177 (26)
Squamous cell carcinoma	106 (16)
Merkel cell carcinoma	9
Others	6

Values in parentheses are percentages determined from the total 676 patients.

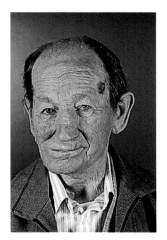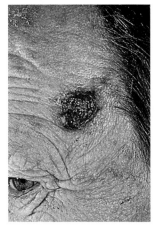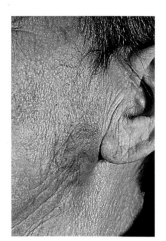

Fig. 20.1 A squamous cell carcinoma of the scalp has given rise to a metastasis in the tail of the parotid gland.

Within the parotid gland, a disjointed tentacular pattern of invasion of SCC was frequently seen, making it difficult to achieve histologically clear margins. Positive margins were present in 40% of patients, and in 47% of cases the metastatic disease was histologically poorly differentiated. In the study, high-risk patients were treated with radiotherapy; however, not all patients received adjuvant radiotherapy. It was also apparent that if the parotid gland was involved and the neck was not treated adequately, there was a high likelihood that disease would recur subsequently in the untreated neck. Equally, among patients with metastatic SCC in cervical lymph nodes where the primary site had the potential to drain to the parotid, treatment of the neck alone was likely to be followed by recurrence of disease in the parotid gland. The disease-specific survival at 2 years was 61%, and survival was significantly worse for those who had metastatic disease in the neck, since this predicted for a higher rate of distant metastatic spread. The patterns of local recurrence with metastatic SCC of the parotid gland can vary, with disease recurring within the parotid bed, in the overlying skin, or in nearby skin due to dermal lymphatic deposits. A multivariate analysis was carried out to determine prognostic factors which predicted for local recurrence: histologically positive surgical margins was the only independently significant factor identified.

It is the author's current practice to treat metastatic SCC in the parotid gland aggressively. Bulky disease should be treated with radical total parotidectomy, even in the presence of normal facial function since a conservative approach has a high likelihood of leading to positive margins which may not be sterilized by post-operative radiotherapy. In addition, it remains our practice to carry out a neck dissection in continuity with the parotidectomy even in the absence of clinically positive lymph nodes. Overall, the incidence of neck involvement, either clinically at the time of presentation or histologically following neck dissection, is 40% in this patient group, and so there is a strong argument for treating the neck. Whether or not this should be done surgically or by radiotherapy is debatable, and individual physicians will need to reach their own conclusions. It should be reiterated, however, that neck involvement in this disease predicts strongly for distant metastases and diminished survival. The use of post-operative radiotherapy should be regarded as being vital, and it is important that the radiotherapy dose to the parotid bed not only penetrates to an adequate depth but also reaches tumoricidal levels at the skin in order to avoid dermal recurrences.

Malignant melanoma

There are approximately 6000 new cases of cutaneous malignant melanoma in Australia each year, with the highest incidence being in Queensland. The incidence of melanoma appears to be flattening, although it is still a major public health problem. Approximately 15% of all cutaneous melanomas involve the skin of the head and neck, the commonest sites of involvement being the scalp and face (O'Brien *et al.* 1991). These sites drain readily to the parotid lymph nodes and so several hundred people in Australia each year are at risk of developing metastatic disease in the parotid gland from malignant melanoma.

Currently, there is no evidence that elective lymphadenectomy confers any survival benefit upon patients with melanoma. In contrast to previous reports recommending the routine use of cervical lymphadenectomy with all parotidectomies for metastatic melanoma (Byers 1986; Vaglini *et al.* 1990), this is now not our practice. However, sentinel lymph node biopsy is being explored as a possible means of identifying patients with microscopic metastatic disease (Uren *et al.* 1994). The role of sentinel lymph node biopsy in the parotid region is controversial, and it remains unclear whether the best technique for treating sentinel nodes at this site should involve superficial parotidectomy or exploration and dissection within the parotid gland to remove individual nodes. It is the author's preference to carry out a parotidectomy when pre-operative lymphoscintigraphy identifies sentinel lymph nodes within the parotid gland. The previous experience of the author in managing the parotid gland in patients with cutaneous melanoma has been published (O'Brien *et al.* 1994). One of the principal findings was that surgery alone may be associated with recurrence within the parotid. The incidence of recurrence in the parotid bed appeared to be significantly reduced among patients who received adjuvant radiotherapy to the parotid gland following a histologically positive parotidectomy (O'Brien *et al.* 1997). The radiotherapy fractionation used in this setting was not standard fractionation but rather a hypofractionated regime using six fractions of 500 cGy. This experience was in contrast to the published experience from the Memorial Sloan-Kettering where surgery alone was associated with only one recurrence among 27 patients (Caldwell and Spiro 1988). Whether or not the cervical lymph nodes should be treated in addition to the parotid gland in cases of metastatic melanoma remains unclear. It is the view of the author that, similarly to SCC, the related cervical lymph node groups should also be treated, and neck dissection has been the preferred option.

The survival of patients who have histological disease in the parotid gland is relatively poor, with approximately 40% surviving 5 years. In the absence of adequate systemic therapy, it is recognized that a high proportion of patients with metastatic melanoma will die of distant disease. Every attempt, however, should be made to maximize control in regional lymph nodes since some of these patients will in fact survive in the long term and the morbidity from uncontrolled regional disease can also be avoided. Whether or not the use of sentinel lymph node biopsy will improve survival remains to be seen. It is the author's opinion, however, that selecting patients for therapeutic dissection based on sentinel node biopsy is a more logical approach than subjecting all patients to elective lymphadenectomy when there is no proof of benefit, and when the node positivity rate from these procedures is low.

Towards preserving the facial nerve   Meirion Thomas

If there is ever a good reason for sacrificing a functioning facial nerve in primary parotid cancer, there is less reason to do so for metastatic disease to parotid lymph nodes. The reason for this is because the nerve is separated from the metastatic disease by the capsule of the involved lymph node, and, therefore, the nerve can only be threatened if there is extracapsular spread. Extracapsular spread is related to the size of the metastasis, and usually a metastatic node would have to reach above 1 cm before the capsule is breached. This group of patients should be 'cancer aware', having already had a primary skin tumour, and also should have been counselled to watch out for new lumps appearing in the pre-auricular region and neck. Because the pre-auricular region is particularly accessible to palpation, for both the patient and the physician, extracapsular spread should be uncommon.

Most parotid lymph nodes are situated in the superficial lobe of the gland, but about 20% of patients with metastatic nodes, from both malignant melanoma and SCC, will have metastatic disease in lymph nodes situated in the deep lobe. As with benign tumours of the deep lobe, the stem and division of the nerve can be displaced. For all patients, a total nerve-preserving parotidectomy is the minimum permissible surgery. As always, malignant melanoma is an unforgiving disease, and inadequate surgical clearance will result in a higher recurrence rate. All patients with SCC to the parotid lymph nodes should be treated with post-operative radiotherapy, but the field does not need to include the course of the facial nerve within the skull, thereby reducing morbidity to the middle ear and limiting the area of depilation. In addition to the unnecessary morbidity produced, there is no evidence that post-operative radiotherapy lowers recurrence rates in malignant melanoma. Similarly, there is no evidence to justify the use of elective parotidectomy with neck dissection in patients with either malignant melanoma or SCC arising in the scalp, pinna, or temporal areas.

With regard to cervical nodes, when enlarged and suspicious, a functional neck dissection or radical neck dissection should be performed. However, when the nodes are not enlarged or suspicious on imaging, we have described the use of per-operative biopsy and frozen section of the jugulo-diagastric node as an indicator for neck dissection (Barr et al. 1994). Equally, one could not quarrel with routine supra-omohyoid neck dissection, or even routine functional neck dissection.

REFERENCES

Byers, R.M. (1986) The role of modified neck dissection in the treatment of cutaneous melanoma of the head and neck. *Arch Surg*, **121**, 1338–41.

Barr, L.C., Skene, A.I., Fish, S., and Thomas, J.M. (1994) Superficial parotidectomy in the treatment of cutaneous melanoma of the head and neck. *Br J Surg*, **81**, 64–5.

Caldwell, C.B. and Spiro, R.H. (1988) The role of parotidectomy in the treatment of cutaneous head and neck melanoma. *Am J Surg*, **156**, 318–22.

Glover, M.T., Niranjan, N., Kwan, J.T., and Leigh, I.M. (1994) Non-melanoma skin cancer in renal transplant recipients: the extent of the problem and a strategy for management. *Br J Plast Surg*, **47**, 86–9.

Khurana, V.G., Mentis, D.H., O'Brien, C.J., Hurst, T.L., Stevens, G.N., and Packham, N.A. (1995) Parotid and neck metastases from cutaneous squamous cell carcinoma of the head and neck. *Am J Surg*, **170**, 446–50.

Marks, R., Staples, M., and Giles, G.G. (1993) Trends in non-melanocytic skin cancer treated in Australia: the second national survey. *Int J Cancer*, **53**, 585–90.

O'Brien, C.J., Coates, A.S., Petersen Schaefer, K., Shannon, K., Thompson, J.F., Milton, G.W. *et al.* (1991) Experience with 998 cutaneous melanomas of the head and neck over 30 years. *Am J Surg*, **162**, 310–4.

O'Brien, C.J., Petersen Schafer, K., Papadopoulos, T., and Malka, V. (1994) Evaluation of 107 therapeutic and elective parotidectomies for cutaneous melanoma. *Am J Surg*, **168**, 400–3.

O'Brien, C.J., Petersen Schaefer, K., Stevens, G.N., Bass, P.C., Tew, P., Gebski, V.J. *et al.* (1997) Adjuvant radiotherapy following neck dissection and parotidectomy for metastatic malignant melanoma. *Head Neck*, **19**, 589–94.

Rowe, D.E., Carroll, R.J., and Day, C.L., Jr (1992) Prognostic factors for local recurrence, metastasis, and survival rates in squamous cell carcinoma of the skin, ear, and lip. Implications for treatment modality selection. *J Am Acad Dermatol*, **26**, 976–90.

Uren, R.F., Howman Giles, R., Thompson, J.F., Shaw, H.M., Quinn, M.J., O'Brien, C.J. *et al.* (1994) Lymphoscintigraphy to identify sentinel lymph nodes in patients with melanoma. *Melanoma Res*, **4**, 395–9.

Vaglini, M., Belli, F., Santinami, M., and Cascinelli, N. (1990) The role of parotidectomy in the treatment of nodal metastases from cutaneous melanoma of the head and neck. *Eur J Surg Oncol*, **16**, 28–32.

Audience discussion

Professor O'Brien: If I may have an opportunity to reply to one of Mr Meirion Thomas' comments. In our practice, the small discrete metastasis to the parotid lymph node is the exception. We see extranodal spread in two-thirds of our cases, and this accounts for the high rate of nerve sacrifice. I am also concerned about intra-operative sampling of jugulo-digastric nodes. There are important nodes (only one of two) at the entry of the spinal accessory nerve to the sternomastoid muscle at the junction of the upper middle third. This is a very common site for metastatic spread from skin, and no matter what parotidectomy or neck dissection you are doing you have got to get these nodes out because this is a site of failure.

Professor McGurk (London, UK): Just to clarify, Professor O'Brien favours superficial parotidectomy with post-operative radiotherapy, while Mr Thomas favours total parotidectomy with nerve preservation?

Professor O'Brien: If the disease is small and localized, I will do a superficial parotidectomy because I am giving it post-operative radiotherapy. A total parotidectomy will add 2–4 more lymph nodes but not alleviate the need for post-operative radiotherapy. With regards to the neck, for SCC, the rules are similar to those for SCC arising within the upper aerodigestive tract. If there is a level II node, for instance, one undertakes a functional neck dissection and not a lymphadenectomy limited to level II.

Mr Thomas: If on the one hand you see 65% of your patients with metastatic disease in the neck, then surely there must be a very high incidence of disease in the deep lobe of the parotid gland as well. Stating that you are going to give them radiotherapy is not a good reason for not taking out the deep lobe. I do not think that this is a very consistent argument.

Mr Watkinson (Birmingham, UK): If I may join the discussion in support of Professor O'Brien's argument. I think there were the studies by McGregor at Glasgow (Lee *et al.* 1985; McKean *et al.* 1985) that actually looked at lymph node numbers in the deep lobe, and there are only two or three. So following on from that, and consistent with what we said earlier about primary parotid cancer, if the disease is not in the deep lobe, then we leave the deep lobe alone.

Professor Snow (Amsterdam, The Netherlands): I ask Professor O'Brien, if one has a small melanoma metastasis in the superficial lobe, do you do the same procedure as in squamous cell carcinoma or do you take the deep lobe, as post-operative radiotherapy is not an effective back-up option?

Professor O'Brien: No. I tend to do a superficial parotidectomy for both malignant melanoma and SCC. Let me use this question to dispel a myth which has been perpetuated for decades and one which I feel strongly about. To state that melanoma is a radioresistant disease is wrong. There are good biological data, for example Bichay *et al.* (1992), demonstrating that melanoma is radiosensitive. However, it is radioresistant at 180 cGy; you need to give it 550 cGy. There is no doubt from our own studies that the addition of radiotherapy to therapeutic neck dissection with a parotidectomy has reduced the recurrence rate from about 28% to 6% in the setting of malignant melanoma.

Question from the floor: You have introduced us to the concept of T stages for metastases to parotid lymph nodes. Could you clarify the distinction from primary parotid cancers and the usefulness of this classification?

Professor O'Brien: The point I was trying to highlight was the inadequacies of the staging system for skin cancer. For example, if it is a parotid metastasis of 6–7 cm with facial nerve involvement, this is termed N1, as is a small discrete parotid node. I was not convinced that that was an appropriate thing, so we applied (in the analysis of the study) the staging system of primary parotid cancers to test for any predictive qualities. As it turned out, this application of the T staging was not very helpful, as other factors, such as neck involvement, confounded the outcome analysis.

Mr Woodward (Manchester, UK): Sticking with metastatic squamous cell carcinoma in the parotid, could Professor O'Brien explain his indications for neck dissection?

Professor O'Brien: In general, we lean towards doing a neck dissection in all cases. In practice, of course, there are some exceptions. For instance, some patients are referred via the radiotherapist, with metastatic disease clinically confined to the parotid. In those circumstances, we agree to do a parotidectomy with subsequent radiotherapy both to the parotid and to the neck.

Bichay, T.J., Feeley, M.M., and Raaphorst, G.P. (1992) A comparison of heat sensitivity, radiosensitivity and PLDR in four human melanoma cell lines. *Melanoma Res*, **2**, 63–9.

Lee, K., McKean, M.E., and McGregor, I.A. (1985) Metastatic patterns of squamous carcinoma in the parotid lymph nodes. *Br J Plast Surg*, **38**, 6–10.

McKean, M.E., Lee, K., and McGregor, I.A. (1985) The distribution of lymph nodes in and around the parotid gland: an anatomical study. *Br J Plast Surg*, **38**, 1–5.

Martin, H. (1952) The treatment of cervical metastatic cancer. *Proc. Roy. Soc. Med.*, **45**, 757–63.

Editorial comment

Essentially, Professor O'Brien is dealing with two separate clinical entities: squamous cell carcinoma and malignant melanoma. The difference between them is that with melanoma, a lymphatic metastasis heralds the likely systematic dissemination of the disease. In squamous cell carcinoma, this principle may not apply. This means that from a clinical view point there is a real prospect of cure in patients with squamous cell carcinoma if the local disease is controlled. This is not necessarily true for melanoma. The significance of a parotid lump in the context of a squamous cell carcinoma is well appreciated in Australia. It is possible that the incidence of such lesions may increase in the European population from travel or perhaps from climate change.

From a practical perspective, the surgical pathology of squamous cell metastasis within the parotid gland is dominated by the fibrinous desmoplastic tissue reaction that seems to follow the earlier surgical excision of the primary tumour of the scalp. This phenomenon was described long ago by Martin (1952) in relation to neck dissection and was the reason for his recommendation that a neck dissection should be done at the same time as the primary tumour. In the parotid gland, it makes the dissection of the facial nerve difficult and this applies especially to the larger lesion. Size is relative. A 2 cm mass in the pre-auricular or mid portion of the parotid is a large lesion! Professor O'Brien, who has an unrivalled experience of lymph node metastasis in the parotid region from scalp or face, came to the same conclusion. He found that up to 70% of parotid metastases had extracapsular spread and that it was difficult to obtain histologically clear margins in this anatomical area. He treats these metastases aggressively, and strongly advocated adjuvant radiotherapy. Whether a total or partial parotidectomy is preferable is an undecidable question on the evidence available. In Professor O'Brien's experience, 40% of patients with parotid gland metastases (from squamous cell carcinoma) developed cervical metastasis, and this argues for an accompanying neck dissection.

CHAPTER 21

Salivary lymphoepithelial lesions and MALT lymphoma

Paul Speight

Introduction

Lymphoepithelial lesions arise within mucosal and glandular tissues and are characterized by dense lymphoid infiltrates which disrupt glandular structures. Classic lymphoepithelial lesions are seen in the stomach, in the context of *Helicobacter pylori* (*H.pylori*)-induced gastritis, and in Hashimoto's thyroiditis. In the salivary glands, lymphoepithelial lesions are seen most commonly in the parotid, although lesions may arise at other sites, including the minor intraoral glands. Lymphoepithelial lesions in the salivary glands have been called *benign lymphoepithelial lesion* (BLEL), *myoepithelial sialadenitis*, or *autoimmune sialadenitis*, but none of these terms are technically correct and the term *salivary lymphoepithelial lesion* (SLEL) is preferred (Speight and Jordan 1994). SLEL is most often seen in the context of primary Sjögren's syndrome where up to 80% of patients may have salivary gland swelling. It may also arise in patients without Sjögren's syndrome.

The classic histopathology of SLEL shows replacement of salivary tissue by dense focal or diffuse lympocytic infiltrates associated with islands of proliferating duct epithelium (Jordan and Speight 1996). The infiltrating lymphocytes are segregated and form normal lymphoid follicles which are often found adjacent to the epithelium. Between the follicle and the epithelium is a well-developed marginal zone of B cells, and the epithelium itself is infiltrated by B cells to form the typical lymphoepithelial lesions which give the disorder its name. Deep to the follicles is a zone of T cells. The overall organization of the lymphoid tissue is similar to that found in normal mucosa-associated lymphoid tissue (MALT) which is typified by the Peyer's patches of the gut. Thus SLEL is an acquired MALT which is most probably a result of persistent antigenic challenge (Fig. 21.1).

Risk of malignant lymphoma

It has been established that Sjögren's syndrome predisposes to lymphoma development with a risk of about 44 times that of the general population (Kassan *et al.* 1978), and an

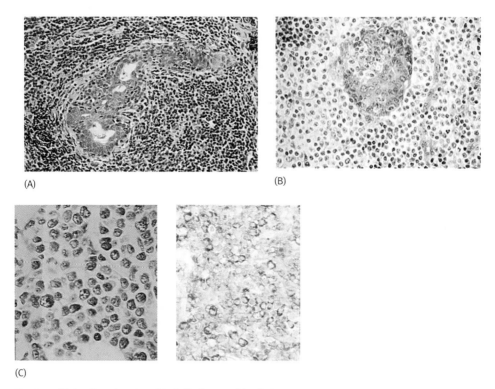

(A)

(B)

(C)

Fig. 21.1 (A) A salivary lymphoepithelial lesion—an island of proliferating epithelial cells infiltrated by lymphocytes.
(B) Early MALT lymphoma—a proliferation of pale centrocyte-like cells expands from the epithelial island. (C) In MALT lymphoma, it is possible to demonstrate that the cells are monotypic or clonal. In this case, all the centrocyte-like cells (left) stain for only the kappa light chain by immunocytochemistry (right).

incidence of 5–10% of patients (McCurley *et al.* 1990; Pavlidis *et al.* 1992; Sutcliffe *et al.* 1998). The main site of lymphoma development is within the parotid gland, and these appear to arise within SLEL. The pathology is similar to that of lymphomas at other MALT sites, and they are designated as MALT lymphomas or extranodal marginal zone B-cell lymphomas (Isaacson and Spencer 1987; Isaacson 1992; Du and Isaacson 1998).

MALT lymphomas appear to arise from the B lymphocytes within the epithelial islands and are first seen as focal proliferations of small to medium lymphocytes with abundant pale cytoplasm. Often they have irregular nuclei and have been called centrocyte-like cells (CCLs), although they may also be monocytoid or plasmacytoid. They first appear as pale staining zones which surround and invade the epithelial islands, but later proliferate and form sheets. Blast cells and plasmacytic differentiation may also be seen. These proliferations of CCLs are monoclonal on the basis of light chain or heavy chain restriction (Schmid *et al.* 1982; Falzon and Isaacson 1991; Jordan *et al.* 1996). Reactive lymphoid follicles almost always accompany a MALT lymphoma and, on occasions, they may be invaded by lymphoma cells (follicular colonization), giving an appearance similar to that of follicular lymphoma (Isaacson *et al.* 1991). The presence of lymphoid follicles is indicative of the lesion's origin in acquired MALT and lends weight to the concept that these lymphomas are antigen driven. This is supported by the demonstration of restricted idiotypes and of a restricted repertoire of VH and CDR3 genes (Lasoto and Miettinen 1997; Bahler and Swedlow 1998), indicating a limited number of antigen recognition sites. Even stronger evidence comes from reports that MALT lymphomas associated with chronic gastritis may resolve after treatment of *H.pylori* infection (Wotherspoon *et al.* 1993). Although *H.pylori* are not found in SLELs (Jordan *et al.* 1997), parotid lesions may resolve after anti-*H.pylori* therapy (Alkan *et al.* 1996). This raises the possibility that the malignant clones found in salivary MALT lymphomas may, in some cases, have arisen in the gut. This is quite feasible since it is well established that MALT lymphomas have a propensity to disseminate to other mucosal sites (Isaacson 1992; Du and Isaacson 1998). This reflects the MALT concept whereby the mucosal lymphoid tissues represent a single organ with cells homing between sites (Fig. 21.2).

MALT lymphomas in the salivary glands appear to be low grade and indolent. Many patients survive for years with no evidence of systemic disease after diagnosis, and many SLELs, even with evidence of *monoclonality*, do not progress to clinically definable lymphomas. Studies have shown that up to 90% of SLELs may have mono-clonal proliferations (Schmid *et al.* 1982; Hyjek *et al.* 1988; Diss *et al.* 1995; Jordan *et al.* 1996). Convention suggests that these lesions thus represent early or established lymphomas. However, clinical experience shows that only a small proportion actually behave as malignant lesions. Recent molecular studies have shown that multiple clones (*oligoclonality*) may be present and that metachronous or synchronous lesions may

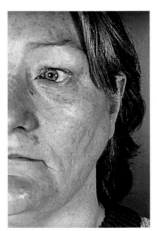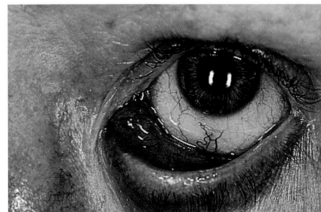

Fig. 21.2 Occasionally, the MALT lymphoma may present simultaneously in the parotid and lacrimal glands.

239

contain two or more dominant clones (De Vita *et al.* 1997; Lasoto and Miettinen 1997). These are seen even in clinically and histologically benign lesions. It is suggested that these clones are small reactive proliferations responding to persistent antigenic stimulation, and provide further evidence that SLEL and subsequent MALT lymphoma are antigen driven. Sensitive methods of detection therefore may identify clonality in a large number of cases and lead to overdiagnosis of lymphoma. This is still a strongly debated issue, but it has implications for the diagnosis of all lymphomas (Savio *et al.* 1996).

Molecular pathology

Current views therefore suggest that SLEL is an antigen-driven lymphoproliferation which may contain oligoclonal or monoclonal B-cell populations (Box 21.1). The persistent antigenic challenge provides a setting for the induction of somatic mutations and other genetic abnormalities. Lymphomas may develop within these proliferating populations as a result of these further molecular events which result in clonal selection and proliferation, and ultimately in malignant transformation. The ongoing genetic abnormalities may include defects in DNA mismatch repair genes, chromosomal translocations, mutations of c-*myc* and *p53*, and loss of heterozygosity (LOH) of tumour suppressor genes (Fig. 21.3). The sequence of events is similar to that described in multistage carcinogenesis for epithelial malignancies.

Management

Because of the indolent nature of the lesions and doubt about criteria for the identification of the malignant transition, management and diagnosis of these lesions is difficult. In the absence of clinical evidence of malignant disease, certain clinical and histological features may be predictive of lymphoma development. In patients with Sjögren's syndrome, the presence of vasculitis and leg ulcers, swollen salivary glands, or lymphadenopathy all have a high odds ratio for risk of lymphoma development

---

Box 21.1 Evidence supporting the hypothesis that SLEL and MALT lymphoma result from persistent antigenic challenge

- Expression of specific antigen-binding sites
- Restricted VH and CDR3 gene repertoire
- Multiple small B-cell clones
- Resolution of lesion after *Helicobacter pylori* eradication

VH gene, immunoglobulin heavy chain gene. CDR3 gene, the third complementarity-determining gene

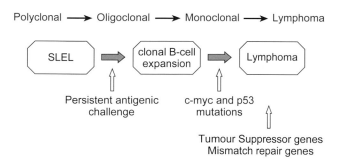

Polyclonal ⟶ Oligoclonal ⟶ Monoclonal ⟶ Lymphoma

Fig. 21.3 Lymphomas arising within a salivary lymphoepithelial lesion (SLEL) may develop through a multistage process. Chronic inflammation results in small reactive B-cell clones, but persistent antigenic challenge provides a setting for further genetic abnormalities with emergence of a dominant clone and malignant transformation. Monoclonal B cells may be found in SLEL even before there is clinical evidence of lymphoma. It is not clear whether this is early lymphoma or only an indication of risk. MMR, mismatch repair defect. (Modified from Du and Isaacson 1998.)

Table 21.1 Clinical features predicting risk of lymphoma in patients with Sjögren's syndrome

Clinical features	Odds ratio (95%CI)
Swollen salivary glands	15.1 (2.1–30.6)
Lymphadenopathy	9.7 (4.5–15.2)
Vasculitis and leg ulcers	21.7 (2.4–39.1)

Data based on 72 patients with Sjögren's syndrome, with five lymphomas (Sutcliffe *et al.* 1998).
CI = Confidence Interval.

(Table 21.1). Labial salivary gland biopsy is a common diagnostic test to confirm salivary gland involvement in Sjögren's syndrome. It has been shown that a proportion of labial glands show monoclonal proliferations of B cells, which is consistent with the immune nature of the disease. Monoclonal B cells were found in up to 18% of labial glands (Jordan *et al.* 1995a,b), and were found to be predictive of future lymphoma development with a predictive value of 31%, with a sensitivity and specificity of 67 and 86%, respectively. Analysis of monoclonality in labial gland biopsies may therefore be a useful method of predicting lymphoma risk in patients with Sjögren's syndrome. However, because of uncertainty about the significance of these findings and the lack of correlation between molecular evidence of monoclonal proliferation and clinical behaviour, treatment must remain empirical.

From the pathologist's viewpoint, a definitive diagnosis of MALT lymphoma in an SLEL can only be made when histology shows proliferating CCLs with evidence of monoclonality detected by immunohistochemistry for immunoglobulin light chains. Recent PCR (polymerase chain reaction) methods for detecting restricted heavy chain gene rearrangements may be too sensitive since they may detect multiple small reactive clones (Jarvis *et al.* 1996). However, when there is evidence of PCR monoclonality, this is an indication of possible lymphoma and of lymphoma risk. From the clinician's point of view, it seems appropriate to instigate treatment for lymphoma only in those cases where there is histological evidence of lymphoma associated with monoclonality and supportive clinical findings. In cases which fall short of these criteria, careful review is essential although preliminary staging procedures may be warranted.

REFERENCES

Alkan, S., Karcher, D.S., Newman, M.A., and Cohen, P. (1996) Regression of salivary gland MALT lymphoma after treatment for *Helicobacter pylori. Lancet*, **348**, 268–9.

Bahler, D.W. and Swerdlow, S.H. (1998) Clonal salivary gland infiltrates associated with myoepithelial sialadenitis (Sjogren's syndrome) begin as nonmalignant antigen-selected expansions. *Blood*, **91**, 1864–72.

De Vita, S., Boiocchi, M., Sorrentino, D., Carbone, A., Avellini, C., Dolcetti, R. *et al.* (1997) Characterization of prelymphomatous stages of B cell lymphoproliferation in Sjogren's syndrome. *Arthritis Rheum*, **40**, 318–31.

Diss, C., Wotherspoon, A.C., Speight, P., Pan, L. and Isaacson, P.G. (1995) B-cell monoclonality, Epstein Barr virus, and +(14;18) in myoepithelial sialadenitis and low-grade B-cell MALT lymphoma of the parotid gland. *Am J Surg Pathol*, **19**, 531–6.

Du, M.Q. and Isaacson, P.G. (1998) Recent advances in our understanding of the biology and pathogenesis of gastric mucosa-associated lymphoid tissue (MALT) lymphoma. *Forum Genova*, **8**, 162–73.

Falzon, M. and Isaacson, P.G. (1991) The natural history of benign lymphoepithelial lesion of the salivary gland in which there is a monoclonal population of B cells. A report of two cases. *Am J Surg Pathol*, **15**, 59–65.

Hyjek, E., Smith, W.J., and Isaacson, P.G. (1988) Primary B-cell lymphoma of salivary glands and its relationship to myoepithelial sialadenitis. *Hum Pathol*, **19**, 766–76.

Isaacson, P.G. (1992) Extranodal lymphomas: the MALT concept. *Verh Dtsch Ges Pathol*, **76**, 14–23.

Isaacson, P.G. and Spencer, J. (1987) Malignant lymphoma of mucosa-associated lymphoid tissue. *Histopathology*, **11**, 445–62.

Isaacson, P.G., Wotherspoon, A.C., Diss, T., and Pan, L.X. (1991) Follicular colonization in B-cell lymphoma of mucosa-associated lymphoid tissue. *Am J Surg Pathol*, **15**, 819–28.

Jordan, R.C. and Speight, P.M. (1996) Lymphoma in Sjogren's syndrome. From histopathology to molecular pathology. *Oral Surg, Oral Med, Oral Pathol Oral Radiol Endod*, **81**, 308–20.

Jordan, R., Diss, T.C., Lench, N.J., Isaacson, P.G., and Speight, P.M. (1995a) Immunoglobulin gene rearrangements in lymphoplasmacytic infiltrates of labial salivary glands in Sjogren's syndrome. A possible predictor of lymphoma development. *Oral Surg, Oral Med, Oral Pathol Oral Radiol Endod*, **79**, 723–9.

Jordan, R.C., Pringle, J.H., and Speight, P.M. (1995b) High frequency of light chain restriction in labial gland biopsies of Sjogren's syndrome detected by *in situ* hybridization. *J Pathol*, **177**, 35–40.

Jordan, R.C., Odell, E.W., and Speight, P.M. (1996) B-cell monoclonality in salivary lymphoepithelial lesions. *Eur J Cancer B Oral Oncol*, **32b**, 38–44.

Jordan, R.C., Diss, T.C., Millson, C., Wilson, M., and Speight, P.M. (1997) Absence of *Helicobacter pylori* DNA in salivary lymphoepithelial lesions. *J Oral Pathol Med*, **26**, 454–7.

Kassan, S.S., Thomas, T.L., Moutsopoulos, H.M., Hoover, R., Kimberly, R.P., Budman, D.R. *et al.* (1978). Increased risk of lymphoma in sicca syndrome. *Ann Intern Med*, **89**, 888–92.

Lasota, J. and Miettinen, M.M. (1997) Coexistence of different B-cell clones in consecutive lesions of low-grade MALT lymphoma of the salivary gland in Sjogren's disease. *Mod Pathol*, **10**, 872–8.

McCurley, T.L., Collins, R.D., Ball, E., and Collins, R.D. (1990) Nodal and extranodal lymphoproliferative disorders in Sjogren's syndrome: a clinical and immunopathologic study. *Hum Pathol*, **21**, 482–92.

Pavlidis, N.A., Drosos, A.A., Papadimitriou, C., Talal, N., and Moutsopoulos, H.M. (1992) Lymphoma in Sjogren's syndrome. *Med Pediatr Oncol*, **20**, 279–83.

Savio, A., Franzin, G., Wotherspoon, A.C., Zamboni, G., Negrini, R., Buffoli, F. *et al.* (1996) Diagnosis and posttreatment follow-up of *Helicobacter pylori*-positive gastric lymphoma of mucosa-associated lymphoid tissue: histology, polymerase chain reaction, or both? *Blood*, **87**, 1255–60.

Schmid, U., Helbron, D., and Lennert, K. (1982) Development of malignant lymphoma in myoepithelial sialadenitis (Sjogren's syndrome). *Virchows Arch Pathol Anat*, **395**, 11–43.

Speight, P.M. and Jordan, R.C. (1994) The molecular pathology of Sjögren's syndrome. In: *Autoimmune Diseases*. pp. 25–42. (D.A. Isenberg and A.C.Horsfall, eds) Bios Scientific Publishers, Oxford.

Sutcliffe, N., Inanc, M., Speight, P., and Isenberg, D. (1998) Predictors of lymphoma development in primary Sjogren's syndrome. *Semin Arthritis Rheum*, **28**, 80–7.

Wotherspoon, A.C., Doglioni, C., Diss, T.C., Pan, L., Moschini, A., de Boni, M. *et al.* (1993) Regression of primary low-grade B-cell gastric lymphoma of mucosa-associated lymphoid tissue type after eradication of *Helicobacter pylori*. *Lancet*, **342**, 575–7.

Audience discussion

Dr Pal (Manchester, UK): In your practice, what tests and investigations help indicate those with SLEL at risk of lymphoma?

Professor Speight: I actually believe that probably all patients with SLEL are at risk of malignant lymphoma, but we have to take a pragmatic approach in the clinic. In the Sutcliffe paper (Sutcliffe *et al.* 1998), we looked at several serum parameters as potential predictive factors. None were as predictive as simple clinical observations. A patient with known rheumatoid arthritis who develops a dry mouth will probably they have Sjögren's and will be at risk of lymphoma. A labial biopsy is helpful and gives clues about lymphoma risk. Serum or urine immunoglobulins are not very useful. A history of persistent or recurrent parotid swelling, or a new swelling on the other side, is an indication for an open parotid biopsy.

Dr Gallo (Florence, Italy): Do you think Epstein–Barr virus (EBV) plays a role in the pathogenesis of Sjögren's and subsequent malignant lymphomatous transformation?

Professor Speight: I think the evidence is lacking for a direct role for EBV. EBV is almost ubiquitous in the parotid glands, and any association is unlikely to be causative. However, to expand the *H.pylori* story a little. I mentioned that this organism is

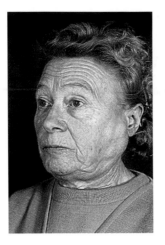 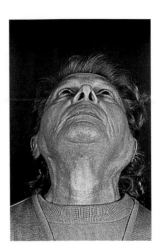

Fig. 21.4 This patient had primary Sjögren's syndrome and an 8-year history of inflammatory swelling of both parotid glands. Slowly she developed a diffuse enlargement of the left parotid which proved to be a MALT lymphoma.

not found in salivary lesions, but that parotid lesions are known to resolve after anti-*H.pylori* therapy. There appear to be at least two different types of salivary MALT lymphomas: one as a consequence of dissemination of *H.pylori*-driven MALT lymphoma in the gut, the other as a consequence of progression of an *in situ* salivary lymphoepithelial lesion, the cause of which is as yet unknown.

I should also point out that *autoimmune sialadenitis* is not synonymous with Sjögren's syndrome, as it may be seen in association with hepatitis C, HDLV and HIV infections. A *sicca*-type syndrome (xerostomia and xerophthalmia) is seen in HIV infection without primary Sjögren's syndrome. In addition, the salivary lymph epithelial lesion associated with HIV disease is a cystic lesion which is not associated with MALT lymphoma. Moreover, it is associated with extranodal lymphomas which may be high grade and may be EBV driven.

Professor McGurk (London, UK): If I may add an observation which I have not seen documented in the literature. We have a Sjögren's clinic at Guy's Hospital and, in preparation for this meeting, I went back and counted 12 cases with salivary MALT lymphomas over the last 4 years. The point I would like to highlight is a clinical one— these lesions present as inflammatory lesions which may fluctuate in size, and respond partially to antibiotics (Fig. 21.4). Previously, as a consequence of one's teaching, I used to consider lymphomas as discrete soft lumps; salivary MALT lymphomas do not present in this way, but rather as a diffuse parotid swelling mimicking a chronic inflammatory disorder.

Editorial comment

A generally accepted model of oncogenesis is one of genetic alteration leading to a growth advantage manifest by selective clonal expansion. This should not be interpreted as meaning a tumour has developed because clonal expansion is mirrored by clonal contraction and so there is a dynamic process of proliferation and involution taking place. It is this background of events (expansion and contraction) against which the neoplastic process develops. The exact initiating or trigger mechanism that causes clonal proliferation and regression for the most part is unknown. What is known is that certain chemicals are carcinogenic, as are some viruses.

The development described by Professor Speight is that in addition to chemical carcinogens and viruses, there is another mechanism which applies to lymphoid tissue, namely antigenic challenge brought about by a bacterium. *Helicobacter pylori* may be the cause of the antigenic challenge in MALT lymphomas.

The particular features of MALT lymphoma arise in a population of lymphocytes that home to the intestinal tract and its related structures, thus creating a mechanism whereby the antigenic challenge may be physically distant from the site of lymphoma manifestation. For example, the antigenic challenge may come from *H.pylori* in the stomach but the MALT lymphoma may arise in the parotid.

The problem of diagnosis of MALT lymphoma arises from two features of its pathology. First, the level of antigen may vary, causing a relapsing inflammatory-like process. This is directly contrary to the normal manifestation of a tumour. A transition into malignancy is a subtle one. Clinically it is manifested by a protracted process resembling chronic inflammation which only after the passage of years becomes recognizably malignant. Thus the object is to obtain early diagnosis, but in present day practice clinicians are prone to manage MALT lymphomas as if they were chronic infective disease. This error is enhanced by MALT lymphomas appearing to respond to antibiotics.

A suggested partial solution to the clinical recognition of MALT lymphoma is a combination of a high suspicion index plus a biopsy of the tail of the parotid, as the tissue changes are not focal within the gland. However, the classical histological appearance of MALT lymphoma is a relatively late event. New molecular techniques can identify expanding lymphoid clones, but the problem remaining is whether the proliferative process represents irreversible neoplastic change. At present, it is not possible to diagnose an early MALT lymphoma reliably on molecular criteria alone. The diagnosis has to be based on a combination of clinical features together with conventional and molecular pathology.

Chronic Salivary Disease and Calculi

CHAPTER 22

Epidemiology and aetiology of salivary calculi

Michael Escudier

Epidemiology

Sialolithiasis is a common finding, accounting for 50% of major salivary gland disease (Epker 1972). Individual experience in managing patients with sialadenitis or sialolithiasis is normally limited, and there are only five series in the literature with over 200 cases (Table 22.1).

There is a male preponderance, and the peak incidence is between the ages of 30 and 60 years (Lustmann *et al.* 1990). As in urolithiasis, the majority are formed from phosphate and oxalate salts (Table 22.2). There seems a clear distinction between submandibular and parotid stones in both frequency and composition (Table 22.3). However, parotid gland stones contain more acidic mineral phases, such as brushite and octacalcium phosphate (Slomiany *et al.* 1983). They also contain about 70% more

Table 22.1 Summary data from five large salivary sialothiasis series (each with >200 patients)

Study	No. of patients	M:F	Submandibular (%)	Parotid (%)	Sublingual (%)	Laterality R:L	Bilateral (%)
Antognini *et al.* (1971)	396	1.8:1	91	8	0.3	1.06:1	–
Yoel (1975)	481	1.2:1	87	12	1	1.08:1	1.9
Mela *et al.* (1986)	215*	1.8:1	100	–	–	0.9:1	0.5
Lustman *et al.* (1990)	245	1:1	94	4.5	0.4	1.05:1	1.2
Escudier and McGurk (1999)	219	1.04:1	72	28	0	1.03:1	1.8

* Limited to submandibular gland cases.

Table 22.2 Comparison of urolithiasis and sialolithiasis

	Urolithiasis	Sialolithiasis
Phosphate salts		90%
Oxalate salts	80%	8%
Urate salts (carbonate apaptite)	18%	2%
Struvite	2%	

Data from Taher *et al.* (1989).

Table 22.3 Composition of salivary calculi

	Submandibular gland	Parotid gland
Organic	18%	51%
Non-organic	82%	49%
Calcium salts	46%	15%

Data from: Haring (1991) and Bodner (1993).

organic matrix, 40% more protein, and 54% more lipids (Slomiany *et al.* 1982). The organic matrix of submandibular stones is richer in protein and has a higher (13%) content of lipids (Slomiany *et al.* 1982). They grow by deposition and range in size from 0.1 to 30 mm (Frame and Smith 1986). The commonest site is the submandibular gland, where 80–90% of calculi are found; 5–10% are found in the parotid gland and approximately 5% in the sublingual and other minor salivary glands (Lustmann *et al.* 1990). Presentation typically is with a painful swelling of the gland at meal times, when the obstruction caused by the calculus becomes most acute (Hardy 1966).

The prevalence of renal calculi is 4–20%, while the annual incidence of hospitalization is estimated at 0.03–0.1% per million (Trinchieri 1996). In contrast, postmortem studies suggest that the prevalence of salivary calculi is approximately 1.2% of the population (Rauch and Gorlin 1970). This represents about 700 000 patients, and it is clear from clinical experience that this is not a true estimate of the problem. We recently have investigated the incidence of symptomatic salivary calculi within a hospital-based population (Escudier and McGurk 1999).

A UK hospital-based prevalence study

In the UK, Hospital Episode Statistics figures held by the Department of Health and based on individual ICD10 code provide a method of assessing the incidence of many diseases. These data relate to the 15 health regions in England and correspond to a population of 48 532 705 based on the 1993 census. The data are corrected at source (DHSS grossing factor) for deficiencies in data collection and refer to all finished consultant episodes (FCEs) for in-patient and day-case admissions in state hospitals. Based on the data for the years 1991–1995 inclusive, the incidence of hospital admis-

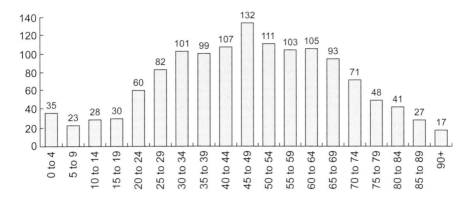

Fig. 22.1 Average number of cases per annum, by age, of sialoadenitis, based on Department of Health Hospital Episode Statistics for the period 1991–1995. The peak incidence was between 30 and 60 years of age. (Reproduced by kind permission of the *British Dental Journal*.)

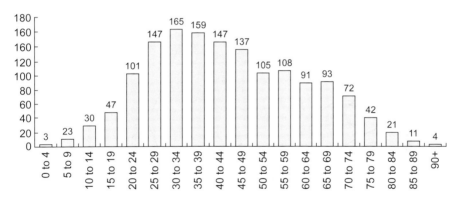

Fig. 22.2 Average number of cases per annum, by age, of sialolithiasis, based on Department of Health Hospital Episode Statistics for the period 1991–1995. The peak incidence was between 25 and 50 years of age. (Reproduced by kind permission of the *British Dental Journal*.)

sion for sialoadenitis and sialolithiasis was 28 (19–46) and 32 (26–37) per million population per annum, respectively (Figs 22.1 and 22.2). A common causal relationship was suggested by the data, as there was a significant correlation in the pattern of incidence between sialadenitis and sialolithiasis [Spearman's correlation coefficient $(r_s) = 0.78, P < 0.01$] when compared by region (Fig. 22.3). This supports the view that an occult calculus is probably the underlying cause of sialoadenitis in the majority of cases. Hence the incidence of symptomatic salivary calculi per annum in the UK is likely to be at least 59 cases per million population per annum or 0.0059% per annum. Based on this figure and assuming the average life expectancy to be 76 years, the pre-

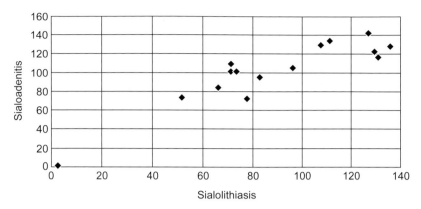

Fig. 22.3 Average number of cases per year, of sialolithiasis and sialoadenitis, by region, based on Department of Health Hospital Episode Statistics for the 15 regions of England during the period 1991–1995. Spearman's correlation coefficient (r_s) = 0.78, P <0.01. (Reproduced by kind permission of the *British Dental Journal*.)

valence for symptomatic sialolithiasis is 0.45%. This latter figure is approximately half that encountered in post-mortem studies.

Aetiology

The aetiology of salivary calculi remains unclear. The requirements for stone formation are shown in Box 22.1. This model may be applied to the various theories of salivary stone formation and gives some insight into the viability of each.

Saturation

The level of saturation may be altered by pH, dehydration, diet, and stagnation. In urolithiasis, a high fluid intake, especially water, is the oldest and still the most powerful means of preventing stone formation (Borghi *et al.* 1999). However, while the supersaturation of saliva with calcium salts is an obvious predisposing factor (Iro *et al.* 1995), it is unlikely to be a precipitating factor as otherwise the disorder would be more common. Further, while experimentally induced hypercalcaemia produced calcified

Box 22.1 **Requirements for stone formation**

- ◆ Saturation
- ◆ Crystal inhibition
- ◆ Crystal nucleation, growth, and aggregation
- ◆ Crystal retention in the ductal system

deposits in the kidneys of rats, the major salivary glands remained normal (Epivatianos and Tsougas 1991).

In particular, strenuous physical exercise or excessive sweating in a hot climate may predispose to stones by salivary concentration and changed salivary pH, but, if they were precipitating factors, the incidence would vary with climate, and this is not so. In the case of diet, unlike urolithiasis, sialolithiasis has not been shown to have any relationship to either calcium or oxalate intake, irrespective of the disease state. Similarly, stagnation does not appear to be a significant factor as the incidence of stones is unchanged in patients with reduced flow. Mucin content is also insignificant, with no increase seen in patients with conditions such as cystic fibrosis.

Crystal inhibition

In urolithiasis, there is evidence that the calcium-binding, acidic glycoprotein nephrocalcin (NC) with molecular weight 14 000 Daltons (Da) may prevent kidney stone formation (Nakagawa 1997). This protein is localized in the proximal tubules of kidneys and occurs in at least four isoforms (NC-A, NC-B, NC-C, and NC-D). Non-stone-forming people excrete more NC-A and NC-B isoforms in urine, while greater quantities of NC-C and NC-D are found in the urine of stone formers. Saliva also contains a family of calcium-binding proteins and it is possible that defects in the function of these proteins may account for some stone formation. However, it cannot be a major cause as bilateral and recurrent stones are uncommon.

Nucleation, growth, and aggregation

Several factors have been implicated in this area, and include bacteria, foreign bodies, cellular debris, and infection. Microorganisms are found commonly on the surface of salivary calculi and occasionally at the interface between lamellae. They may therefore provide an organic matrix and be an important factor in the later phase of the pathogenesis of salivary calculi. Foreign bodies have also been found within salivary calculi but are uncommon, and as such unlikely to be of any great significance. Cellular debris may also play a role and is commonly evident on endoscopy of infected salivary ducts. Harrison and colleagues (1993) have provided convincing evidence for the continual and spontaneous formation of microcalculi in the salivary glands through calcification of cellular debris shed into ducts. This observation is not the complete answer because the presence of microcalculi increases with age whereas the peak incidence of sialoliths is in middle age. These authors also feel that infection is an important aetiological factor, with subclinical disease acting as the initiating factor. The order of events is unclear as the peak incidence of sialadenitis post-dates that for sialolithiasis, suggesting that it is a sequel rather than the cause.

Retention in the ductal system

Crystallization processes alone cannot explain the pathophysiology of stone disease. In recent years, evidence has emerged that cells lining the renal tubules have an active role in creating the conditions under which stones may develop. In particular, the roles, in urolithiasis, of transepithelial oxalate transport and crystal–cell interactions have been investigated *in vitro* (Verkoelen *et al.* 1997). While the former is unlikely to be a significant factor in sialolithiasis, the latter may well contribute. In addition, simple anatomical factors, such as the mylohyoid bend and the long course of the submandibular duct, and the fact that the saliva is secreted against gravity should not be overlooked.

At present, no single theory appears to explain fully the aetiology of salivary calculi. Hence, it is likely that several factors, working in parallel or in series, contribute to the development of a sialolith.

REFERENCES

Antognini, F., Guiliani, R., Magagnoli, P.P., and Romagnoli, D. (1971) [Clinico-statistical study on sialolithiasis]. *Mondo Odontostomatol*, **14**, 38–55.

Bodner, L. (1993) Salivary gland calculi: diagnostic imaging and surgical management. *Compendium*, **14**, 572, 574–6, 578 passim.

Borghi, L., Meschi, T., Schianchi, T., Briganti, A., Guerra, A., Allegri, F. *et al.* (1999) Urine volume: stone risk factor and preventive measure. *Nephron*, **81 Suppl 1**, 31–7.

Epivatianos, A. and Tsougas, M. (1991) [The effect of hypercalcaemia on the major salivary glands of the rat]. *Stomatol Athenai*, **47**, 306–13.

Epivatianos, A., Harrison, J.D., Garrett, J.R., Davies, K.J., and Senkus, R. (1986) Ultrastructural and histochemical observations on intracellular and luminal microcalculi in the feline sublingual salivary gland. *J Oral Pathol*, **15**, 513–7.

Epker, B.N. (1972) Obstructive and inflammatory diseases of the major salivary glands. *Oral Surg Oral Med Oral Pathol*, **33**, 2–27.

Escudier, M.P. and McGurk, M. (1999) Symptomatic sialoadenitis and sialolithiasis in the English population, an estimate of the cost of hospital treatment. *Br Dent J*, **186**, 463–6.

Frame, J.W. and Smith, A.J. (1986) Large calculi of the submandibular salivary glands. *Int J Oral Maxillofac Surg*, **15**, 769–71.

Haring, J.I. (1991) Diagnosing salivary stones. *J Am Dent Assoc*, **122**, 75–6.

Harrison, J.D., Triantafyllou, A., and Garrett, J.R. (1993) Ultrastructural localization of microliths in salivary glands of cat. *J Oral Pathol Med*, **22**, 358–62.

Iro, H., Zenk, J., and Benzel, W. (1995) Minimally invasive therapy for sialolithiasis—the state of the art. In: *Advances in Otolaryngology—Head and Neck Surgery*, Vol. 9. pp. 31–48. Mosby, St Louis.

Lustmann, J., Regev, E., and Melamed, Y. (1990) Sialolithiasis. A survey on 245 patients and a review of the literature. *Int J Oral Maxillofac Surg*, **19**, 135–8.

Mela, F., Berrone, S., and Giordano, M. (1986) [Clinico-statistical considerations of submandibular sialolithiasis]. *Minerva Stomatol*, **35**, 571–3.

Nakagawa, Y. (1997) Properties and function of nephrocalcin: mechanism of kidney stone inhibition or promotion. *Keio J Med*, **46**, 1–9.

Rauch, S. and Gorlin, R.J. (1970) Diseases of the salivary glands. In: *Oral Pathology*, 6th edn. pp. 997–1003. (R.J. Gorlin and H.M. Goldman, eds) Mosby, St Louis.

Slomiany, B.L., Murty, V.L., Aono, M., Slomiany, A., and Mandel, I.D. (1982) Lipid composition of the matrix of human submandibular salivary gland stones. *Arch Oral Biol*, **27**, 673–7.

Slomiany, B.L., Zdebska, E., Murty, V.L., Slomiany, A., Petropoulou, K., and Mandel, I.D. (1983). Lipid composition of human labial salivary gland secretions. *Arch Oral Biol*, **28**, 711–4.

Taher, A.A. (1989) The incidence and composition of salivary stones (sialolithiasis) in Iran: analysis of 95 cases—a short report. *Singapore Dent J*, **14**, 33–5.

Trinchieri, A. (1996) Epidemiology of urolithiasis. *Arch Ital Urol Androl*, **68**, 203–49.

Verkoelen, C.F., van der Boom, B.G., Schroder, F.H., and Romijn, J.C. (1997) Cell cultures and nephrolithiasis. *World J Urol*, **15**, 229–35.

Yoel, J., ed. (1975) *Pathology and Surgery of the Salivary Glands*. pp. 854–901. C.C. Thomas, Springfield, Ilinois.

Editorial comment

The recent work described in this chapter has provided a clearer picture of the incidence of salivary stones that cause illness and disability. The incidence of stones present at post-mortem examination is a different entity from the clinical incidence of symptomatic calculae.

There is profuse evidence concerning the aetiology of salivary stones although a unifying theory has not been propounded. Payling Wright (Guy's Hospital) outlined aetiological agents as 'initiators or triggering factors' and 'contributing or predisposing causes'. He stated that antecedent circumstances relating to disease may be difficult to draw into a coherent order. Clearly the nearer the change approaches the final event, the more influential the factors become. The final link or terminal event is usually a unique causal agent. Aetiological agents of this kind can be considered initiating. Those less immediately connected play a role and can be considered contributing agents. They are of a secondary class in the aetiological process. In the context of salivary gland calculi, a wide range of contributing agents has been identified, but no clear triggering agent. The fact that bilateral stones are so rare militates against general or systemic factors playing an initiating role. It suggests that there is some unknown local or anatomical cause for stone formation. However, the fact that recurrent stones are so rare suggests that there may be some element of pure chance in the development of this disease.

Wright, G.P. (1952) *An Introduction to Pathology*. Longman, Green and Co., London.

CHAPTER 23

Extracorpeal lithotripsy for salivary calculi: results and future roles

Michael Escudier, Philippe Katz, and Pasquale Capaccio

Introduction Michael Escudier

There is a growing public demand for the introduction of minimally invasive procedures as an alternative to conventional surgery. Extracorporeal shock wave lithotripsy is one such technique which was introduced originally for the treatment of renal calculi (Marberger *et al.* 1988), and later used in the management of biliary calculi (Zwergel *et al.* 1987; Ell *et al.* 1990). Further developments in this field made it possible to extend the technique to salivary calculi as was first reported by Iro and colleagues (Iro *et al.* 1989).

Imaging

The introduction of minimally invasive techniques in the management of salivary calculi has been intimately related to the development of the newer imaging modalities. In the case of extracorporeal shock wave lithotripsy, this has involved the use of ultrasound to locate the stone and monitor the progress of treatment peroperatively.

Ultrasound does not require ionizing radiation and has been shown to be a safe, simple, and well-tolerated technique for the detection of salivary calculi. The density and inorganic content of salivary calculi ensure a difference in acoustic impedance compared with adjacent soft tissues. Salivary calculi can be readily identified sonographically as highly reflective echogenic interfaces accompanied by marked posterior acoustic shadowing. Thus a large calculus may not always be fully demonstrated since its medial surface lies within the acoustic shadow. This does not prevent the whole of its lateral surface from being seen, and hence a measurement of its antero-posterior or vertical dimension can be taken. Ultrasound is able to detect radiolucent stones (which account for 20–43% of submandibular stones) (Yune and Klatte 1972; Blair 1973), although the acoustic shadow is not as marked (Traxler *et al.* 1992).

It also enables confirmation of the diagnosis during acute inflammation and depicts ductal morphology, the extent of glandular enlargement, changes in internal structure, and the relationship with surrounding tissues (Gritzman 1989; Yoshimura *et al.* 1989a; Angelelli *et al.* 1990).

Calculi detection rates vary between 63 and 94% (Escudier 1998), and are equal to those for sialography (van den Akker and Busemann Sokole 1983). The distal portion of the submandibular and parotid ducts can be difficult to visualize using extraoral ultrasound. However, the use of small, high-frequency intraoral probes can overcome this limitation (Brown *et al.* 1997). In view of the advantages of this imaging technique and the fact that stones smaller than 2 mm are unlikely to cause symptoms, ultrasound is becoming the diagnostic modality of choice for the detection of sialoliths, in addition to its role in their treatment.

Development of salivary extracorporeal shock wave lithotripsy

Initially, both the piezoelectric and third generation electromagnetic renal lithotripters were used to treat salivary calculi. There were however, inherent difficulties with these machines. Targeting of these relatively small salivary calculi was difficult using a 3.5 MHz ultrasound transducer. In the head and neck, the procedure was painful because the large focal area of the shock wave (~20 mm × 20 mm) always encountered bone, causing periosteal irritation.

Recently, a dedicated sialolithotripter (Minilith SL1, Storz Medical, Kreuzlingen, Switzerland) has been introduced (Fig. 23.1) with an improved 7.5 MHz ultrasound imaging system (Sigma 1AC; Kontron Instruments, St Quentin en Yvelines, France) and a smaller shock wave focus (2.4 mm wide by 25 mm long) which has removed

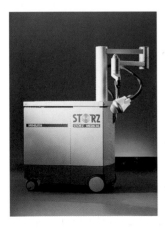
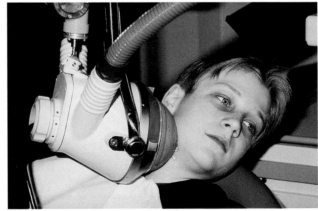

Fig. 23.1 A Storz Minilith SL1 extracorporeal lithotripter for salivary stones. The therapy head positioned to target a submandibular stone.

the need for analgesia. The shock wave is generated within an electromagnetic, small diameter, cylindrical source and focused using a parabolic reflector. It is then transmitted to the patient via a latex coupling cushion filled with water and covered with ultrasound jelly. The aim is to fracture the stone into fragments, with a diameter of less than 2 mm, which will then pass spontaneously.

Shock wave generation and mechanism of action

The shock waves can be generated by electrohydraulic, electromagnetic, and piezo-electric mechanisms, and the resultant waves are brought to a focus through acoustic lenses. They then pass through a water-filled cushion to the targeted stone where two mechanisms, stress and cavitation, act to fracture the stone. Water and soft tissue have equal acoustic impedance, so that the shock wave has a reflection-free passage into the body. At the sialolith–water interface, a compressive wave is propagated through the substance of the stone, subjecting it to stress. Cavitation is the second mechanism of degradation. Reflected energy at the sialolith–water interface results in a rebounding tensile or expansion wave, inducing cavitation bubbles. When these bubbles collapse, a jet of water is projected through the bubble onto the surface of the stone. This force is sufficient to pit the stone and eventually break it.

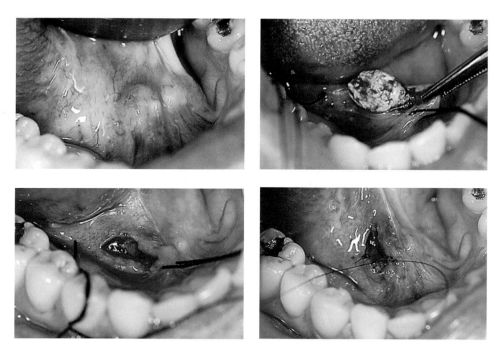

Fig. 23.2 A large stone impacted at the orifice of the submandibular duct is released by a simple intraoral procedure. The incised duct wall is sutured to the oral mucosa to ensure duct patency.

Patient selection

The stone must be readily identified by ultrasound. Acute sialoadenitis if present, should be treated prior to commencing treatment. In general, parotid stones and sub-mandibular stones in the gland, or proximal third of the duct, are easily imaged. Those in the middle third of the submandibular duct are closely related to the mandible and it is difficult to position the therapy head of the lithotripter adequately. Stones in the distal two-thirds of the submandibular duct are therefore best managed surgically (Fig. 23.2).

If the salivary duct is too small on sialography (<1 mm diameter) to allow the evacuation of salivary stone fragments, the only treatment available is surgery. Any blood dyscrasia or haemostatic abnormality is a contraindication to extracorporeal shock wave lithotripsy.

Technique and results

Several studies have been published using either electromagnetic or piezoelectric sialolithotripters. In each case, the results are similar, and a summary is provided in Table 23.1. However, a number of other factors have been investigated by specific groups, and these are presented in the following sections.

The Paris experience Philipe Katz

Extracorporeal shock wave lithotripsy of salivary stones has been undertaken for the past 4 years (Katz 1993). This has used electromagnetic shock waves produced by a dedicated sialolithotripter (Minilith SL1, Storz Medical, Kreuzlingen, Switzerland) specially adapted for use in salivary calculi.

The treatment is practically painless, requiring no anaesthesia or analgesia. The patient sits in a semi-reclining position. The shock waves are generally fired at 120/min, but this can be reduced to 90 or 60 shocks/min. A total of 1500 ± 500 shocks are delivered per session, the sessions being 1 month apart. In view of the extreme fragility of the salivary gland parenchyma, salivary lithotripsy should not be attempted using renal lithotripters as this may cause irreversible damage.

Between July 1995 and April 1999, 400 patients were treated, consisting of 198 males (49%) and 202 females (51%). The age of the patients ranged from 6 to 85 years, with a mean age of 45.5 years. Of these, 262 (65.5%) presented with single or multiple stones in the submandibular gland and 138 (34.5%) with a parotid calculus. Extracorporeal shock wave lithotripsy, either alone or with adjuvant techniques, suc-cessfully removed 252 stones (63%) consisting of 164 submandibular calculi (41%) and 88 parotid calculi (22%). The remaining stones, 148 (37%), were reduced in volume with residual fragments of between 3 and 5 mm. The vast majority of patients, 388 (97%), were rendered asymptomatic.

The salivary fragments were either passed spontaneously, in the saliva, or removed with a micro-basket probe catheter under endoscopic guidance and an associated sphincterotomy. A small number, eight (2%), required removal of the submandibular gland which revealed a blockage secondary to multiple fragments at the junction of Wharton's duct with the gland's pelvis. In addition, four (1%) were placed on a combination of analgesics, antibiotics, and corticosteroids until their symptoms resolved. In this group, all the salivary calculi were fragmented, irrespective of their size.

Some transient side effects were observed in the course of the lithotripsy. These included petechiae at the point of entry of the shock wave (144 patients; 36%), slight pain associated with swelling of the treated gland (90 patients; 22.5%), and ductal haemorrhage which resolved spontaneously (258 patients; 64%). In the 2 weeks following treatment, 36 cases of glandular infection were observed. These were treated with antibiotics and corticosteroids. No permanent or temporary facial nerve lesion was observed.

The Milan experience Pasquale Capaccio

Extracorporeal shock wave lithotripsy of salivary stones has been performed at our centre since 1993 (Ottaviani *et al.* 1996). A dedicated sialolithotripter (Minilith SL1, Storz Medical, Kreuzlingen, Switzerland) has been used, as above, to produce electromagnetic shock waves.

The shock wave energy levels used were 9–12 kV (mean 11 kV) and the frequency of shock wave pulses was 0.5–2.0/s. No more than 2100 shock waves per session were administered, with a mean of 1200 per session. The duration of a typical session of extracorporeal shock wave lithotripsy for salivary calculi was 30 min. Sessions were repeated at weekly intervals. If no fragmentation of the stone had occurred by the sixth session, the patients underwent sialoadenectomy. Follow-up ultrasound was performed 1 week after completion of the course of lithotripsy, and thereafter at 1, 3, 6, and 12 months.

Between December 1993 and September 1996, 80 consecutive, symptomatic outpatients with single or multiple calculi underwent extracorporeal shock wave lithotripsy. These consisted of 37 males and 43 females whose ages ranged from 6 to 81 years (mean 46.8 years, median 47.0 years). The submandibular gland was the affected site in 56 patients and the parotid gland in 24 patients (Ottaviani *et al.* 1997).

Complete disintegration was achieved in 37 (46%) patients consisting of 23 (19%) submandibular and 14 (37%) parotid stones (Table 23.1). In 24 (30%) patients (14 submandibular stones and 10 parotid stones), residual fragments with a diameter of less than 2 mm, measured by ultrasound, were detected. These fragments either passed spontaneously or with the use of citric acid-induced salivation. In seven patients with submandibular stones, palpable fragments migrated to the distal third of the duct and were removed surgically via an intraoral approach. In the remaining 19 patients (all with stones in the submandibular gland), fragments greater than 2 mm in diameter were detected. Five of this group eventually underwent sialoadenectomy either because of the difficulty in obtaining adequate fragmentation or because of persistent disease in the affected gland.

Table 23.1 Results of extracorporeal shock wave lithotripsy

Authors	No. of stones	Stone-free (%)	Residual fragments (%)
Iro *et al.* (1992)	51*	53	47
Schlick *et al.* (1993)	33†	18	82
Kater *et al.* (1994)	104‡	39	62
Gutman *et al.* (1995)	46‡	35	65
Ottoviani *et al.* (1996)	52‡	46	54
Escudier *et al.* (1998)	65‡	31	69
Katz (see above)	400‡	63 [#]	37

* Piezoelectric lithotripter.
† Modulith electromagnetic lithotripter.
‡ Minilith electromagnetic lithotripter.
[#] Includes adjutant techniques.

Overall treatment was more successful for parotid stones than for submandibular calculi. There was also a statistically significant relationship between a stone diameter of less than 7 mm and a successful outcome.

All of the successfully treated patients were followed-up both clinically and with ultrasound for 2–20 months (median 12 months). None had a recurrence of the calculus or reported any salivary dysfunction. In those patients where complete stone clearance was achieved, the parenchymal echotecture returned to a normal, homogenous appearance. There was also clinical recovery of secretory function. In patients with residual fragments, the recovery was less marked.

In the 448 extracorporeal shock wave sessions performed, immediate side effects such as mild pain, swelling of the gland, self-limiting ductal haemorrhage, or cutaneous petechiae were observed in 19 (24%) patients.

The London experience Michael Escudier

The technique utilizes the dedicated sialolithotripter and is undertaken on an out-patient basis with a rest period of a week between treatment sessions (Escudier 1998). If the patient travels a great distance, then treatment on consecutive days may be undertaken but with an associated increase in morbidity. The duration of each session is largely dependent on the number and rate of delivery of the shock waves. However, it is usually between 50 min and 1 h. Ultrasound jelly is applied between the therapy head membrane and the skin that overlies the affected gland to prevent energy loss during transduction of the shock waves. Earplugs are inserted and teeth guards placed on the treatment side. Continuous sonographic monitoring using the in-line ultrasound transducer positioned along the longitudinal axis of the reflector enables both exact positioning of the calculus within the shock wave focus and monitoring of the disintegration of the stone during treatment (Fig. 23.3). The shock wave energy levels

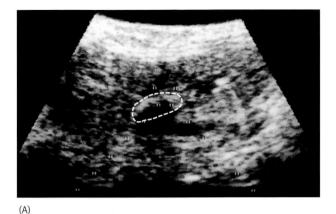

(A)

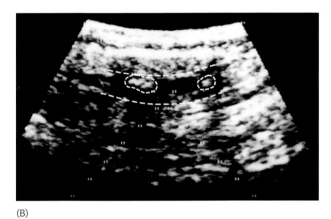

(B)

Fig. 23.3 Ultrasound scan of (A) a large hilar parotid stone (white dotted shape) pre-lithotripsy treatment, and (B) showing fracture of the stone and distal movement of fragments with Stenson's duct (white dashed lines).

used vary between 9 and 14 kV and the frequency of shock wave pulses is 2/s. The number of shocks per session is variable, but up to 5000 per session are possible. If the stone persists after 15 000 shock wave applications, alternative treatment options should be considered as also advocated by the Milan group.

Between September 1994 and September 1998, 65 consecutive, symptomatic salivary calculi were entered into a minimally invasive treatment protocol. Of these, 38% of patients were rendered asymptomatic and stone-free, as demonstrated by ultra-sound and sialography. In the remaining 62%, residual fragments were identifiable within the ductal system although 42% of these were asymptomatic, presumably because the stone had fractured and the obstruction was released. A stone-free, or symptom-free, outcome is felt by some to be more likely in parotid sialolithiasis, and this series confirmed this, with 33% of submandibular cases and 50% of parotid cases rendered both stone- and symptom-free. This may be related to the easier positioning of the therapy head or the physiological characteristics of the parotid gland, including the regular course of the main secretory duct and the characteristics of the serous saliva.

Several studies have reported a statistically significant correlation between a stone diameter of less than 7 mm and the efficacy of extracorporeal electromagnetic shock wave lithotripsy (Ottaviani *et al.* 1996, 1997; Kater *et al.* 1994; Yoshizaki *et al.* 1996). Recently, a prospective randomized clinical trial was undertaken to assess the effect of stone size, stone duration, intended number of shock waves, and pressure of shock wave on outcome. This confirmed that stone size and, to a lesser degree, duration of stone are statistically significant (P <0.05) in predicting a stone-free outcome. This relationship is probably related to the smaller stones representing an earlier stage in the natural history of sialolithiasis with a relatively preserved glandular function.

In those cases with residual fragments, the number of shocks is significant in predicting a symptom-free outcome, while stone size is not significant. Hence, patients with larger sialoliths may be rendered symptom-free, rather than stone-free, although a large number of shocks at a high pressure may be required. In cases where sialolithiasis has existed over several years and been complicated by infective episodes, it is likely that some irreversible damage will have occurred to the gland function. This hypothesis is supported by the observation, of the Milan group, that pre-existing abscess cavities in the affected glands, detected on ultrasound, are related to an unsuccessful outcome for shock wave lithotripsy. At present, it has not been established if the function of the successfully treated glands returns to normal. However, animal studies have shown that cell death is extremely rare after ligation of the main salivary duct (Tamarin 1971a,b). Furthermore, when the ligature is removed, the gland structure returns to normal. Using scintigraphic methods in humans, function of the salivary glands can be assessed. Scintigraphy before and after removal of a submandibular calculus has shown that the gland can recover (Yoshimura *et al.* 1989b). With extracorporeal electromagnetic shock wave lithotripsy, the Milan group have reported a return to a normal echostructural appearance in those cases rendered stone-free. In addition, a return to a normal sialographic appearance of the gland is seen in many of the stone-free cases, and further supports the possibility of functional recovery. Also, the duration of obstructive symptoms may not influence the amount of recovery.

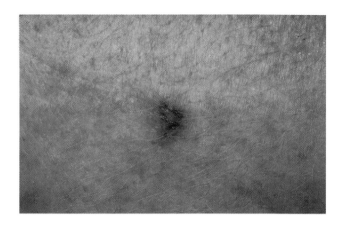

Fig. 23.4 Petechial skin haemorrhage associated with the use of extracorporeal shock wave lithotripsy.

The technique has a very low morbidity. Complications include localized petechial skin haemorrhage (Fig. 23.4), temporary gland swelling, and tenderness, as reported by all groups. In addition, self-limiting ductal haemorrhage occurs, especially when treating ductal stones. Further, patients with chronically infected glands are at risk of an acute infection, and these patients may benefit from the use of prophylactic antibiotics. The passage of fragments is usually associated with mild obstructive symptoms, which resolve once the fragment has passed. In up to 15% of cases, fragments become impacted at the ostium and require surgical removal. There is no adverse effect on hearing or local nerve function.

The role of extracorporeal shock wave lithotripsy in the management of salivary calculi

During the past decade, several minimally invasive techniques for the treatment of salivary calculi have been developed. However, it is only recently that the results of studies of efficacy have been available to enable the development of indications for the use of each.

On the current evidence, extracorporeal lithotripsy is indicated for those stones not amenable to simple intraoral surgery, basket retrieval, or intracorporeal lithotripsy. As such, it represents the treatment of choice where the alternatives are either intraoral surgical removal under general anaesthesia, or sialoadenectomy.

REFERENCES

Angelelli, G., Favia, G., Macarini, L., Lacaita, M.G., and Laforgia, A. (1990) [Echography in the study of sialolithiasis]. *Radiol Med Torino*, **79**, 220–3.

Blair, G.S. (1973) Hydrostatic sialography. An analysis of a technique. *Oral Surg, Oral Med Oral Pathol*, **36**, 116–30.

Brown, J.E., Escudier, M.P., Whaites, E.J., Drage, N.A., and Ng, S.Y. (1997) Intra-oral ultrasound imaging of a submandibular duct calculus. *Dentomaxillofac Radiol*, **26**, 252–5.

Ell, C., Kerzel, W., Schneider, H.T., Benninger, J., Wirtz, P., Domschke, W. *et al.* (1990) Piezoelectric lithotripsy: stone disintegration and follow-up results in patients with symptomatic gallbladder stones. *Gastroenterology*, **99**, 1439–44.

Escudier, M. (1998) The current status and possible future for lithotripsy of salivary calculi. In: *Atlas of The Oral and Maxillofacial Surgery Clinics of North America*, Vol. 6. pp. 117–32. W.B. Saunders, Philadelphia.

Gritzmann, N. (1989) Sonography of the salivary glands. *AJR Am J Roentgenol*, **153**, 161–6.

Gutman, R. Ziegler, G., Leunig, A. *et al.* (1995) Die endoscopie und extrakorporale Stosswellen-Lithotripsie vo Speichelsteinen. *Laryngo-Rhino-Otogoie*, **74**, 249–53.

Iro, H., Nitsche, N., Schneider, H.T., and Ell, C. (1989) Extracorporeal shockwave lithotripsy of salivary gland stones. *Lancet*, **2**, 115.

Kater, W., Meyer, W.W., Wehrmann, T., Hurst, A., Buhne, P., and Schlick, R. (1994) Efficacy, risks, and limits of extracorporeal shock wave lithotripsy for salivary gland stones. *J Endourol*, **8**, 21–4.

Katz, P. (1993) [New treatment method for salivary lithiasis]. *Rev Laryngol Otol Rhinol Bord*, **114**, 379–82.

Marberger, M., Turk, C., and Steinkogler, I. (1988) Painless piezoelectric extracorporeal lithotripsy. *J Urol*, **139**, 695–9.

McGurk, M., Prince, M.J., Jiang, Z.X., and King, T.A. (1994) Laser lithotripsy: a preliminary study on its application for sialolithiasis. *Br J Oral Maxillofac Surg*, **32**, 218–21.

Nakagawa, Y. (1997) Properties and function of nephrocalcin: mechanism of kidney stone inhibition or promotion. *Keio J Med*, **46**, 1–9.

Ottaviani, F., Capaccio, P., Campi, M., and Ottaviani, A. (1996) Extracorporeal electromagnetic shock-wave lithotripsy for salivary gland stones. *Laryngoscope*, **106**, 761–4.

Ottaviani, F., Capaccio, P., Rivolta, R., Cosmacini, P., Pignataro, L., and Castagnone, D. (1997) Salivary gland stones: US evaluation in shock wave lithotripsy. *Radiology*, **204**, 437–41.

Schlick, R.W., Hessling, K.H., Djamilian, M.H. *et al.* (1993) ECSWL in patients suffering from sialolithiasis. *Minimal Invas Ther*, **2**, 129–33.

Tamarin, A. (1971a) Submaxillary gland recovery from obstruction. I. Overall changes and electron microscopic alterations of granular duct cells. *J Ultrastruct Res*, **34**, 276–87.

Tamarin, A. (1971b) Submaxillary gland recovery from obstruction. II. Electron microscopic alterations of acinar cells. *J Ultrastruct Res*, **34**, 288–302.

Traxler, M., Schurawitzki, H., Ulm, C., Solar, P., Blahout, R., Piehslinger, E. *et al.* (1992) Sonography of nonneoplastic disorders of the salivary glands. *Int J Oral Maxillofac Surg*, **21**, 360–3.

van den Akker, H.P. and Busemann Sokole, E. (1983) Submandibular gland function following transoral sialolithectomy. *Oral Surg Oral Med Oral Pathol*, **56**, 351–6.

Yoshimura, Y., Inoue, Y., and Odagawa, T. (1989a) Sonographic examination of sialolithiasis. *J Oral Maxillofac Surg*, **47**, 907–12.

Yoshimura, Y., Morishita, T., and Sugihara, T. (1989b) Salivary gland function after sialolithiasis: scintigraphic examination of submandibular glands with 99mTc-pertechnetate. *J Oral Maxillofac Surg*, **47**, 704–10.

Yoshizaki, T., Maruyama, Y., Motoi, I., Wakasa, R., and Furukawa, M. (1996) Clinical evaluation of extracorporeal shock wave lithotripsy for salivary stones. *Ann Otol Rhinol Laryngol*, **105**, 63–7.

Yune, H.Y. and Klatte, E.C. (1972) Current status of sialography. *Am J Roentgenol Radium Ther Nucl Med*, **115**, 420–8.

Zwergel, T., Neisius, D., and Zwergel, U. (1987) [Extracorporeal shockwave lithotripsy: extracorporeal piezoelectric shockwave therapy (EPL) using the Piezolith 2200]. *Krankenpfl J*, **25**, 61–5.

Audience discussion

Dr Kim (Wisconsin, USA): Do you routinely perform a papillotomy when carrying out lithotripsy? If so, when is it performed? How do you overcome the problem of strictures anterior to the stone?

Dr Capaccio: We used to perform a papillotomy after lithotripsy to allow the fragments to pass; however, this is no longer routine. The presence of strictures anterior to the stone does not preclude the use of lithotripsy. Our practice is to prescribe anti-inflammatory drugs and antibiotics prior to lithotripsy in those cases with inflammatory stenosis of the duct.

Dr Katz: We carry out a papillotomy for every patient who undergoes lithotripsy of a stone in the submandibular gland. This is performed at the initial visit. Parotid papillotomy though is only performed if a fragment becomes lodged at the distal end of the duct. Incidentally, papillotomy is always required in those cases that require basket retrieval of residual fragments.

Professor van den Waal (Amsterdam, The Netherlands): Have you had any recurrence of salivary calculi after lithotripsy?

Dr Capaccio: In the 5 years we have been performing lithotripsy, we have not had recurrence if the calculus was completely fractured and passed. There have been three cases of recurrence in patients who had small residual fragments remaining after treatment. Long-term follow-up of all these patients is required to establish whether our patients will remain stone-free.

Dr van den Akken (Amsterdam, The Netherlands): Surgical removal of stones located in the distal aspect of the duct is straightforward and there is no risk of leaving residual fragments. As it is possible that these fragments may be the seeds for future calculi, would it not be better to treat these surgically in the first instance?

You have said that the ideal size of a stone treated by lithotripsy is one less than 7–8 mm in diameter. The majority of patients have stones larger than this at the hilum of the gland. What is your advice for these patients?

Dr Escudier: We would only treat those patients who had calculi that were not amenable to simple intraoral stone removal, and where sialadenectomy would have been the only other alternative. We have treated patients with calculi larger than 7 mm. If after lithotripsy there is a residual calculus at the hilum of the gland which is symptomatic, then we do offer the patient surgery. However, the surgery is less radical and the calculus is removed via an intraoral approach, leaving the gland.

Dr Capaccio: We treated all patients with calculi whatever the location in order to evaluate lithotripsy. As regards size of the stone, we have shown statistically that a stone less than 7 mm is the ideal for lithotripsy to be successful. However, we have achieved good results in some patients with larger stones. I would consider a formal adenectomy if there was a large stone associated with gross destruction of the gland as demonstrated by sialography.

Dr Katz: Size of stone is not an important factor. More significant is the state of the gland architecture as shown on ultrasound or sialography. I have treated a patient with a 3 cm stone. Although I was unable to break the stone completely, the patient is now symptom-free and is pleased because he has not had to have surgery. We always have the option of offering the patient surgery at a later date if required.

Mr Baraka (Lancaster, UK): How would your results compare with those patients with kidney stones who have been treated using lithotripsy? Why do you not perform a CT prior to lithotripsy?

Dr Escudier: Our results are not as good as those for kidney stones at the present time. However, one would expect our results to improve as the technique is refined, since this was the case with kidney stones. Also, the development of intracorporeal lithotripsy and adjuvant techniques such as basket retrieval of stones will improve our success rate. There will still be cases in which you will remove the gland for various reasons, but each technique will find its own niche within the marketplace, much as it has in the case of kidney stones. We do not use CT because sialograms give better detail of the duct system in the gland. The duct may have a stricture downstream of the stone which negates the use of extracorporeal lithotripsy until it is dilated.

Dr Katz: There are inherent differences between the two areas of interest that make comparison difficult. In the kidney, complete anaesthesia can be obtained with local anaesthetic; therefore, significantly more shocks can be delivered per session. Perhaps if we were able to give more shocks per visit our results would be similar.

Mr Carter (London, UK): Is there any danger to the teeth when performing extra-corporeal lithotripsy?

Dr Escudier: It has generally been possible to avoid pain in the teeth. In the case of the submandibular gland, it is easy to adjust the angle of the shock wave to avoid the teeth. In the case of the parotid, if cottonwool is placed in the buccal sulcus, the shock wave is unable to propagate any further and so the teeth are protected.

Dr Katz: We have had some problems with dental pain during lithotripsy. These seem to be patients who have existing dental disease. We get our patients 'dentally fit' prior to lithotripsy to minimize these symptoms.

Mr Cvijtiec (Kings Lynn, UK): How many visits does the treatment take and how long is each individual session? How much does a course of lithotripsy cost?

Dr Escudier: We generally provide treatment over three visits, each visit being 1 hour long. The machine delivers 120 shocks per minute and we give 5000 shocks per visit. The additional time is needed to allow for repositioning of the head which is inevitably required to make sure the stone is targeted accurately. Cost is fixed by the Trust, and currently a course of treatment costs around £1500, which is significantly less than sialadenectomy. This price includes the initial outlay for the equipment.

Mr Cvijtiec: The success rate in surgery is not 30% as it is in lithotripsy, therefore do you allow for this in your calculation of cost?

Dr Escudier: The success rate is not 100% as it is in surgery. Making a direct com-parison of cost between the two treatments is difficult because the end-points are dif-ferent. In surgery, you have no stone but you also have no gland. The patients are keen to avoid surgery and, therefore, from a quality of life viewpoint are happy so long as they are asymptomatic even if the stone has not been totally removed.

Mr Bailey (London, UK): Do you think that with the smaller calculi located in the submandibular duct that it is actually papillotomy that is giving you the success rather than the lithotripsy itself?

Professor McGurk (London, UK): We have not routinely performed papillotomies on all our patients. If the papillotomy were accounting for the success of the technique, one would expect to see all the fragments damming up at the ostium in our patients. This is not what is seen, so I am sure that the papillotomy is not responsible for the success.

Mr Bailey: If you look at the results that you presented this morning, your series seems to be less successful than that of your colleague. The only difference between treatments is that one is doing a papillotomy and you are not. It seems reasonable to assume that this is the reason why the difference in success can be attributed to the papillotomy.

Dr Escudier: My feeling is that this is not the reason. The only way to determine this would be to carry out a prospective randomized clinical trial.

Dr Gertzéen (Örebro, Sweden): Have you evaluated your treatment by scintigraphy?

Dr Escudier: We have not routinely performed scintigraphy. However, in terms of anatomical improvement on the basis of sialography, there is, in a number of patients, significant improvement in the anatomical appearance of the gland

Editorial comment

Although extracorporeal lithotripsy is a well-established technique for renal stones, it is a new development for the treatment of salivary calculae. Only a small number of centres are using the method (probably no more than 5–6), and now five centres have published their results. They are very similar. Approximately a third of unselected patients will be cured of their calculi.

Improved results are probably only obtainable by better initial selection of cases; namely stones 7–8 mm or less in diameter. Large stones are probably best treated by intracorporeal lithotripsy (Chapter 24). The principal factor driving the practice of extracorporeal lithotripsy is its low morbidity when compared with the incidence of complications following sialoadenectomy.

Lastly, there is a group of patients characterized by enhanced consciousness of health issues who do not want to submit to surgery but agree to lithotripsy in the full knowledge of its limitations.

Salivary gland endoscopy

Salivary gland endoscopy and intracorporeal
lithotripsy
Emilio Arzoz

Development and application of microsalivary
gland endoscopy
Oded Nahleili

Salivary gland endoscopy and intracorporeal lithotripsy
Emilio Arzoz

It has become apparent that with the advances occurring in both optical technology
and instrument miniaturization, it would eventually be possible to examine salivary
glands directly with mini-endoscopes. This is now a reality (Arzoz *et al.* 1994, 1996).
The techniques described in this chapter for sialolithiasis are an adaptation of those
employed in urology for removal of ureteric calculi.

The advantage of the mini-uroscopes is the availability of a working channel which
allowed instrumentation of both the parotid and submandibular duct system under
direct vision. With this facility, endocorporeal fragmentation of the stone became a
reality. Since 1992, substantial improvements have been made in the technique and it
is now a reliable method of managing salivary calculi.

Technique: sialoendoscopy using a mini-endoscope

In our hands, the method has two stages carried out over two consecutive days. The
first step is to provide easy access to the duct system and the second entails the actual
instrumentation of the salivary glands. Both procedures are carried out under local
anaesthesia. On the first day, a Teflon™ guide wire is introduced into the duct orifice
and 1.5–2.7 mm dilators used to enlarge the orifice. A papillotomy is performed over
the dilator with the guide wire *in situ*. An 18 G Alocath™ canula is introduced over the
guide wire and is sutured into position for 24 h.

On the second day, the area is anaesthetized and an endoscope introduced with irrigation through the working channel. The duct has to be flushed manually to inflate the
lumen and provide adequate vision. If the channel is occupied by an instrument, additional pressure is required to maintain irrigation. Care must be taken not to puncture
the duct wall otherwise fluid will extravasate into the floor of the mouth. The duct

normally is navigated easily and as the tip of the endscope approaches the hilum, the kink in the duct is straightened by elevating the submandibular gland with finger pressure. Once the stone is identified, the appropriate instruments are introduced into the working channel and the stone extracted. If the stone lies in a diverticulum or is too large to extract along the duct, then intracorporeal shock waves are applied to its surface under direct vision to fragment the stone. Haemorrhage must be avoided as it limits vision. If the stone does not fragment, the alocath is left in position and a further attempt is made at 24–72 h. The procedure is covered by a course of antibiotics to prevent acute sialoadenitis. Anti-inflammatory drugs are also prescribed.

Endoscopes

Rigid endoscopes are used and have the advantage that one can guide them along the duct system. The 2.1 mm scope is the largest and has a 1 mm operating channel. The advantage of this particular scope is that it will accommodate the 0.8 mm pneumobalistic probe or electrohydraulic wire used to provide intracorporeal lithotripsy. The limitation is that the 2.1 mm scope may be too large to navigate the duct successfully. Both lithotripsy systems convey significant energy, and the electrohydraulic system can cause significant damage if it is not positioned accurately.

A second small (1.5 mm) endoscope is available with a 0.8 mm angled working channel. The smaller dimension means that all ducts can be negotiated by the endoscope. However, only the electrohydraulic wire and laser fibre will pass through the lumen successfully.

A set of forceps is available to work with the large 2.1 mm endoscope. They are easy to use and can be used in a narrow compartment, and they have a surprisingly good grip. They do not fit the smaller endoscope, but a second instrument shaped like a trident can be used. It is easy to manipulate and grips the stone readily. It is the best instrument to use but is expensive and difficult to open in a confined space.

Likewise, the Dormia basket can be used with the smaller endoscope. It is a very useful device but, once a stone is captured, it cannot be released. The basket is not robust enough to crush the stone. The Dormia basket should be used with caution if the stone is larger than the duct that the stone has to be pulled through, since it is possible for the basket to become lodged and require surgical removal.

Intracorporeal energies

Pneumobalistic and electrohydraulic intracorporeal lithotripters are the most effective shock wave generators. However, again the large endoscope with a 1.2 mm working channel is required for access. Hard stones fragment easily but, if the cortex is soft, then complete fracture is delayed, and the process can become tedious. It is essential to work under direct visual control to avoid damage to the duct walls and prevent impaction of stone fragment into the duct walls. The electrohydraulic device which generates a shock wave by an electric spark is traumatic to the tissues and is not recommended as it produces severe glandular contusion and impaction of fragments. Experience with the laser has been disappointing (Fig. 24.1), and the Alexandrita™ laser has since been

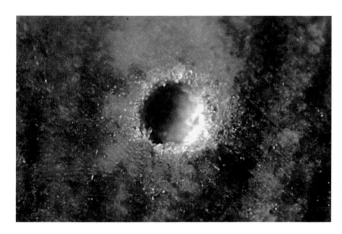

Fig. 24.1 A microscopic pit produced in a salivary stone by a pulse of laser energy.

abandoned. It was slow, expensive, and difficult to apply. The potential advantage of the laser system was that the 1.5 mm endoscope could be used.

Complications

A false passage can be created and fluid extravasated into the floor of the mouth. The duct endothelium can be traumatized or torn and one may fail to extract the stone fragments. The electrohydraulic intracorporeal device is indiscriminate in its energy distribution and can cause violent fragmentation of the stone together with glandular contusion and impaction of stone fragments. This damage can be controlled if the technique is performed carefully. On one occasion, the Dormia basket became trapped in the pelvis of the gland holding a calculus. The stone would not fracture and eventually the basket broke. It is important to maintain adequate drainage after treatment by leaving the stent in position, otherwise oedema causes symptoms of obstruction.

Contradictions

Endoscopy cannot be performed without patient cooperation and is also to be avoided when there is a long history of repeated sialoadenitis or radiological or clinical evidence of advanced chronic infection. These are features that suggest poor function of the gland.

Surgical extraction of the stone is the treatment of choice when the calculus lies in the distal third of the duct. When the stone is large (>1 cm), multiple endoscopic sessions are required and this is therefore not recommended.

Outcome

The technique of endoscopy and the instruments have been refined over the last 8 years. It is now a reliable technique, whereas in 1995 we had a 33% failure in performing endoscopy. In contrast, the results of intracorporeal lithotripsy have not improved. The energy source is still not ideal. Pneumobalistics in combination with an Alexandrita™ laser gave the best results. However, residual stone persisted in 40–50% of cases, and this figure has not improved with time. We have now abandoned the Alexandrita™ laser and the incidence of residual fragments of stone has increased. We currently are gaining experience with a holmium laser, and the results are promising. The future of sialolithotripsy resides in the use of a combination of minimally invasive technique based around extra- and intracorporeal lithotripsy.

Development and application of microsalivary gland endoscopy   Oded Nahleili

Obstructive sialadenitis, with or without sialolithiasis, is the main cause of inflammatory disease of the major salivary glands (Chapter 22). Satisfactory treatment depends on a precise diagnosis and, in the case of sialoliths, the accurate location of the obstruction. This can be difficult due to the limitation of current imaging techniques. In terms of treatment, obstruction can be divided into those which can be reached by the intraoral route, i.e. the length of Wharton's duct to the posterior edge of the mylohyoid and the portion of Stensen's duct distal to the masseter muscle.

Other sites of obstruction require sialadenectomy or removal via an external approach. A significant advance in the management of salivary obstruction has occurred in the last 8 years with the introduction of salivary gland endoscopy (Arzoz *et al.* 1994). It provides an accurate method of both locating the obstruction and treating it by minimally invasive intraductal techniques (Arzoz *et al.* 1996). This section summarizes experience gained on 236 salivary gland endoscopies over a period of 5 years (Nahlieli and Baruchin. 2000).

History of sialoendoscopy

Katz (1991) was the first to use a mini-flexible endoscope (0.8 mm diameter) to extract a calculus with a Dormia basket. Later, Konigsberger *et al.* (1993) combined this technique with an intracorporeal lithotripter to fragment calculi. The flexible endoscope had no working channel and the manipulation of the stone was undertaken blind. Arzoz *et al.* (1996) described a different technique; they used a 2.1 mm mini-rigid urethroscope with a working channel of 1 mm. This allowed fragmentation of the calculi under direct vision by intracorporeal pneumobalistic lithotripter and laser lithotripter. This approach has been adopted by others (Baurmash and Dechiara 1991; Gundlach *et al.* 1994), and to date 12 publications report its application.

Instruments

There are three types of mini-endoscopes suitable for instrumentation of the parotid and submandibular salivary glands—flexible, rigid, and semi-rigid. The rigid endoscope is less fragile and provides a better image than the flexible endoscope. Its disadvantage lies in its stiffness and inability to turn sharp corners. The semi-rigid

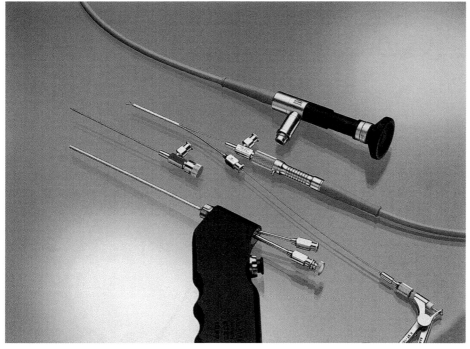

(A)

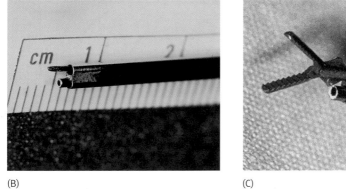

(B)

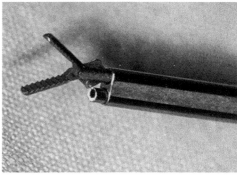

(C)

Fig. 24.2 The Nahleili sialoendoscope system manufactured by Storz (A), The introducer has two channels (B), one for the endoscope, the other for an instrument (C)

endoscope, on the other hand, combines the acceptable properties of both, and, at present, is the instrument of choice. The various forceps and other miniaturized surgical tools can be introduced easily through the rigid and the semi-rigid endoscopes, an advantage not possible with the flexible endoscope.

We initially used a mini-rigid arthroscope (2 mm in diameter), then a rigid 2.5 mm paediatric urethroscope with a working channel of 1 mm (Neder *et al.* 1996; Ziegler *et al.* 1999). We have now progressed to a semi-rigid, moderately flexible device (Nahlieli Sialoendoscope™, Karl Storz Co, GmbH, Germany) designed for salivary gland endoscopy. It is 1 mm in diameter and can be used with two types of outer sleeve: (i) an exploration unit with an outer sleeve of only 1.3 mm and (ii) a treatment unit with an outer sleeve of 2.3 mm × 1.3 mm. The latter has three channels: one for the endoscope, one which will accept a surgical device up to 1 mm in diameter, and the third is an irrigation port (Fig. 24.2). Useful microinstruments include grasping forceps, wire baskets, graspers, intracorporeal lithotripter probes, balloon-like Fogarty or Lacricath×™ (Atrion Medical Products, Birmingham, AL) catheter, and biopsy forceps. The object is to work under direct vision but if there is a problem with space and the multichannel endoscope cannot be inserted, then the diagnostic unit and the surgical endoscope can be used side by side. The last option is to work using a semi-blind technique to identify the obstruction with the 1.3 mm diagnostic unit, then to remove the 1 mm telescope from the channel, replacing it with a working instrument through the sleeve.

Indications and contraindications

The indications for sialoendoscopy are given in Box 24.1. The only absolute contraindication to minimally invasive sialolithiasis is acute sialadenitis. Relative contraindications or technical limitations are a ductal lumen that cannot be enlarged to 1.3 mm; calculi larger than 10 mm, which are difficult to crush and remove; and intraparenchymal stones.

Endoscopic technique

Pre-treatment sialography is used to investigate the ductal system for possible anatomical variation and to determine if the duct will inflate and enable an endoscope to pass along its lumen. There are four possible methods for introducing the endoscope into the ductal lumen: (i) simple dilatation and introduction of the exploration unit

Box 24.1 Indications for sialoendoscopy

◆ Calculi in the proximal portion of Wharton's and Stensen's ducts
◆ Screening the ductal system for residual calculi (32% of stones in the submandibular gland and 63% in the parotid gland were undetectable prior to endoscopy)
◆ Positive evidence of ductal dilatation or stenosis on sialography or ultrasound
◆ Recurrent episodes of major salivary gland swellings without obvious cause.

(1.3 mm) through the punctum; (ii) a papillotomy performed surgically or with a CO_2 laser immediately behind the punctum; (iii) exploration of the duct ('a ductal cutdown') which involves surgical dissection and opening the duct along its length. If there are any difficulties introducing the endoscope into the distal portion of the duct or a stricture is encountered, it may be necessary to expose the duct proximally until the lumen is wide enough to accommodate the endoscope; and (iv) after sialolithotomy, the endoscope can be inserted through the same opening in the duct where the stone was extracted in order to search for residual stones.

Irrigation

Irrigation is crucial in every endoscopy procedure. The duct lumen must be filled with fluid to allow free movement of the instrument and to permit good visualization. Two millilitres of 2% lidocaine are also injected through the irrigation port to provide anaesthesia of the entire ductal system. A 500 ml bag of isotonic saline is then connected to the irrigation port and the endoscope is moved forward accompanied by a gentle flow of saline.

Technique of endoscopic sialolithomy

When a sialolith is encountered, its diameter is estimated by comparison with the endoscope and, if small, it may be removed in one piece with a grasper forceps, basket, or suction apparatus (Fig. 24.3). If this is not possible, the stone may be crushed

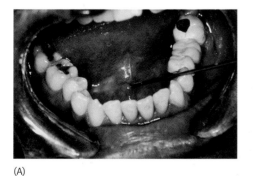

(A)

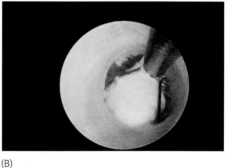

(B)

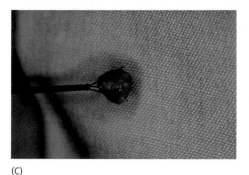

(C)

Fig. 24.3 Introducing the endoscope into Wharton's duct (A), grasping the stone with the duct under direct endoscopic vision (B), and retrieval of the stone (C).

277

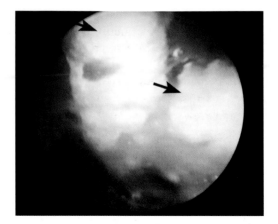

Fig. 24.4 The view of calculus (arrows) in the submandibular gland being broken up by intracorporeal lithotripsy.

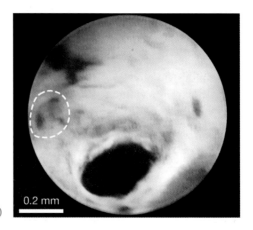

(A)

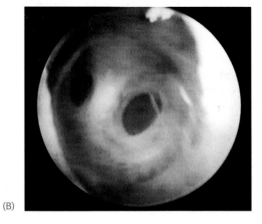

Fig. 24.5 A case of chronic sialadenitis without lithiasis (A). Following copious lavage with isotonic saline, the proximal duct (dotted line in upper panel) was rendered patent again (B).

(B)

with forceps and then removed in pieces by suction. Large or hard stones can be fragmented with an intracorporeal lithotripter (Calcultrip™, Karl Storz, GmbH, Germany) (Fig. 24.4), and finally all these methods can be combined in the recalcitrant case.

If lithotripsy is used or multiple sialoliths are encountered, a second course of sialoendoscopy may be required to clear the obstruction. In cases of chronic sial-adenitis without lithiasis, copious lavage with isotonic saline may be used as a therapeutic measure (Fig. 24.5).

Choice of instrument

If an instrument can be passed behind a calculus, it is usually best retrieved with a Dormia basket. If the lumen is too narrow, a grasping forceps may be used. The stone can be held and manoeuvred easily by this instrument. Lithotripter probes are used to fragment the calculus when other techniques fail. Balloons are used for strictures and for soft small calculi. Biopsy forceps are used to remove polyps.

Post-operative management

Following endoscopy, a 2 mm diameter polyethylene tube is left in the duct, ideally for 2 weeks, to prevent obstruction through post-operative oedema and to allow any residual calculus to be washed out of the duct system. It also acts to reduce stenosis. Marsupialization of the duct through suturing its incised margins to the overlying mucosal margins ensures patency.

Results

Over 5 years (1994–1999), we performed 236 salivary gland endoscopies, of which 170 cases were for obstructive sialadenopathy (Table 24.1). Seven patients had bilateral submandibular sialoliths. In 56 glands (25%), sialadenitis alone was identified, 37 (66%) instances of which were in the parotid; the remaining 19 were in the submandibular gland.

Endoscopy technique failure due to inability to intubate the duct or from ductal perforation before beginning sialoendoscopy occurred in 10/236 cases (4%). Intra-operative failure to remove or eliminate the obstruction occurred in only 18/170 (10%) of cases, and late failures due to recurrent obstruction in 12/170 (7%). The overall success rate was thus 83%. The reasons for intra-operative or late failures were either large calculi or stones sited in the gland parenchyma. There were only four cases of sialolith recurrence; these all occurred 2 years after the procedure and were located near the orifice of the submandibular duct. Their subsequent removal was routine.

Table 24.1 The Tel Aviv sialoendoscopic experience with 170* obstructive glands (1994–1999)

	No. of glands	Submandibular gland	Parotid gland
Sialolithiasis	139	103	34
Duct stricture	18	12	6
Duct polyps†	10	4	6
Foreign bodies‡	3	3	–
Anatomic malformations	2	2	–
Total	170	124	46

* In total, sialoendoscopy was performed on 236 glands (149 submandibular, 86 parotid, and one sublingual), of which 170 were obstructive cases. In the total group, there were 122 males and 114 females (age range 5–85 years). All patients underwent pre- and post-operative screening with routine radiography, sialography, and ultrasound. Post-operative examination was repeated 1 month after treatment, and patients were followed-up until 40 months. The majority of the procedures were performed under local anaesthesia on an out-patient basis, and the duration of the procedure was 30–60 min. In the first week post-treatment, patients are prescribed an antibiotic as a prophylaxis against infection.

† All the polyps showed up as a filling defect on the sialogram and were not evident on ultrasound; they were extracted by miniature biopsy forceps or basket.

‡ Hair accounted for four cases, plant debris for the other two. Five foreign bodies were associated with calculi; three of them were in children. Sialolith formation around a hair shaft was observed in two cases.

Complications

Treatment is followed by significant swelling of the affected gland, but if patency of the duct is maintained, swelling subsides spontaneously after a few hours. One patient suffered from temporary lingual nerve paraesthesia (caused by iatrogenic perforation), two patients developed a ranula, and six patients had a post-operative infection. Seven patients suffered from ductal strictures; five of these underwent successful dilatation, but required sialadenectomy. No other major post-operative complications were noted in a follow-up period of 6–40 months.

Endoscopic observations and treatment

Anatomical observations

Mason and Chisholm (1975) in their book described the presence of smooth muscle strands around the walls of Wharton's duct, and Katz (1991) remarked on them in his article. We have also observed this structure (Nahlieli et al. 1994; Nahlieli and Baruchin 1997). Although a sphincter-like mechanism has not been reported in the parotid duct, such a structure has been seen. The difference between the sphincter-like system in the parotid and that in the submandibular gland is in their location. In Wharton's duct, the sphincter-like system begins near the papilla and runs proximally; in Stensen's duct, it is located proximally in the vicinity of the duct hilum.

The sublingual gland (Bartholin's duct) opens into Wharton's duct in about 15% of cases and this was seen occasionally. This opening was 0–5 mm posterior to the papilla.

Duct abnormalities

Duct abnormalities were detected in 18 cases; four kinks (three submandibular and one parotid) and 14 strictures (nine submandibular and five parotid). Dilatation was accomplished by pressure of the saline wash if the stricture was less than 5% of the lumen diameter. In more severe strictures, a balloon was inserted—either a Fogarty™ 3 F or Lacricath™ 3 F (Atrion Medical Products, Birmingham, AL) and inflated to 9 atmspheres for 90 s and repeated for a further 60 s. The duct was then washed with a 100 mg hydrocortisone solution via the irrigation port and a polyethylene stent left *in situ*. In the management of kinks, balloon dilatation and stenting was followed by advancement ductoplasty with the object of straightening out the kink. Again hydrocortisone was used to limit the inflammatory response. Both procedures were performed under local anaesthetic on an out-patient basis.

In a 10-year-old child, where two calculi were extracted from Wharton's duct, an invagination in the duct wall was noted. It obstructed the ductal lumen and appeared to be the cause of the formation of calculi. It is assumed that the invagination is a form of anatomical malformation.

Alteration in duct appearance with disease

In chronic sialadenitis or with long-standing calculi, the mucosal lining of the ductal system develops a matted appearance with ecchymoses and reduced blood vessels. The healthy duct has a shiny appearance with numerous blood vessels evident.

Attachment between calculi and the ductal wall was observed in the submandibular and parotid glands. In Wharton's duct, these formed when the stone was proximal to the bifurcation (the point where the duct divides into the inner and the outer lobes), whereas in the parotid gland, they were proximal to the masseter. No such connections were detected anterior to these regions.

REFERENCES

Arzoz, E., Santiago, A., Garatea, J., and Gorriaran, M. (1994) Removal of a stone in Stensen's duct with endoscopic laser lithotripsy: report of a case. *J Oral Maxillofac Surg*, **52**, 1329–30.

Arzoz, E., Santiago, A., Esnal, F., and Palomero, R. (1996) Endoscopic intracorporeal lithotripsy for sialolithiasis. *J Oral Maxillofac Surg*, **54**, 847–50.

Baurmash, H. and Dechiara, S.C. (1991) Extraoral parotid sialolithotomy. *J Oral Maxillofac Surg*, **49**, 127–32.

Gundlach, P., Hopf, J., and Linnarz, M. (1994) Introduction of a new diagnostic procedure: salivary duct endoscopy (sialendoscopy) clinical evaluation of sialendoscopy, sialography, and X-ray imaging. *Endosc Surg Allied Technol*, **2**, 294–6.

Iro, H., Waldfahrer, F., Gewalt, K., Zenk, J., and Altendorf Hofmann, A. (1995) Enoral/transoral surgery of malignancies of the oral cavity and the oropharynx. *Adv Otorhinolaryngol*, **49**, 191–5.

Katz, P. (1991) [Endoscopy of the salivary glands]. *Ann Radiol Paris*, **34**, 110–3.

Konigsberger, R., Feyh, J., Goetz, A., and Kastenbauer, E. (1993) Endoscopically-controlled electrohydraulic intracorporeal shock wave lithotripsy (EISL) of salivary stones. *J Otolaryngol*, **22**, 12–3.

Lustmann, J., Regev, E., and Melamed, Y. (1990) Sialolithiasis. A survey on 245 patients and a review of the literature. *Int J Oral Maxillofac Surg*, **19**, 135–8.

Mason, D.K. and Chisholm, D.M. (1975) *Salivary Gland: In Health and Disease*. p. 10. W.B. Saunders, London.

Nahlieli, O. and Baruchin, A.M. (1997) Sialoendoscopy: three years' experience as a diagnostic and treatment modality. *J Oral Maxillofac Surg*, **55**, 912–8; discussion 919–20.

Nahlieli, O. and Baruchin, A.M. (1999) Endoscopic technique for the diagnosis and treatment of obstructive salivary gland diseases. *J Oral Maxillofac Surg*, **57**, 1394–401.

Nahlieli, O. and Baruchin, A.M. (2000) Long-term experience with endoscopic diagnosis and treatment of salivary gland inflammatory diseases. *Laryngoscope*, **110**, 988–93.

Nahlieli, O., Neder, A., and Baruchin, A.M. (1994) Salivary gland endoscopy: a new technique for diagnosis and treatment of sialolithiasis. *J Oral Maxillofac Surg*, **52**, 1240–2.

Ziegler, C.M., Nahlieli, O., and Muhling, J. (1999) [Video-endoscopy of the major salivary glands]. *Mund Kiefer Gesichtschir*, **3**, 320–4.

Audience discussion

Mr Foster (Manchester, UK): Apart from calculi, what else have you seen in the ducts using endoscopy?

Dr Arzoz: We have seen and retrieved foreign bodies, an example of which was a calcified fish bone. We have also identified in several patients valve-like structures in the submandibular duct.

Professor McGurk (London, UK): We have also used a flexible endoscope to visualize stones. It is too long and flexible which makes manipulation of the fibre difficult. The technique involves using both hands, therefore losing any ability to retrieve the stone. Would you agree a shorter semi-rigid or rigid endoscope would be a better system to use, especially if you are considering therapy?

Dr Katz (Paris, France): Yes, unfortunately the manufacturers will not modify their equipment for me. I presently use a long endoscope and I agree it is quite difficult to control at the same time as performing laser lithotripsy.

Dr Capaccio (Florence, Italy): The optimal endoscope should be rigid or semi-rigid, so the endoscope can be manipulated precisely and enable operative techniques to be performed.

Editorial comment

Endoscopy has gained popularity and is accepted as a minimal invasive technique in most surgical fields. Owing to the rapid development in optical technology together with illumination, digitalization, and miniaturization, it is now possible to perform diagnostic and surgical procedures in the salivary ductal system. Endoscopy is capable of identifying radiolucent stones, polyps, stenoses, mucous plugs, foreign bodies, and anatomic abnormalities not evident with conventional imaging techniques.

It is also possible to obtain information on the status of the glandular tissue from the appearance of the ductal lining. More importantly, endoscopy provides a means of removing stones by minimally invasive surgery rather than traditional sialo-adenectomy. Also of major benefit is the ability to demonstrate radiolucent stones especially those in the parotid duct and gland. Until the introduction of sialo-endoscopy, the clinical impression was that submandibular stones far exceeded those found in the parotid, but the present consecutive series for cases suggests that 25% of stones occur in the parotid. Approximately 60% of these parotid calculi were not detected by conventional means. They were probably of lower density and masked in the sialogram by the 'ductal sausageing' (areas of stenosis adjacent to ductal dilatation) or the dense flocculent saliva that is characteristic of chronic recurrent parotitis. Many cases of sialolithiasis in the parotid occur subsequent to pre-existing long-term history of chronic recurrent parotitis.

It remains to be determined if the results of minimally invasive treatment of salivary obstruction will be permanent and whether normal function will be restored to the affected gland. However, sialoendoscopy is a promising new method for use in diagnosing, removing, and post-operatively managing sialolithiasis and sialadenitis. It is an out-patient procedure, utilizing local anaesthesia and without major complications. It appears to be the future investigative tool for the management of perplexing inflammatory salivary gland pathology.

As more clinicians become involved with endoscopy, more findings and innovations will be forthcoming, adding to its effectiveness.

CHAPTER 25

Interventional radiological techniques for the treatment of benign salivary obstruction

Jacqueline Brown and Nicholas Drage

Introduction

Recurrent salivary gland swelling is a common clinical complaint. This is usually caused by obstruction through the presence of a salivary calculus or duct stenosis. Salivary stones are more common in the submandibular gland (70–90%) compared with the parotid gland (5–20%) (Lustmann *et al.* 1990; Escudier and McGurk, 1999). Strictures may be identified at sialography and are more common in the parotid gland where they account for 23–30% of recurrent swellings in the parotid compared with only 3% of recurrent submandibular swellings (Patey 1965; Rose 1954). Duct strictures are believed to result from epithelial duct injury or secondary calculi (Manashil 1978).

Calculi in the anterior third of Wharton's duct in the submandibular gland system or near the orifice of Stenson's duct in the parotid duct system are amenable to simple surgical removal via an intraoral approach, and this remains the most efficient method of treating them. Stenoses in this region of the duct may be dilated with lacrimal duct dilators via the duct papilla; stones and strictures located more proximally present a greater problem. The traditional options have included a conservative approach, either using stimulated salivary flow to dislodge a small calculus or waiting for gland atrophy. The final option is surgery. This may involve duct reimplantation (for osteal lesions), duct ligation, sialoductoplasty, sialolithectomy, and ultimately gland removal. The latter offers a permanent solution but may be accompanied by the attendant complications of surgery, including infection, neurological damage, facial scarring, and Frey's syndrome. The costs of a surgical procedure must also be borne in mind and, together, these negative factors may outweigh the benefits of surgical treatment if the symptoms are mild.

New minimally invasive techniques now offer a realistic alternative to surgery in the treatment of obstructive conditions in suitable cases. Innovations include extracorporeal and intracorporeal shock wave lithotripsy (Iro *et al.* 1992; Escudier 1998), and interventional radiological techniques for both the removal of calculi (Briffa and Callum 1989; Kelly and Dick 1990; Yoshino *et al.* 1996) and the dilation of ductal strictures (Buckenham *et al.* 1992; Brown *et al.* 1997). An added advantage is that treatment is possible on an out-patient basis and post-treatment morbidity is minor (Buckenham *et al.* 1994). Thus it is possible to relieve symptoms (meal time syndrome and infection) by removing the obstruction without the complication or cost associated with surgery. Also, the reduced morbidity associated with minimally invasive techniques means they can be considered in situations where surgical intervention would not be justified. Patients with less acute clinical presentations may be offered treatment.

The use of interventional radiology for relief of obstruction has not been thoroughly investigated, the literature consisting of many small series or case reports. This chapter builds on previous work (Drage *et al.* 2000) and reports on the progress of research into the efficacy of interventional radiological techniques in the treatment of obstruction by salivary calculi and benign strictures. The study is being run to a trial of extracorporeal salivary stone lithotripsy at Guy's Dental Hospital, London. These two techniques are complementary since, following lithothripsy, a significant number of patients have retained stone fragments that do not vent spontaneously and have to be retrieved manually.

Application and evidence of technique

In this study, 62 patients attending the Salivary Gland Clinic at Guy's Dental Hospital were recruited between October 1995 and June 1999. There were 27 males and 35 females, with an age range from 13 to 69 years. All had major salivary gland obstruction which was confirmed on sialography. Forty-four patients had salivary calculi (parotid, 13; submandibular, 31) and 18 patients had duct strictures (parotid, 14; submandibular, four).

Those patients with calculi were treated by fluoroscopically guided stone retrieval using a 3.5 F helical stone extractor (Captura™, Cook® Urological). Strictures were dilated using a 3.5 F 2 cm balloon dilatation catheter (Symmetry, Meditech®, Boston Scientific Corp.) to 3.5 mm (parotid duct) or 5 mm diameter (submandibular duct) at 15 Atmospheres pressure. In the majority of cases, the device was introduced directly into the duct orifice without the aid of an introducer. In a small number of submandibular procedures, a 3.5 F introducer set was first placed within the narrow opening to Wharton's duct to facilitate the insertion of the interventional device. Digital subtraction imaging at a rate of one frame every 2 seconds, in a modified occipito-mental position, supplemented lateral views of the parotid duct system. The procedures were carried out under local anaesthesia on an out-patient basis. Local anaesthetic is administered as a local infiltration around the duct orifice and, in addition, the solution was mixed 50:50 with the contrast agent for improved intraductal topical anaesthesia. In the case of submandibular procedures, anaesthesia was improved by an inferior dental nerve block. A minimal papillotomy usually was required to deliver stones of greater than 2 mm diameter. Sialograms were performed immediately after treatment to gauge success and to act as a baseline for subsequent comparison. All patients were given a questionnaire in order to record post-treatment symptoms and complications. Those patients who underwent stone retrieval were reviewed at 3 months or, if not possible, contacted by telephone. Ductoplasty cases were reviewed with a sialogram at 3 months and again at 1–2 years. The maximum follow-up period was 2.5 years.

In the group of patients undergoing stone removal ($n = 44$), all stones were removed successfully in 21 (48%) patients. In 10 patients (23%), the procedure was partially successful, with some stones or part of a stone removed; and in the remaining 13 patients (29%), the procedure was unsuccessful. In the half of the study group where the procedure was successful, 17 of the 21 (80%) were symptom-free at follow-up (3 months to 2.5 years). Surprisingly, 90% of the partially successful cases were also symptom-free or had alleviation of symptoms.

In those patients where balloon dilatation was performed ($n = 18$), the stricture was navigated successfully in 15 (83%). In three patients, the procedure was abandoned due to failure to get passed the stricture. No cases had to be abandoned through inadequate pain control. Five of the 15 were sialographically normal, and 10 were symptom-free, despite some residual stricture, at review (3 months–2.5 years).

The usual post-operative complications included tenderness and swelling of the instrumented gland for 1–7 days (100%); low-grade sialadenitis was induced that required antibiotic therapy (14/59 or 24%), and, in one case, a basket secured a stone but became impacted in the duct on retrieval and the instrument had to be released surgically from the parotid (Fig. 25.1). The questionnaire revealed a very high acceptance rate for minimally invasive procedures.

The Guy's series and the rest of the literature

Stone removal by interventional radiological techniques

Over the past 10 years, many case reports and small studies have reported on the use of interventional techniques in the treatment of salivary stones and strictures, and indicated that in selected cases, it was an effective alternative to surgery. The techniques have evolved since Briffa and Callum (1989) first reported the successful removal of a salivary calculus from the proximal portion of the submandibular duct using an inflated angioplasty balloon. This was followed by other case reports and small series (Guest et al. 1992; Marchbank and Buckenham 1993; Blaine and Frable 1994; Sharma et al. 1994; North 1998; Nixon and Payn, 1999) of stones being removed from the submandibular and the parotid duct using angioplasty balloons, Dormia baskets, and a vascular snare. The larger of these series are summarized in Table 25.1—notably the success rates varied from 40 to 100%. The present series of 44 patients, as far as we are aware, is the largest published study of salivary stones removed using interventional radiological techniques. It was possible to remove all evidence of salivary stones completely in 48% of cases, and to alleviate symptoms by the partial removal of calculi in a further 28% of cases. This group of patients was unselected and the study appeared to identify factors that predict for successful stone removal as previously proposed. Stone

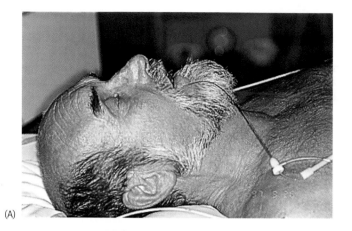

(A)

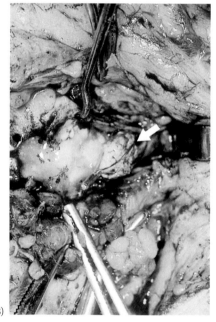

(B)

Fig. 25.1 Once a stone is secured by a basket, it cannot be released. Prior to attempting this technique, it should be established that no stricture is present and that the stone is not too big to pass down the duct. A patient is shown with a basket impacted around a stone in the parotid gland (A). It had to be released surgically. The stone is shown in the parotid duct caught by the basket (arrow) (B).

mobility was the most important factor in predicting outcome, with stones found to be fixed to the duct wall being impossible to capture (Fig. 25.2). Other factors influencing success included the position of the stone—those located in a position where the basket could not be passed beyond the stone proved impossible to engage. Stones lodged in the hilum are difficult to engage for this reason, and those located at or proximal to the submandibular duct genu were difficult to capture. Those located within side branches and diverticula off the main duct were impossible to remove. From this experience, our criteria for the selection of cases is shown in Box 25.1.

Table 25.1 Salivary gland stone removal by interventional radiological techniques

	No. of patients	Gland	Method	Complete stone removal	Alleviation of symptoms*
Buckenham and Guest (1993)	2	P	Balloon	100%	Not recorded
Buckenham et al. (1994)	5	2P; 3SM	Vascular snare	40%	100%
Kim et al. (1996)	9	3P; 6SM	Basket and grasping forceps	78%	100%
Yoshino et al. (1996)	16	5P; 11SM	Baskets	63%	100%
Davies et al. (1997)	7	5P; 2SM	Basket and balloon	86%	57% asymptomatic 43% some improvement
Present series	44	13P; 31SM	Baskets, forceps, balloons	48%	80% asymptomatic

P, parotid gland; SM, submandibular gland.

* Rates of 'alleviation of symptoms' based on successfully completed cases.

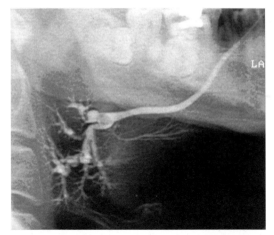

(A)

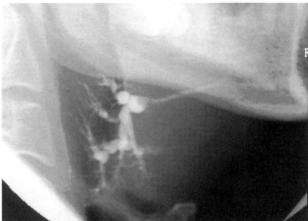

(B)

Fig. 25.2 Sialogram of a stone at the proximal end of the submandibular duct (A). The sialogram shows movement of the stone anteriorly within a short section of the submandibular duct (B). This makes the stone available to basket retrieval.

Box 25.1 Selection criteria for stone removal with interventional radiological techniques

- ◆ Mobile stone
- ◆ Submandibular gland: stone located within lumen of main duct distal to bend of duct over posterior border of mylohyoid muscle
- ◆ Parotid gland: stone located within lumen of main duct distal to hilum
- ◆ Patent main duct to allow passage of stone under traction. If not, consider duct dilation prior to stone removal and use of an angioplasty balloon to remove the stone

Treatment of ductal strictures by interventional radiological techniques

Buckenham and colleagues (1992) first reported the successful dilation of a parotid ductal stenosis using an angioplasty balloon. Further case reports followed (Fernando 1994; Waldman *et al.* 1998), and other series which are summarized in Table 25.2. The most extensive study to date was undertaken by Brown *et al.* (1997) including 30 patients undergoing balloon dilation for salivary duct stenoses. They reported that immediate success was achieved in 87% of cases. This rate is similar to our own results of 83% but, on further follow-up (and without sialogram), only 56% of patients reported complete resolution of symptoms, 36% reported improvements in symptoms, while 8% remained unchanged. In our study, the patients were assessed both by clinical criteria and by sialography. The radiological images showed that 33% of cases were sialographically normal but it was notable that 66% continued to show some stricture at review. It is interesting that in all these cases there had been failure to eliminate the stricture completely at the time of dilatation. Some strictures appeared to be densely fibrotic, showing necking of the fully dilated balloon even at 15 Atmospheres pressure. It was observed that this was found most commonly in strictures of long standing in more elderly patients who also showed significant ductal dilatation proximal to the stricture. Strictures normally dilated completely in younger patients and in those with a short history of obstruction. Our selection criteria for dilatation are shown in Box 25.2.

A new technique must possess both low morbidity and good long-term success if it is to merit consideration as an alternative to traditional treatment methods. Postoperative complications described in the literature following intervention included a case with transient local pain for 24 h, some swelling for 48 h, and one with mild discomfort on eating for 1 month. In our study, a patient questionnaire revealed that all suffered some tenderness and swelling of the affected gland for 1–7 days and that 9% developed low-grade sialadenitis requiring antibiotic therapy. Patients suspected of harbouring low-grade infection should be treated prophylactically by a short course of antibiotics. The questionnaire revealed that the procedures were well tolerated by the patients, and a strong preference was expressed for minimally invasive treatment.

The most serious complication was the impaction within the duct of a basket containing a captured large stone—this required surgical release. In cases which are judged sialographically to demonstrate a large calculus, which may need to be delivered down a length of considerably narrower duct, the use of an angioplasty balloon as opposed to a Dormia basket is advised. Dilation of the duct distal to the stone may then be performed and the balloon may then be used as the retrieval device. A balloon may be deflated and removed easily, while it is not possible to disengage a basket once a stone is captured.

The long-term success of these procedures is encouraging—improvement or complete resolution of symptoms has been reported in 71–100% following stone removal and 66–100% following balloon ductoplasty. This study found that 90% were symptom-free or improved following stone or partial stone removal, and 100% had

Table 25.2 Result of treatment of salivary ductal strictures by interventional radiological techniques

	No. of patients	Gland	Method	Technical success rate	Alleviation of symptoms*
Buckenham and Guest (1993)	3	3P	Balloon	100%	Third improved
Buckenham et al. (1994)	8	5P; 3SM	Balloon	63%	100%
Roberts et al. (1995)	3	3P	Balloon	100%	66% asymptomatic
					33% improved
Kim et al. (1996)	4	2P; 2SM	Balloon	100%	100%
Davies et al. (1997)	10	8P; 1SM	Balloon	90%	60% asymptomatic
					30% some improvement
Brown et al. (1997)	30	24P; 6SM	Balloon	87%	56% complete resolution
					36% some improvement
					8% unchanged
Present series	18	14P; 4SM		83%	33% asymptyomatic
					66% some improvement

P, parotid gland; SM, submandibular gland.

* Rates of 'alleviation of symptoms' based on successfully completed cases.

Box 25.2 Selection criteria for duct dilatation

◆ Stricture located within main duct

◆ Main duct patent both distal to and through stricture on sialogram

alleviation of symptoms following ductoplasty, although only 33% showed a totally normal duct on review sialogram. In those not responding to minimally invasive techniques, surgery remains an option.

REFERENCES

Blaine, D.A. and Frable, M.A. (1994) Removal of a parotid duct calculus with an embolectomy catheter. *Otolaryngol Head Neck Surg*, **111**, 312–3.

Briffa, N.P. and Callum, K.G. (1989) Use of an embolectomy catheter to remove a submandibular duct stone. *Br J Surg*, **76**, 814.

Brown, A.L., Shepherd, D., and Buckenham, T.M. (1997) Per oral balloon sialoplasty: results in the treatment of salivary duct stenosis. *Cardiovasc Intervent Radiol*, **20**, 337–42.

Buckenham, T. and Guest, P. (1993) Interventional sialography using digital imaging. *Australas Radiol*, **37**, 76–9.

Buckenham, T.M., Page, J.E., and Jeddy, T. (1992) Technical report: interventional sialography—balloon dilatation of a Stensen's duct stricture using digital subtraction sialography. *Clin Radiol*, **45**, 34.

Buckenham, T.M., George, C.D., McVicar, D., Moody, A.R., and Coles, G.S. (1994) Digital sialography: imaging and intervention. *Br J Radiol*, **67**, 524–9.

Davies, R.P., Whyte, A.M., and Lui, C.L. (1997) Interventional sialography: a single-center experience. *Cardiovasc Intervent Radiol*, **20**, 331–6.

Drage, N.A., Brown, J.E., Escudier, M.P., and McGurk, M. (2000) Interventional radiology in the removal of salivary calculi. *Radiology*, **214**, 139–42.

Escudier, M.P. and McGurk, M. (1999) Symptomatic sialoadenitis and sialolithiasis in the English population, an estimate of the cost of hospital treatment. *Br Dent J*, **186**, 463–6.

Escudier, M. (1998) The current status and possible future for lithotripsy of salivary calculi. In: *Atlas of Oral and Maxillofacial Surgery Clinics of North America*. pp. 117–32. (L.A. Asseal and M.A. Pogrel, eds) W.B. Saunders, Philadelphia.

Fernando, C.C. (1994) Balloon dilatation of a parotid duct stricture. *Australas Radiol*, **38**, 221.

Guest, P., Maciag, A., and Buckenham, T. (1992) Non-operative removal of a parotid duct stone with a balloon angioplasty catheter. *Br J Oral Maxillofac Surg*, **30**, 197–8.

Iro, H., Schneider, H.T., Fodra, C., Waitz, G., Nitsche, N., Heinritz, H.H. *et al.* (1992) Shockwave lithotripsy of salivary duct stones. *Lancet*, **339**, 1333–6.

Kelly, I.M. and Dick, R. (1991) Technical report: interventional sialography: dormia basket removal of Wharton's duct calculus. *Clin Radiol*, **43**, 205–6.

Kim, R.H., Strimling, A.M., Grosch, T., Feider, D.E., and Veranth, J.J. (1996) Nonoperative removal of sialoliths and sialodochoplasty of salivary duct strictures. *Arch Otolaryngol Head Neck Surg*, **122**, 974–6.

Lustmann, J., Regev, E., and Melamed, Y. (1990) Sialolithiasis. A survey on 245 patients and a review of the literature. *Int J Oral Maxillofac Surg*, **19**, 135–8.

Manashil, G.B., ed. (1978) *Clinical Sialography*. pp. 46–73. C.C. Thomas, Springfield, Ilinois.

Marchbank, N.D. and Buckenham, T.M. (1993) Removal of a submandibular duct calculus with a vascular snare. *Dentomaxillofac Radiol*, **22**, 97–8.

Nixon, P.P. and Payne, M. (1999) Conservative surgical removal of a submandibular duct calculus following interventional sialography. *Clin Radiol*, **54**, 337–8.

North, E.A. (1998) Submandibular sialoplasty for stone removal and treatment of a stricture. *Br J Oral Maxillofac Surg*, **36**, 213–4.

Patey, D.H. (1965) Inflammation of the salivary glands with particular reference to chronic and recurrent parotitis. *Ann R Coll Surg Engl* **36**, 26–44.

Rose, S.S. (1954) A clinical and radiological survey of 192 cases of recurrent swellings of the salivary glands. *Ann. R. Coll Surg Engl*, **15**, 374–401.

Roberts, D.N., Juman, S., Hall, J.R., and Jonathan, D.A. (1995) Parotid duct stenosis: interventional radiology to the rescue. *Ann R Coll Surg Engl*, **77**, 444–6.

Sharma, R.K., al Khalifa, S., Paulose, K.O., and Ahmed, N. (1994) Parotid duct stone—removal by a dormia basket. *J Laryngol Otol*, **108**, 699–701.

Waldman, D.L., Westesson, P.L., and Hengerer, A.S. (1998) Balloon dilation of parotid duct stenosis. *J Vasc Interv Radiol*, **9**, 167–8.

Yoshino, N., Hosokawa, A., Sasaki, T., and Yoshioka, T. (1996) Interventional radiology for the non-surgical removal of sialoliths. *Dentomaxillofac Radiol*, **25**, 242–6.

Audience discussion

Dr Katz (Paris, France): What is the diameter of the balloon you use to dilate the ducts. We inflate our balloon for about 30 minutes at each stricture, how does that compare with your timings?

Dr Brown: For the parotid gland, we use a balloon with a diameter of 3.5 mm when inflated. For the submandibular gland, a larger diameter may be required, such as 5 mm. The balloon is inflated twice at each stricture for 5 minutes. Total inflation time is 10 minutes.

Mr Boyd (Dublin, Ireland): Have you ever considered using real-time video recording of you sialography?

Dr Brown: Yes, we video all our interventional cases.

Mr Boyd: I have been surprised that many of the speakers have not mentioned ultrasound as an investigation for salivary gland disease. Have you considered using ultrasound guidance for any of this work?

Dr Brown: In the future, ultrasound may become an alternative to fluoroscopy as a method of guidance of the balloons or baskets. Unfortunately, up to now, we have had limited access to an ultrasound machine. We shall be acquiring a machine imminently and this is an aspect of the technique I would like to pursue further.

Professor Langdon (London, UK): What is the best way of assessing residual function of the salivary glands? Is recovery of function best shown on sialograms by a return to normal anatomical structure, or is scintigraphy a more reliable method?

Dr Brown: I am not sure that there is a 100% reliable method of assessing post-treatment function. You have to rely on a combination of symptoms, clinical examination, and special tests to provide an overall impression of function.

Dr Sheltna (London, UK): Are there any other ways of assessing gland recovery following treatment apart from these methods?

Mr Bailey (London, UK): Clear saliva expressed from the gland is good evidence of recovery. A post-operative sialogram will demonstrate the ductal structure. The emptying film will illustrate, to a degree, whether the gland is functioning

Mr Davies (Kent, UK): It is important to remember why we are treating these glands, which is largely for the patient's symptoms of obstruction. Dry mouth is not normally a problem after one gland has been removed. So I dispute whether any assessment of function is required, so long as the patient is asymptomatic.

Mr Shaheen (London, UK): As well as volume and colour of the saliva, I find that consistency of saliva is also a good indicator of the state of the gland. A thick jelly-like secretion indicates the gland is unlikely to recover.

Dr Capaccio (Florence, Italy): Sialography is important in two respects. If there is gross destruction of the gland on sialography, the chances of recovery are remote. Parotid sialography is useful even if the decision to remove the gland has already been made, since the degree of destruction can be assessed. Consequently, the amount of fibrosis of the gland can be judged and therefore the degree of difficulty of removing the parotid gland without detrimental effects to the facial nerve. This information is useful when warning the patient pre-operatively about the risks of parotid surgery. Total conservative parotidectomy is the operation of choice, since a further operation at a later date to remove a symptomatic deep lobe is very difficult because of the scarring associated with the initial operation.

Editorial comment

Until recently, the minimally invasive approach to salivary calculi has been by interventional radiology using fluoroscopic control of instruments (basket, snares, or dilators). In this chapter, two areas have been investigated: stone retrieval and stricture release (dilatation).

Success depends on case selection, and the criteria are: a mobile stone in a salivary duct that is wide enough to allow the passage of a stone once it has been snared. To this may be added a third limitation, namely the presence of a space sufficient to allow the snare to be passed beyond the stone.

Strictures create more of a problem. Some strictures are so densely fibrotic that attempts at dilatation using a balloon fail to make any impression on the stricture. Even in the best of circumstances, the duct may not revert to normal and some residual narrowing of the duct is still present. Nevertheless, and despite its limitations, dilatation has a real role to play when dealing with strictures of the parotid duct as it improves symptoms and here the likely overriding wish of the clinician is to avoid interventional surgery in the parotid. The current radiological instruments can be applied through the working channel of the new endoscopes. Where there are two techniques that are equally effective but one avoids radiation, then the latter is likely to become the treatment of choice.

CHAPTER 26

Treatment for non-neoplastic disease of the submandibular gland

Sialadenectomy

Oreste Gallo, Pasquale Berloco, and Luca Bruschini

A conservative approach to the removal of hilar stones

Mark McGurk

Sialadenectomy
Oreste Gallo, Pasquale Berloco, and Luca Bruschini

Sialolithiasis is the most common cause of salivary gland obstruction and occurs mainly (90%) in the submandibular gland (Chapter 22). Salivary gland stones, whose exact mechanism of formation remains unclear, are invariably associated with chronic inflammation of the gland. Salivary gland stones may be single or multiple and can lie within the duct or gland. At least a third of calculi of the submandibular gland lie in the distal third of the duct where they can be removed simply through an incision in the floor of the mouth (McGurk and Escudier 1995). This approach is generally complication-free; however, it may not modify the course of chronic sialoadenitis affecting the gland. It is taught that the risk of recurrent stones is high in such circumstances, and often a more extensive surgical procedure is required for recurrent disease (Ellies *et al.* 1996).

The standard treatment for calculi in the proximal duct or in the submaxillary gland is submandibular gland removal or sialoadenectomy (Norman 1995). This procedure is normally straightforward but significant morbidity may be encountered. Moreover, although sialodenectomy is a relatively standard procedure, it is uncommon for any one individual to accumulate a large experience. It is evident from current trends (Chapter 23–25) that sialoadenectomy is likely to become a less common method of managing sialoadenitis in the future. This chapter reports on a large series treated for submandibular gland disease at the University Institute of Otolaryngology Head and Neck Surgery in Florence, and updates a previous report (Gallina *et al.* 1990). Clinical and pathological analysis as well as follow-up studies were undertaken on these patients with the aim of identifying the indications for surgery. This study, together with an extensive review of the literature, holds as a baseline against which minimally invasive techniques may be judged.

The Florence experience

The records of 130 consecutive patients treated between January 1989 and December 1995 were reviewed retrospectively. Relevant factors in the patients' history such as tobacco and alcohol habits, as well as clinical and radiological findings, histopathological diagnosis, and post-operative morbidity were recorded. Prior to surgery, the function of the lingual, facial, and hypoglossal nerves was checked by clinical evaluation of facial movements, the appearance and the movement of the tongue, and by enquiry into the presence of lingual paraesthesia. Post-operative assessment was performed in the same fashion usually on the first post-operative day or the day of discharge (mean 3.9 days). If nerve injury was identified and the nerve had not been sectioned intentionally, the patient was re-evaluated at regular intervals thereafter until weakness had resolved. Pre-operatively, the majority of patients were evaluated with radiographs and ultrasonography.

The basic characteristics of the 130 patients are shown in Table 26.1. The major indication was the clinical impression of chronic sialoadenitis secondary to the presence of salivary stones. Importantly, all but one of the patients, who was treated by

Table 26.1 Descriptive details of a consecutive series of submandibular sialadenectomies performed in Florence (1989–1995)

	Pre-operative diagnosis	Histological diagnosis
No. of patients	130	
Males:females	70:60	
Median age (range)	49 (15–78) years	
Chronic sialadenitis in the presence of:		
Salivary calculi (symptomatic)	67 (52)	48/67 (72) (stone confirmed)
(non-symptomatic)		8/42 (19) (stone confirmed)
No sialolithiasis	42 (33)	
Unknown origin	18 (14)	10 immuno-sialadenitis
		2 pleomorphic adenoma
		1 dermoid cyst
Abscess	3	

Values in parentheses are percentages.

The primary clinical symptom was a painful swelling in 99 patients (sialolithiasis, 79%; without calculi, 89%; and three subjects with a salivary gland abscess). In contrast, only 50% of patients with a gland swelling of uncertain origin reported pain. Twenty-five (19%) patients had a painless swelling and the remaining seven presented with pain as the only symptom. Symptoms were related to food ingestion (meal time syndrome) in 81 patients (63%) but was more prevalent in those patients with sialoadenitis, 68% of whom had calculi. Those patients who had swelling of uncertain origin or had an abscess had meal time syndrome in 33% of cases. The difference between these groups was significant (P = 0.017).

medical therapy following the intraoral removal of a stone, underwent a surgical excision of the submandibular gland with a classic cervical approach. After surgery, salivary
gland stones were confirmed in 48 out of the 67 patients thought to have a stone at
presentation. In 38 of the patients, a history of previous calculi removed through an
incision of the floor of the mouth was documented. This was also true in eight out of
42 patients with an initial diagnosis of sialoadenitis without any clinical and radiological signs of calculi. Overall, histological reports were not available in 43 cases.
In the remaining 87 patients, chronic sialoadenitis was present alone in 34 cases,
associated with fibrosis in 37 cases, four cases of gross infection, 10 cases of immuno-
sialoadenitis, two pleomorphic adenomas, and a dermoid cyst.

When the age of patients presenting with sialoadenitis either with or without stones
was compared, there was no difference between the groups (49.6 versus 45.1 years,
respectively) but there was a slight preponderance of males in both groups. More
operations were undertaken on the right side compared with the left (61% versus
39%), with no differences according to the presence or absence of sialolithiasis
($P = 0.66$). A careful revision of clinical records showed that a history of tobacco
exposure was reported in 70 out of 130 patients (54%), while only 31.5% of patients
were alcohol drinkers. In both cases, no statistically significant difference was found
with regard to the presence or absence of calculi in inflamed glands ($P = 0.94$ and
$P = 0.57$, respectively).

The interval between the onset of symptoms and the surgery was recorded in
all patients. The shortest interval was seen in patients with suspected sialoadenitis
characterized by a gland swelling of uncertain origin (mean 16.3 months; range
0.7–39 months). Interestingly, patients with sialolithiasis showed a longer interval
(mean 46; range 0.5–120 months) when compared with patients with sialoadenitis
without calculi (mean 28.5; range 1–160 months) ($P = 0.01$).

Complications

Minor and major complications following salivary gland removal were present in 28
(22%) patients. Nerve injury occurred in the remaining 12 cases principally affecting
the *mandibular branch* of the facial nerve. The incidence of injury to this nerve in our
series was 7% (9/130 resections) but, over a period of 3 months, five of these nine had
a full spontaneous recovery of function; the remaining four patients had a permanent
deficit. The incidence of facial nerve weakness did not correlate with either the presence or the absence of calculi in the excised gland. Temporary *lingual nerve* paraesthesia
occurred in two resections (1.5%) when a large fibrotic salivary gland was excised.
Finally, *hypoglossal nerve* paralysis was seen in one patient (0.8%) but disappeared
spontaneously within 2 weeks of surgery. Additional complications included: subjective
xerostomia (three cases), temporary neck swelling (four cases); wound infection (six
cases), and obvious scarring (three cases).

A total of 94 patients could be traced for follow-up evaluation. The follow-up period
varied from 1 month to 15 years (mean 73 months). The only reported late complication was recurrent calculus formation. In two patients, calculi reformed in
Wharton's duct at 18 and 24 months after submandibular gland excision.

Morbidity following submandibular sialoadenectomy: a literature search

During the preparation of this chapter, we also undertook a comprehensive search of the literature (MEDLINE 1966–1999) examining specifically for complications following submanbidular sialadenectomy. We found 14 studies which, combined with our own series and the unpublished series from the Christie Hospital, Manchester, resulted in 16 reports totalling almost 1800 patients. The complications are tabulated in Tables 26.2 and 26.3.

The first observation is the great variance in reported morbidity. This may reflect differences in patient age, medical status, previous history of gland infection, and surgical experience. Injuries to the nerves cause the greatest concern both to the surgeon and to the patient. Overall, temporary injury to the *ramus mandibularis* branch of the facial nerve is approximately 10%, with permanent injuries at 3%. These contrast with those following parotid surgery for benign disease (Chapter 6). Overall, injuries to the lingual and hypoglossal nerves are uncommon (<4%) but where they occur, the literature suggests that over half of these may be permanent. Multiple nerve injury may also occur. Immediate post-operative problems are due mainly to haemorrhage (0–14%) and infection (0–14%), usually delaying hospital discharge rather than threatening life, but serious haemorrhage has been reported. Another frequent complaint (but not always thoroughly reported in studies) is dissatisfaction with an unsightly scar.

Recurrent stone formation in the remnants of Wharton's duct is reported in 0–7% of patients and probably relates to the sublingual gland in many instances. In the main, the complications do not prevent the patient living an apparently normal life. Submandibular gland removal is not a taxing operation and is frequently delegated to the trainee surgeon, which may explain the relatively high incidence of neuropraxia. Similarly in the case of the parotid gland, the risk to these nerves increases significantly with the indurated and fibrosed gland where the lingual nerve can become welded to the gland by scar tissue and difficult to identify.

Remarks

Sialolithectomy or sialoadenectomy are the traditional methods of treating sialolithiasis. The former is undertaken for ductal stones, especially those located in the anterior portion of the salivary gland. The technique is well established and is amenable to laser dissection (Azaz *et al.* 1996). Many surgeons advocate an immediate sialolithectomy, even in the acute stage, because most of the symptoms develop from obstruction to salivary flow. Sialoadenectomy of the submandibular gland constitutes the last method of treatment and is justified in a non-functioning gland. The problem is that there is no definitive way of assessing salivary gland function in patients with sialolithiasis, or of predicting recovery. However, recent studies have suggested that salivary gland function can recover after sialoadenectomy (Yoshimura *et al.* 1989), with regeneration of glandular parenchyma (Bhaskar *et al.* 1966). The contrary view, held by the majority of surgeons, is that chronic inflammation of the salivary gland (infective or immuno-

Table 26.2 Nerve morbidity following submandibular sialoadenectomy from 16 series

Author	No. of patients	Permanent			Transient		
		Ramus mandubularis	Lingual	Hypoglossal	Ramus mandubularis	Lingual	Hypoglossal
Yoel (1975)	179	1	4 (2)	0	13 (7)	2	1
Gallois (1978)	55	0	0	0	5 (9)	4	0
Goudal and Bertrand (1979)	83	1	4 (5)	1	5 (6)	10	1
Coumel et al. (1979)	50	0	2	0	11 (22)	1	1
Panzoni et al. (1984)	50	10 (20)	0	15 (30)	0	0	0
Milton et al. (1986)	137	10 (7)	4 (3)	0	15 (11)	0	1
Kennedy and Poole (1989)	76	6 (8)	0	0	7 (9)	0	0
Berini Aytes and Gay Escods (1992)	206	16 (8)	3	6 (3)	8 (4)	0	1
Smith et al. (1993)	92	0	0	0	33 (36)	0	0
Hald and Andreassen (1994)	159	1	4 (3)	0	29 (18)	8	0
Ellies et al. (1996)	233	1	5 (2)	0	0	0	0
Bates et al. (1998)	41	5 (12)	0	0	0	0	0
Goh and Sethi (1998)	87	0	0	0	2	0	0
Turco et al. (1998)	50	9 (18)	3	3	0	0	0
Florence series (2000)	130	4 (3)	0	0	5 (4)	2	1
Christie series (2000)*	170	2	0	0	40 (23)	7 (5)	3
Totals	1798	60 (3.3)	29 (1.6)	25 (1.4)	173 (9.6)	34 (1.9)	9 (0.5)

Values in parentheses are percentages.

* The Christie series are unpublished data. The surgery was performed by three surgeons (1960–1992). The histologies were: pleomorphic adenomas, 21; chronic sialadenitis with calculi, 82; chronic sialadenitis without calculi, 46; salivary lymphoepithelial lesion, four; fatty changes, three; toxoplasmosis, tuberculosis, and venous congestion, one each.

Table 26.3 Non-neural complications following submandibular sialoadenectomy from 16 series

Author	No. of Patients	Haemorrhage	Fistula	Infection	Cysts	Altered sensation	Xerostomia	Scar	Recurrent stone
Yoel (1975)	179	2	–	3	3	–	–	4	–
Gallois (1978)	55	1	2	5	3	3	–	5	3
Goudal and Betrand (1979)	83	1	3	3	5	3	–	–	2
Coumel et al. (1979)	50	7 (14)	1	2	–	2	–	6	1
Panzoni et al. (1984)	50	6 (12)	–	–	–	–	–	8 (16)	–
Milton et al. (1986)	137	14 (10)	4	12 (9)	–	–	–	6 (4)	3
Kennedy and Poole (1989)	76	2	–	–	–	–	–	–	–
Berini Aytes andGay Escoda (1992)	206	8 (4)	–	15 (7)	–	–	–	10 (5)	15 (7)
Smith et al. (1993)	92	5 (5)	–	7 (8)	–	–	–	5 (5)	–
Hald and Andreassen (1994)	159	5 (3)	2	22 (14)	–	25 (16)	–	9 (6)	8 (5)
Ellies et al. (1996)	233	0	0	–	7 (3)	–	–	8 (3)	–
Bates et al. (1998)	41	1	1	–	–	–	–	1	–
Goh and Sethi (1998)	87	0	–	2	–	–	–	–	–
Turco et al. (1998)	50	0	–	–	–	–	–	–	–
Florence series (2000)	130	0	0	6 (5)	4	0	3	3	2
Christie series (2000)	170	0	1	14 (8)	1	0	6 (4)	8 (5)	8 (5)
Totals (ranges %)	1798	(0–14)	(0–4)	(0–14)	(0–3)	(0–16)	(0–4)	(0–16)	(0–7)

(–) denotes that details were not recorded. Values in parentheses are percentages.

logical) inevitably leads to fibrosis and a repeating cycle of infection, with progressive destruction of the gland often complicated by stone or abscess formation. This scenario is the justification for a definitive surgical approach.

Many of our patients who underwent a sialoadenectomy had a history of multiple calculi. More than half of those with sialolithiasis at the time of surgery had a stone removed on a previous occasion through an oral incision. This finding suggests that simple sialolithectomy may not always be a curative procedure. Traditionally, no alternative to adenectomy has existed in patients with chronic sialoadenitis without salivary stones. In our series, many patients had a history of multiple medical therapies; most of them reported recurrent painful swelling with food ingestion but sometimes without any clinical and radiological evidence of calculi. These 'non-sialolithiases' frequently are due to duct stenosis (19% in our series) or microcalculi formation in the saliva (Harrison *et al.* 1997).

The incidence of post-operative complications in our series was comparable with that of others. We documented subjective xerostomia in three patients. This sequela is uncommon; however, higher rates have been reported recently following a unilateral submandibular gland excision (Laskawi *et al.* 1996; Cunning *et al.* 1998). Likewise, a facial nerve weakness occurred in 7% of our cases, of which five subsequently resolved. Similarly, the injuries to the lingual and hypoglossal nerves were temporary. None-theless, the permanent facial weakness rate was 3%, a figure similar to that quoted following parotidectomy (Chapter 6). With this sobering thought comes the suggestion that perhaps complications have been underestimated in the past literature.

A conservative approach to the removal of hilar stones
Mark McGurk

Traditional surgical practice

Dr Escudier has already pointed out (Chapter 22) that approximately 3700 patients in the UK are admitted to hospital annually with salivary obstruction or infection and, of these, an estimated 2000 patients undergo sialoadenectomy. The main factor determining this surgical policy is the widely held view that the obstructed and/or infected salivary gland is permanently damaged by these events, and the structural damage within the gland predisposes it to recurrent disease. Conservative measures less than sialoadenectomy only postpone the gland excision. Both clinical and experimental evidence point to the conclusion that good recovery can be achieved even in glands with evidence of severe damage (Isacsson *et al.* 1981; van der Akker and Busemann-Sokole 1983; Yoshimura *et al.* 1989; Kim *et al.* 1996). The degree of histological change does not appear to correlate with the duration of symptoms but rather with the size of the stone (Isacsson *et al.* 1981). Factors affecting the patients' choice of treatment are the morbidity encountered with surgery, personal preference, and the effectiveness of alternative management methods.

Salivary lithotripsy has brought about an alteration in perspective for the treatment of salivary calculi. The rationale for a conservative approach is that once the stone is released, the majority of salivary glands become asymptomatic and appear to regain normal function, with the proviso that there is no accurate method to access salivary function except salivary flow or through scintigraphy. Secondly, there is pressure from the patient to avoid surgery. Once patients enter a minimally invasive programme, they are reluctant to revert to adenectomy. A similar situation occurred in the management of renal stones, where surgical treatment is now restricted to 5% of cases (Chaussy and Fuchs 1989).

This section describes the management of 209 patients with salivary calculi treated at Guy's Hospital, London, and provides a rationale for a conservative surgical approach to treatment. The technique for removal of a calculus from the hilum of the submandibular gland is described.

Intraoral removal of the submandibular hilar stone

Failure of conservative treatment presents either as the persistence of a large stone in the hilum of the submandibular gland or as a persistently infected salivary gland. In this 4-year study, a hilar stone was the more common problem. Chronic infection was mainly in the submandibular gland, and only one parotidectomy was performed. Large stones (>1 cm diameter) are resistant to lithotripsy. They invariably lie at the junction of Wharton's duct and the submandibular gland wedged below the posterior margin of the mylohyoid muscle.

The successful execution of an intraoral approach to the hilum of the submandibular gland depends on a small number of factors (Seward 1968). First, the stone should be discernible on bimanual palpation. Secondly, successful surgery depends on scrupulous haemostasis. Thirdly, as access to the posterior border of the mylohyoid muscle is difficult, an experienced surgical assistant makes an important contribution both by elevating the gland through manual pressure in the submandibualr triangle and by helping with retraction of oral tissue.

The surgeon is positioned on the contralateral side to the stone, the floor of the mouth is infiltrated with 4 ml of 1:200 000 lignocaine and adrenaline, and the tongue is retracted antero-medially. This latter action exposes the floor of the mouth which usually resembles a narrow gutter. An oblique incision is made from the punctum of the submandibular salivary duct (Wharton's duct) along the floor of the mouth towards the third molar tooth. After the incision parts the mucosa, the loose areolar tissue of the floor of the mouth is opened by blunt dissection (Fig. 26.1). This dissection should start proximal to the body of the sublingual gland because this gland is difficult to dissect and bleeds easily. The submandibular duct can be difficult to identify within the sublingual gland but it can be seen as it descends through the loose areolar tissue proximal to the gland. Identification of the duct can be aided by cannulating it prior to surgery. The lingual nerve runs obliquely from the tongue, beneath the duct to the submandibular ganglion laterally. The submandibular ganglion is bound down to the surface of the submandibular gland as it curls over the mylohyoid. The nerve then ascends medially, crossing over the submandibular duct as it enters the gland. It is here that the stone is situated. The lingual nerve must be mobilized from the duct and

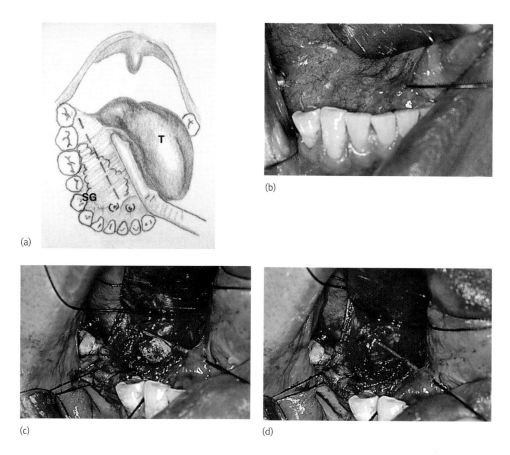

Fig. 26.1 The surgical approach to the removal of a stone in the hilum of the submandibular gland (a). The submandibular gland is cannulated (b) and the floor of the mouth carefully dissected to expose the duct. The stone is located at the junction of the duct and gland (c). The duct is subsequently repaired with multiple sutures (d) T, tongue; SG, sublingual gland.

retracted medially to visualize the stone in the hilum of the gland. It is at this point that manual pressure is used to elevate the submandibular gland, the duct is incised, and the stone delivered. The duct is irrigated with normal saline in order to remove additional stone debris and the incision is closed with fine resorbable sutures. The duct system is decompressed by a ducto-plasty in the distal third of the duct to avoid leakage of saliva from the hilum into the floor of the mouth.

The results of a conservative approach to salivary calculi

In the period 1995–1999, 209 patients with proven salivary calculi were referred to the Salivary Gland Clinic at Guy's Hospital and entered prospectively into a research programme to determine the application of lithotripsy (Table 26.4). Stones in the distal third of the submandibular duct or near the punctum of Wharton's or Stenson's duct

Table 26.4 Results of a conservative approach to the treatment of salivary calculi at the Guys Salivary Gland Service (1995–1999)

Treatment	Salivary calculi	Failures
Minimally invasive (lithotripsy and basket retrieval)	182	28*
Hilar removal of stone	22	
Submandibular sialoadenectomy	5	
Total	209	

* Persistent symptoms after minimally invasive treatment but patient refused surgery. Adenectomy was required for 3 hilar stones that failed to respond to intraoral surgery and two patients who had repeated acute onchronic infections after lithotripsy.

were removed surgically under local anaesthesia. Otherwise it was policy for all cases of stone to be treated by lithotripsy.

As experience was gained with radiological techniques, a number of small mobile stones were treated by basket retrieval (Chapter 25). This method of stone removal proved particularly useful as an adjunct to lithotripsy for removing stone fragments from the duct system. Patients with asymptomatic calculi were treated expectantly; minor symptoms normally prompted another course of lithotripsy. Experience shows that stone fragments not causing obstruction can remain asymptomatic and apparently dormant for years. Surgery was held in reserve for symptomatic cases that failed to respond to these conservative measures.

Failure occurred in the form of a large symptomatic stone at the hilum of the submandibular gland or from a chronically infected salivary gland. A small group of 25 patients (males, 12; females, 13) had stones at the hilum of the submandibular gland removed intraorally. With a follow-up of 3–18 months, this technique has failed in three instances, and these glands subsequently were removed. Of the remaining 22 patients, 18 (78%) remain symptom-free and four have mild symptoms of obstruction. In 18 patients, the function of the gland was assessed by scintigraphy 3 months after treatment. All glands demonstrated evidence of active secretion but in only half did the flow match that in the contralateral gland. Temporary parasthesia occurred in all cases due to retraction of the lingual nerve, but normal function returned within 3 weeks of surgery.

The results of this conservative approach are quite different from traditional practice. Of the 209 patients with proven stones, 182 (87%) were rendered symptom-free by minimally invasive therapy. Approximately half of these patients had evidence of residual stone but the fragments were insufficient to obstruct the flow of saliva and most patients declined further treatment. It remains to be seen how long these patients remain asymptomatic. A further 28 (13%) patients had persistent symptoms but not sufficiently severe for them to request further intervention. One parotidectomy was performed during this period as a result of repeated infection. The aetiology was unknown and not due to a stone.

The initial results are promising, but not conclusive. There is still the possibility that these patients may develop recurrent stones or infection in the years to come.

REFERENCES

Azaz, B., Regev, E., Casap, N., and Chicin, R. (1996) Sialolithectomy done with a CO_2 laser: clinical and scintigraphic results. *J Oral Maxillofac Surg*, **54**, 685–8.

Bates, D., O' Brien, C.J., Tikaram, K., and Painter, D.M. (1998) Parotid and submandibular sialadenitis treated by salivary gland excision. *Aust NZ J Surg*, **68**, 120–4.

Berini Aytes, L. and Gay Escoda, C. (1992) Morbidity associated with removal of the submandibular gland. *J Craniomaxillofac Surg*, **20**, 216–9.

Bhaskar, S.N., Lilly, G.E., and Bhussry, B. (1966) Regeneration of the salivary glands in the rabbit. *J Dent Res*, **45**, 37–41.

Chaussy, C.G. and Fuchs, G.J. (1989) Current state and future developments of noninvasive treatment of human urinary stones with extracorporeal shock wave lithotripsy. *J Urol*, **141**, 782–9.

Coumel, C., Vesse, M., Perrin, L., and Rouaux, J.P. (1979) [50 submandibular gland resections]. *Rev Stomatol Chir Maxillofac*, **80**, 344–8.

Cunning, D.M., Lipke, N., and Wax, M.K. (1998) Significance of unilateral submandibular gland excision on salivary flow in noncancer patients. *Laryngoscope*, **108**, 812–5.

Ellies, M., Laskawi, R., Arglebe, C., and Schott, A. (1996) Surgical management of nonneoplastic diseases of the submandibular gland. A follow-up study. *Int J Oral Maxillofac Surg*, **25**, 285–9.

Gallina, E., Gallo, O., Boccuzzi, S., and Paradiso, P. (1990) Analysis of 185 submandibular gland excisions. *Acta Otorhinolaryngol Belg*, **44**, 7–10.

Goh, Y.H. and Sethi, D.S. (1998) Submandibular gland excision: a five-year review. *J Laryngol Otol*, **112**, 269–73.

Goudal, J.Y. and Bertrand, J.C. (1979) [Complications of surgical treatment for submandibular calculi]. *Rev Stomatol Chir Maxillofac*, **80**, 349–50.

Hald, J. and Andreassen, U.K. (1994) Submandibular gland excision: short- and long-term complications. *ORL J Otorhinolaryngol Relat Spec*, **56**, 87–91.

Harrison, J.D., Epivatianos, A., and Bhatia, S.N. (1997) Role of microliths in the aetiology of chronic submandibular sialadenitis: a clinicopathological investigation of 154 cases. *Histopathology*, **31**, 237–51.

Isacsson, G., Ahlner, B., and Lundquist, P.G. (1981) Chronic sialadenitis of the submandibular gland. A retrospective study of 108 cases. *Arch Otorhinolaryngol*, **232**, 91–100.

Kennedy, P.J. and Poole, A.G. (1989) Excision of the submandibular gland: minimizing the risk of nerve damage. *Aust NZ J Surg*, **59**, 411–4.

Kim, R.H., Strimling, A.M., Grosch, T., Feider, D.E., and Veranth, J.J. (1996) Nonoperative removal of sialoliths and sialodochoplasty of salivary duct strictures. *Arch Otolaryngol Head Neck Surg*, **122**, 974–6.

Laskawi, R., Ellies, M., Arglebe, C., and Schott, A. (1995) Surgical management of benign tumors of the submandibular gland: a follow-up study. *J Oral Maxillofac Surg*, **53**, 506–8.

McGurk, M. and Escudier, M. (1995) Removing salivary gland stones. *Br J Hosp Med*, **54**, 184–5.

Milton, C.M., Thomas, B.M., and Bickerton, R.C. (1986) Morbidity study of submandibular gland excision. *Ann R Coll Surg Engl*, **68**, 148–50.

Norman, J.E. de B. (1995) Salivary calculus disease. In: *Colour Altas and Text of Salivary Gland Disease, Disorders and Surgery*. (J. de Burgh Norman and M. McGurk, eds) Mosby-Wolfe, London.

Panzoni, E., Marchesi, A., and Lippi, L. (1984) [Submandibular sialoadenectomy: surgical technique, surgical case study and remote results]. *Riv Ital Stomatol*, **53**, 121–30.

Seward, G.R. (1968) Anatomic surgery for salivary calculi. 3. Calculi in the posterior part of the submandibular duct. *Oral Surg, Oral Med Oral Pathol*, **25**, 525–31.

Smith, W.P., Peters, W.J., and Markus, A.F. (1993) Submandibular gland surgery: an audit of clinical findings, pathology and postoperative morbidity. *Ann R Coll Surg Engl*, **75**, 164–7.

Turco, C., Nisio, A., and Brunetti, F. (1988) [Submandibular sialoadenectomy and long-term results]. *Minerva Stomatol*, **37**, 329–34.

van den Akker, H.P. and Busemann Sokole, E. (1983) Submandibular gland function following transoral sialolithectomy. *Oral Surg, Oral Med Oral Pathol*, **56**, 351–6.

Yoel, J., ed. (1975) *Pathology and Surgery of the Salivary Glands*. C.C. Thomas, Springfield, Ilinois.

Yoshimura, Y., Morishita, T., and Sugihara, T. (1989) Salivary gland function after sialolithiasis: scintigraphic examination of submandibular glands with 99mTc-pertechnetate. *J Oral Maxillofac Surg*, **47**, 704–10.

Audience discussion

Mr Webb (Bristol, UK): I can raise a point on the technique of removing the sub-mandibular salivary gland. Most textbooks will tell you to make a transverse incision through the platysma around 4 cm below the horizontal body of the mandible. I cannot remember the last time I did it that way. I always separate the platysma in the line of its fibres over the gland and then, with the aid of a facial nerve stimulator, identify the cervical branches and mandibular branches of the facial nerve. If you do not identify these branches, then you will cut them very easily with the traditional technique. If you know where the branches are, you can split the platysma safely. I have not had any weakness, transient or otherwise, since I have been doing it

Professor O' Brien (Sydney, Australia): We do not try to identify the nerve during the operation. We make a transverse incision through the platysma and, although I have a 10% incidence of temporary nerve weakness, they all recover. The patient though has to be warned of the possibility of facial nerve weakness following the operation.

Dr Gallo: We also use a transverse incision and do not try to identify the nerve during surgery.

Professor Speight (London, UK): How do you close the duct at the end of the procedure and have you had complications such as stenosis or ranula?

Professor McGurk: I use 5/0 dexon and place two sutures at the hilum. I then decompress the duct distally to prevent any pressure build-up that could force saliva into the soft tissues forming a ranula. I have not had any problems with the formation of strictures.

Question from the floor: We have heard that we really do not understand the aetiology of stones and thus, by implication, we cannot understand their natural history. We have had evidence to show that the average age of presentation is in the mid to late 40s and that this corresponds well with sialoadenitis. It is likely that the two are causally related.

Therefore, are we looking at a long period for the stones to develop? In treating the stones with a minimally invasive technique, we have done nothing to alter what causes that stone to form in the first place. Presumably then, the patient is at risk of forming further stones. If the stone takes 20 years to form, are we merely delaying surgery by 20 years? If we performed conventional surgery in the first instance, at least the patients are younger and more likely to be fit for surgery.

Professor McGurk: This is one of the most important questions, but one that no one can answer at the moment. I am intending to follow these patients up for as long as is possible. Only time will tell if we are delaying the need for surgery.

Dr van den Akker (Amsterdam, The Netherlands): To Professor McGurk, with the different techniques available for the treatment of salivary stones, what is the therapy protocol for a stone located at the hilum of the gland?

Professor McGurk: After examining the patient, I send the patient for a sialogram. If the stone is fixed at the hilum, lithotripsy is normally arranged. If on sialography the stone is proven to be mobile and the duct anterior to the stone is sufficiently wide, basket retrieval of the stone is performed. Basket retrieval is also performed after lithotripsy if there are mobile fragments present that fail to pass spontaneously. With the advent of short rigid endoscopes with narrow working channels, our protocol is likely to be modified. We are likely to use intracorporeal lithotripsy to treat larger stones located within the main duct, which cannot be treated by either of the above techniques. Surgical removal is a third option, with adenectomy reserved for failed cases. However, our referrals are often from other centres, and these patients are determined to avoid surgery. They have heard about these minimally invasive techniques and are willing to try these options, in the knowledge that they are no worse off if the technique is unsuccessful.

Editorial comment

Dr Gallo has presented what are probably the best results likely to be obtained by conventional treatment of submandibular sialoadenectomy, with facial nerve damage (ramus mandibularis branch) at 3% and no permanent damage to the lingual or hypoglossal nerves. These results compare favourably with a review of complications from other series which put the incidence of permanent facial nerve damage at 1–6%, and permanent injury to lingual or hypoglossal nerves at 2–3%. However, these figures probably under-represent the complication rate because only good centres have enough self-confidence to be candid about complication rates. At present, there is a low threshold for submandibular sialoadenectomy and the question that must be asked is whether a more conservative approach can be undertaken in the future. A partial answer to this question is provided by Professor McGurk. His paper reports both a method for removing recalcitrant stone from the hilum of the submandibular gland, and the results obtained. They are favourable, with only a small number of patients reporting persistent symptoms and requiring sialoadenectomy.

This chapter describes a major shift in current practice toward a conservative approach. The Guy's series shows submandibular sialoadenectomy was necessary in only five cases in a consecutive series of 209 patients with salivary complaints. Whether this is the pattern of the future remains to be determined, as it is possible that a conservative approach may store up problems for the future and only delay surgery. Whether this is so or not is still within the womb of time.

CHAPTER 27

Surgical management of chronic sialadenitis

The clinical problem

Malcolm Bailey

Surgical treatment and results

Christopher O'Brien

The clinical problem   Malcolm Bailey

Chronic sialadenitis is a condition characterized by recurrent swelling, pain, and a muco-purulent discharge, giving rise to a bad taste. The more severe cases may develop abscess or fistula formation. The incidence of this problem is difficult to determine.

The present overview will concentrate on adult management. When this problem affects children, it almost exclusively affects the parotid gland and usually responds to conservative measures. The symptoms generally disappear by puberty, and surgery is rarely indicated (Cohen *et al.* 1992).

Local abnormalities associated with chronic parotid sialadenitis include radiolucent stones, stricture of the anterior portion of the duct or orifice, external pressure on the main duct, congenital duct abnormalities, and foreign bodies (Zou 1992). Conversely, often the only identifiable cause of submandibular sialadenitis is a radio-opaque stone, or a duct stricture following removal of a calculus (Isacsson *et al.* 1981; Smith *et al.* 1993).

It is important to note that parenchymal inflammation is also associated with a number of other conditions, including lymphoepithelial lesions, tuberculosis, actinomycosis, HIV infection, and tumours. This group will not be considered further. If treatment is indicated, it is directed towards the underlying disease process.

The natural history of sialadenitis of unknown cause is that if seen during the early presentation, up to 20% of cases may undergo spontaneous remission (Maynard 1965). With increasing episodes of obstruction and where sialographic investigation reveals ductal and acinar changes, treatment may become necessary.

Clinical features

Clinical evidence of sialadenitis occurs when there is a degree of obstruction of salivary output leading to gland enlargement (Batsakis 1979). Infection may result from this chain of events or indeed may cause it. When present, it increases the discomfort felt and, if left untreated, may lead to abscess or fistula formation.

The clinical diagnosis can often be made on the history and clinical examination alone. The likely factors associated with the problem may be elucidated by plain radiographs and sialography. Plain radiographs may reveal evidence of tuberculosis, radio-opaque stones, or foreign bodies. Sialography produces additional information on the detection and localization of stones, differentiating between strictures and stones, and revealing the extent of damage to both ducts and acini (Adam *et al.* 1983; Morgan *et al.* 1985). In addition to the diffuse gland enlargement generally produced by this disease, a localized lump may be palpated in the chronic state. Ultrasound, computed tomography (CT), or magnetic resonance imagine (MRI) may be useful to differentiate the localized lump from a tumour (Chitre and Premchandra 1997). In clinical practice, however, this situation is unusual and these latter investigations are therefore rarely indicated (Maynard 1988).

Treatment

The treatment of sialadenitis should be tailored to any known cause or related disease process. In the submandibular gland, this is usually a stone or a stricture following stone excision. The clinician will make a judgement as to whether calculus extraction or gland excision is more appropriate, depending on such factors as stone size and anatomical position. Submandibular gland excision is straightforward and produces minimal morbidity in experienced hands, and there is little current controversy surrounding its management (Isacsson *et al.* 1981).

The same cannot be said of the management of parotid sialadenitis. The general principle of addressing the treatment to the known cause or disease process applies. Unlike the submandibular gland, however, the bulk of cases have no known and identifiable cause and the gland cannot be excised cleanly, owing to its relationship to the facial nerve. Where local factors exist, such as a stone or stricture in the anterior portion of the duct, these may be addressed with some success. However, for the majority of patients, excision of sufficient parenchymal tissue to produce a cure with the least morbidity is required.

The factors leading the clinician to advise the patient to undergo a surgical solution are failure of non-surgical measures, and the incidence, length of history, and severity of episodes of parotitis. In addition to the severity of the symptoms, sialographic findings aid guidance to likely prognosis if left untreated. Non-surgical options include massage, antibiotics, flushing of the gland, sialogogues, and radiation (Ericson *et al.* 1991; Mandel and Kaynar 1995).

In a recent study by the author (Tighe *et al.* 1999), an attempt was made to relate gradations of pre-operative sialographic findings (Wang *et al.* 1992) to the final histopathology grading (Seifert and Donath 1997), and also to relate the length of history to the histological outcome. The results showed that in the parotid gland the sialograms suggested rather greater architectural damage than the final histology revealed. The longer the duration of symptoms, the greater the sialographic and histopathological findings.

In the submandibular gland, there was a closer correlation between the sialographic and histopathological findings. There was also a positive correlation between a short history and the severity of histopathological grade.

Numerous surgical procedures have been advocated for parotid sialadenitis. Denervation and duct ligation have been tried and abandoned, owing to poor outcomes (Nichols 1977). There has been a general reluctance to advocate superficial or subtotal parotidectomy owing to a perceived risk to the facial nerve, yet both procedures have now been shown to be safe and effective.

The criteria by which we can measure the success or otherwise of these two procedures should include cure of the presenting symptoms and signs, achieved by surgery that produces the least likely morbidity to the facial and great auricular nerves, retention of functioning parenchymal tissue, and cosmesis. The author would suggest that for the small number of patients presenting with near total obstruction from stenosis or stone, not amenable to local surgery, together with patients who have widespread end-stage parenchymal disease with abscess or fistulae, subtotal parotidectomy is indicated. For the majority, a superficial parotidectomy, with preservation of the main duct, a pressure dressing for 24 h, and suction drainage, will produce highly successful results (Arriaga and Meyers 1990; Sadeghi *et al.* 1999). Long-term follow-up of these patients being undertaken currently shows symptom-free patients, with clear saliva issuing from the duct and post-operative sialograms suggesting near-normal duct structure of the remaining gland, but with continuing dilatation and stenosis of the main duct.

Surgical treatment and results   Christopher O'Brien

Sialadenitis is a relatively common clinical problem due principally to an obstruction to salivary flow. When the primary cause is a calculus, removal of the stone usually leads to resolution of the problem. Primary calculus formation is uncommon in the parotid gland and so chronic parotitis is not well understood. There are cyclical bouts of swelling and discomfort related to salivary stasis and secondary infection. Patients presenting with this clinical problem are best treated conservatively with massage, mouth washes, sialogogues, and antibiotics when necessary. Local interventions to the parotid duct opening by means of probing or meatoplasty can also be beneficial when this is found to be the cause of obstruction. In a small proportion of patients, however, symptoms persist despite conservative measures and, in this setting, there is a definite role for surgical removal of the parotid gland.

The role of parotidectomy in the management of sialadenitis is controversial, with some workers claiming that parotidectomy really has no role. Other surgeons recognize a limited role for parotidectomy but do so grudgingly, demanding that patients accept the attendant risk of the procedure. The technical difficulties of the operation and potential risk to the facial nerve have probably influenced this point of view.

It is the view and experience of the author that parotidectomy is very useful in the treatment of sialadenitis in selected patients. The decision to operate is, in general, a clinical one, supported by radiological findings wherever possible. Sialography is a useful investigation for patients with recurrent parotitis. A symptomatic patient with a normal sialogram should be encouraged to persist with conservative measures. A patient with a very abnormal sialogram, demonstrating stenoses, duct narrowing, or sialectasis, can be advised that recurrent bouts of parotitis are probably inevitable, and a surgical option may be taken earlier, if symptoms warrant it.

In an initial report (O'Brien *et al.* 1993) from the author, 17 patients had parotidectomy for chronic sialadenitis. The incidence of post-operative facial weakness was approximately 30%, and all but two patients had complete resolution of their presenting symptoms. Patients in this study were treated with both superficial and near-total parotidectomy, with the latter procedure being used increasingly as the experience of the author developed. The two operations, however, appeared to have equal efficacy in controlling symptoms in the long term. In a subsequent study (Bates *et al.* 1998), the treated group had reached 49 in number, comprising 14 superficial and 35 near-total parotidectomies. The incidence of temporary facial nerve weakness remained at about 30% and, interestingly, stones were implicated in the disease process in 24% of patients.

In that study, a range of pathological processes were identified. A total of 12 patients had histological evidence of benign lymphoepithelial lesion with acinar atrophy, epithelial islands, and a lymphocytic infiltrate. The remaining patients had evidence of chronic inflammation and fibrosis. To date, a total of 73 parotidectomies have been carried out for sialadenitis. Two patients have undergone bilateral procedures, and near-total conservative parotidectomy is now the preferred operation, the aim being to remove as much parotid tissue as possible. Facial nerve morbidity remains at approximately 26%; however, normal function invariably is re-established in this group within 3–6 months of surgery. Minor recurrent bouts of discomfort may occur after surgery, but in general the patient satisfaction level is very high. Appropriate patient selection and careful pre-operative counselling are important if the beneficial role of parotidectomy is to be maximized in the setting of chronic recurrent parotitis.

REFERENCES

Adam, E.J., Willson, S.A., Corcoran, M.O., and Hobsley, M. (1983) The value of parotid sialography. *Br J Surg*, **70**, 108–10.

Arriaga, M.A. and Myers, E.N. (1990) The surgical management of chronic parotitis. *Laryngoscope*, **100**, 1270–5.

Bates, D., O' Brien, C.J., Tikaram, K., and Painter, D.M. (1998) Parotid and submandibular sialadenitis treated by salivary gland excision. *Aust NZ J Surg*, **68**, 120–4.

Batsakis, J.G. (1979) *Tumors of the Head and Neck*, 2nd edn. Williams and Wilkins, Baltimore.

Chitre, V.V. and Premchandra, D.J. (1997) Recurrent parotitis. *Arch Dis Child*, **77**, 359–63.

Cohen, H.A., Gross, S., Nussinovitch, M., Frydman, M., and Varsano, I. (1992) Recurrent parotitis. *Arch Dis Child*, **67**, 1036–7.

Ericson, S., Zetterlund, B., and Ohman, J. (1991) Recurrent parotitis and sialectasis in childhood. Clinical, radiologic, immunologic, bacteriologic, and histologic study. *Ann Otol Rhinol Laryngol*, **100**, 527–35.

Isacsson, G., Ahlner, B., and Lundquist, P.G. (1981) Chronic sialadenitis of the submandibular gland. A retrospective study of 108 case. *Arch Otorhinolaryngol*, **232**, 91–100.

Mandel, L. and Kaynar, A. (1995) Recurrent parotitis in children. *NY State Dent J*, **61**, 22–5.

Maynard, J.D. (1965) Recurrent parotid enlargement. *Br J Surg*, **52**, 784–9.

Maynard, J.D. (1988) Solitary cysts of the parotid. *Br J Surg*, **75**, 1043.

Morgan, R.F., Saunders, J.R., Jr, Hirata, R.M., and Jaques, D.A. (1985) A comparative analysis of the clinical, sialographic, and pathologic findings in parotid disease. *Am Surg*, **51**, 664–7.

Nichols, R.D. (1977) Surgical treatment of chronic suppurative parotitis. A critical review. *Laryngoscope*, **87**, 2066–81.

O'Brien, C.J., Malka, V.B., and Mijailovic, M. (1993) Evaluation of 242 consecutive parotidectomies performed for benign and malignant disease. *Aust NZ J Surg*, **63**, 870–7.

Sadeghi, N., Black, M.J., and Frenkiel, S. (1996) Parotidectomy for the treatment of chronic recurrent parotitis. *J Otolaryngol*, **25**, 305–7.

Seifert, G. and Donath, K. (1997) Zur Pathogenese des Kuttner—Tumors der Submandibularis. *HNO*, **21**, 81–92.

Smith, W.P., Peters, W.J., and Markus, A.F. (1993) Submandibular gland surgery: an audit of clinical findings, pathology and postoperative morbidity. *Ann R Coll Surg Engl*, **75**, 164–7.

Tighe, J.V., Bailey, B.M., Khan, M.Z., Stavrou, M., and Todd, C.E. (1999) Relation of preoperative sialographic findings with histopathological diagnosis in cases of obstructive sialadenitis of the parotid and submandibular glands: retrospective study. *Br J Oral Maxillofac Surg*, **37**, 290–3.

Wang, S.L., Zou, Z.J., Wu, Q.G., and Sun, K.H. (1992) Sialographic changes related to clinical and pathologic findings in chronic obstructive parotitis. *Int J Oral Maxillofac Surg*, **21**, 364–8.

Zou, Z.J. (1992) [Chronic obstructive parotitis: a report of 92 cases]. *Chung Hua Kou Chiang Hsueh Tsa Chih*, **27**, 200–2, 255.

Editorial comment

If chronic sialoadenitis of the submandibular gland does not resolve with conservative treatment, it is easily dealt with by adenectomy. There is no debate on this point.

In the parotid, treatment options are not as clear. If surgery is required, what is the best option—a near-total or partial parotidectomy? The question is unresolved. What is clear is that once the surgery is undertaken, no further surgery is possible without considerable risk to the nerve.

Professor O'Brien reports an initial series of 17 patients with chronic parotitis treated mainly by superficial parotidectomy with a symptomatic success rate of about 90%. He also reports a larger series (which included the 17 patients described above) of 73 cases, with a large majority being successful in significant abolition of symptoms. It does not report any permanent facial nerve palsy. Interestingly, the results were equally good with near-total or superficial parotidectomy.

The Guy's Hospital experience amounts to 23 cases with a median follow-up of 12 years who answered a questionnaire. This disclosed symptomatic success in 21 cases. Again it was found that there was no difference in terms of success between superficial and total partotidectomy (Table 27.1).

Table 27.1 Outcomes following parotidectomies for chronic sialadenitis – Guy's Hospital series, 1994–1999

	No. of patients	Success	Failures
Superficial parotidectomy	17	16	1
Total parotidectomy	6	5	1

Surgical problems of parotidectomy (superficial or total) reside in the scarring of the gland which can make dissection of the gland extremely difficult. There appears to be a case to be made for early surgery rather than postponement, since the latter presumably means a more scarred and densely fibrosed gland. A possible part solution to the problem of whether to advocate early surgery or advise delay because spontaneous resolution may take place may come with the use of fibre-optic inspection of the parotid duct. It is hoped that endoscopy may offer a more objective assessment of the disease process than current investigative techniques.

Index